Ethical and Philosophical Aspects of Nursing Children and Young People

Edited by

Dr Gosia M. Brykczyńska

and

Dr Joan Simons

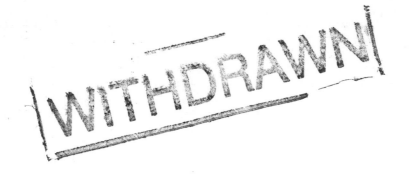

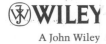WILEY

A John Wiley

Library of Congress Cataloging-in-Publication Data

Ethical and philosophical aspects of nursing children and young people / edited by Gosia M. Brykczyńska and Joan Simons.
    p. ; cm.
Includes bibliographical references and index.
ISBN 978-1-4051-9414-3 (pbk. : alk. paper)
    1. Pediatric nursing–Moral and ethical aspects.   2. Pediatric nursing–Philosophy.   I. Brykczyńska, Gosia M., 1947–
II. Simons, Joan (Joan M.)
    [DNLM: 1. Pediatric Nursing–ethics. 2. Adolescent. 3. Child. 4. Ethics, Nursing. 5. Philosophy, Nursing. WY 85]
RJ245.E77 2011
618.92′00231–dc22
                                          2010031134
A catalogue record for this book is available from the British Library.

Set in 9.5/11.5 Palatino by Spi Publisher Services, Pondicherry, India

Printed and bound in Malaysia by Vivar Printing Sdn Bhd

1   2011

Contents

Notes on Contributors   v
Foreword   ix
Preface   x
Acknowledgements   xii

**Part I The Philosophical
Foundations of Caring for Children
and Young People**   **1**

1 Histories and Philosophies
of Childhood   3
Gosia M. Brykczyńska

2 Theories of Moral Philosophy
Applied to Paediatric Nursing   23
Gosia M. Brykczyńska

3 A Review of Children's Rights
as Applied to Paediatric Nursing   36
Jim Richardson

**Part II Ethical Aspects of the
Continuum of Care**   **45**

4 Beginning of Life: Ethical Issues
in Neonatology Nursing   47
Amanda Williamson and Julie Mullett

5 Ethical Issues in Caring for Toddlers
and School Age Children: Ethical
Aspects of the Role and Work of
the Health Visitor   55
Monica Davis

6 Promoting the Health of School-Aged
Children: An Ethical Perspective   66
Gill Coverdale

7 'To Be Like the Others':
Children's Views of Nursing in
Community Settings   77
Duncan Randall

8 Care of the Severely Disabled Child:
A Moral Imperative   88
Vicki Rowse

9 Ethical Aspects of Care of
the Adolescent   100
Yvonne Dexter

10 Ethical and Legal Aspects of Working
with Children and Young People
with Emotional and Psychiatric
Health Needs   112
Tim McDougall

Part III Ethical Issues in the Acute Care Setting   **125**

11 Children's Experience of Hospitalisation and Their Participation in Health-Care Decision-Making   127
Imelda Coyne

12 The Ethics of Family-Centred Care for Hospitalised Children   144
Linda Shields

13 Above All Else do No Harm: An Ethical Evaluation of Paediatric Nurses Management of Children's Pain   155
Joan Simons

14 Ethical Aspects in Children's and Young People's Cancer Care: Professional Views   164
Faith Gibson

15 Withholding and Withdrawal of Treatment: Ethical, Legal and Philosophical Aspects of Paediatric Intensive Care Nursing   173
Karen Harrison-White

16 Palliative Care of Children: Some Ethical Dilemmas   187
Vicki Rowse and Martin Smith

Part IV Philosophical Considerations in Professional Practice   **199**

17 Researching Children and Young People: Exploring the Ethical Territory   201
Bernie Carter

18 Philosophical and Epistemological Aspects of Children's Spirituality   220
Rita Pfund

19 'Are you Sitting Comfortably?' Storytelling and the Power of Narratives – A Philosophical Analysis   237
Gosia M. Brykczyńska

20 Who is Shaping Children's Nursing?   251
Duncan Randall

Appendices

Appendix I
Summary of Possible Situations for Withdrawal and Withholding Treatment in Children According to the *Royal College of Paediatrics and Child Health* Guidelines   261

Appendix II
United Nations Convention on the Rights of the Child (Abridged)   262

Appendix III
Summary of the International Council of Nurses Ethical Code   265

Appendix IV
Summary of the Principles for the Ethical Conduct of Medical Research Involving Children   267

Index   268

Notes on Contributors

Dr Gosia M. Brykczyńska PhD, BA, BSc, Post-graduate Diploma in Public Health, PGDE; RN/RSCN, RNT Gosia M. Brykczyńska is a humanities graduate, obtaining a degree in nursing from Columbia University in New York City and children's nursing qualifications from Great Ormond Street Hospital for Sick Children (GOS). She is a specialist in paediatric oncology nursing. Her clinical work has been both in the USA and the UK. Since 1985, she has been involved in the education of nurses in the UK at the pre- and post-registration levels. She was the Royal College of Nursing (RCN) paediatric nurse representative on the RCPCH Ethics Advisory Committee 1989–2000. More recently, she has worked as an international officer at the RCN and as RCN refugee nurses' project coordinator. She is the editor and author of several books on nursing, including *Ethics in Paediatric Nursing* published in 1989. Currently, she works part-time as senior lecturer in child health at Thames Valley University.

Dr Bernie Carter, PhD, PGCE, BSc, RSCN, SRN Bernie Carter is a children's nurse who is passionate about research. She sees research as an important means of enhancing the care and life experiences of children and their families. Her research is participative, narrative, appreciative, collaborative and arts-based in its approach. She is particularly interested in children's pain and the illness experiences of marginalised children or those with uncertain diagnoses. Her research also encompasses work focusing on community children's nursing. Bernie believes that the ethical researcher requires an ongoing commitment to being critically aware of the micro- and macro-ethical issues that can create challenges throughout a research study.

Currently, Bernie Carter is a professor of children's nursing at the University of Central Lancashire and director of the Children's Nursing Research Unit at Alder Hey Children's NHS Foundation Trust. She is also the editor of the *Journal of Child Health*.

Gill Coverdale, MPH, BSc (Hons), Cert. Ed, RNT, RSCPHN, RGN Gill Coverdale has more than 20 years experience in health promotion, public health and health-related research both in the UK and internationally. Her nursing practice has included delivering adult and midwifery services in hospital, community, GP practice and primary care, before moving into children and young people's services as a school nurse, including work as a specialist community public health nurse. She has advised the government on the development of health services for children and young people ensuring a health-promoting approach for all and has worked with the Nursing and Midwifery Council (NMC)

in the development of nurse education programmes. Since 2001, she has also been working
as a senior lecturer. She is currently working as a
lecturer in public health and primary care whilst
enrolled as a PhD student at the Institute of
Family, Maternal and Community Health, School
of Healthcare, University of Leeds.

Dr Imelda Coyne, PhD, BSc (Hons) with Education,
Dip N, RSCN, RGN, RNT, FEANS   Imelda
Coyne is a research associate at the Children's
Research Centre, Trinity College, Dublin; a post-
doctoral fellow of Lund University, Sweden; and
a fellow of the European Academy of Nursing
Science. She has over 20 years experience in children's nursing, firstly as a practising nurse and
then as a lecturer. Her programme of research
includes children's participation in consultation
and decision-making, family-centred care, young
people's experiences of mental health service
provision, parenting practices, transition process,
nurses' contribution to care, ethics of researching children and advanced practice. Professor
Imelda Coyne is currently working as head of
children's discipline/director of children's
research at Trinity College, Dublin.

Monica Davis, BSc (Hons), MA (education), PGDE,
RHV, RGN, NP   Monica Davis is a lecturer-
practitioner. She has had a long-standing interest in child protection and domestic violence
and was a former chair of Women's Aid in
Harrow which is now part of *Hestia Housing and
Support*. Hestia is a registered charity which
delivers a range of housing, care and support
services across London, including for cases of
domestic violence. She is a co-opted trustee on
Hestia's board. Currently, she is working as a
health visitor for Ealing and Harrow PCT. She is
also a lecturer with Thames Valley University,
where she is a member of the Faculty of Health
and Human Sciences, School of Community
Health.

Yvonne Dexter, RGN/RSCN, RCNT, RNT, BSC
(Hons) Open University   Yvonne Dexter gained
her paediatric nursing and nurse education
experiences at GOS, London, and the Royal
Berkshire Hospital, Reading, and Wycombe
General Hospital. She has a particular interest in
adolescent health, loss, bereavement and grief in
children, and safeguarding children and child
protection. She is currently a senior lecturer in

the Child Health Nursing Department at Thames
Valley University in Slough.

Dr Faith Gibson, PhD, MSc, Cert Ed, RGN/RSCN,
RNT, ENB237   Faith Gibson has over 25 years
experience in children's cancer nursing that
includes clinical practice, education and research.
Her main fields of research and supervision
include:

- Improving process and outcomes of care for
  children/young people with cancer and their
  families;
- Improving assessment and management of
  symptoms;
- Improving skills of the nursing workforce to
  deliver cancer care.

She has been influential in the expansion of the
research evidence base for children's cancer
nursing. She has presented at national and international conferences, has edited three textbooks
and has over 70 publications to her credit. Since
2009, she has been a clinical professor of children's and young people's cancer care at Great
Ormond Street Hospital for Children NHS Trust
and London South Bank University.

Karen Harrison-White, BSc (Hons), Post-Grad
Diploma in Health Care Ethics, PGDE; MSc in
Paediatric Critical Care, RN (Child), RGN   Upon
qualifying, Karen Harrison-White worked in
adult wards and then moved into adult intensive care. Many infants and children were being
cared for in adult intensive care units; therefore,
in 1994, she decided to gain specialist experience
in a paediatric intensive care nursing. Since then
she has held a variety of posts in this speciality
including senior sister, clinical nurse educator
and research nurse. Since 2004, she has taught
paediatric high dependency/paediatric intensive care at Thames Valley University in West
London. Currently, she is working at Bucks New
University in Uxbridge, Middlesex.

Tim McDougall, RMN, BSc (Hons), PG Dip,
Specialist Practitioner (Mental Health), ENB
603   Tim McDougall has worked in a range of
CAMHS settings, including community child
mental health teams, adolescent inpatient services and secure adolescent forensic services.
With a national profile in CAMHS and with
over 80 book and journal publications, he has

spoken at national and European conferences about the mental health of children and adolescents. Tim was formerly nurse advisor for CAMHS in the Department of Health in England and is primarily interested with the strategic development and leadership of CAMHS and nursing. Tim was an expert witness for the national inquiry into self-harm by young people and is currently a member of the National Advisory Council for Children's Mental Health and Psychological Wellbeing. He has edited the textbook *Child and Adolescent Mental Health Nursing* (2006) by Wiley/Blackwell. Tim McDougall is currently working as a part-time nurse consultant (Tier 4 CAMHS) and lead nurse (CAMHS) at the Cheshire & Wirral NHS Foundation Trust and is part of the North West NHS Children and Families Programme Team.

Julie Mullett, RGN, RM, MSc Health Sciences Julie Mullett is a qualified midwife and advanced neonatal nurse practitioner who has been working with neonates for 15 years. She was previously an operational manager at the Norfolk and Norwich University NHS Hospital Foundation Trust but has recently returned to work as an advanced neonatal nurse practitioner.

Rita Pfund, MA, BSc (Hons), PGDEA, RN (child, adult)   Rita Pfund has extensive experience in general children's nursing and palliative care of children and young people both from a clinical and educational perspective. She has a particular professional interest relating to how children make sense of adverse life events which has led to an interest in how professionals can best nurture a child's spirituality, as well as how professionals can best support families through adverse life events. She has recently co-edited a book with Susan Fowler-Kerry entitled *Perspectives on Palliative Care for Children and Young People* (2010) by Radcliffe Publishing. She is currently a lecturer in child health at the Division of Nursing, Midwifery and Physiotherapy at the University of Nottingham, UK.

Dr Duncan Randall, RGN, RSCN, RHV, RNT, BSc (Hons), CHN, PGCE, MSc, PhD Duncan Randall's clinical experience includes nursing children in hospitals and as a community children's nurse. He has also practiced as a health visitor. In 2006, he was awarded a *Leading Practice*

Through Research award from the Health Foundation. This award funded research into children's perceptions of receiving nursing care at home, which was the doctoral study he had undertaken at the University of Warwick. Duncan is the honorary secretary for the Association of British Paediatric Nurses. He lectures on complex health needs and children's nursing at the University of Birmingham, and has written on how children's views can influence the education of nurses. He currently works as a lecturer at The University of Birmingham.

Dr Jim Richardson   Jim Richardson undertook a bachelor of arts (humanities) at the University of Strathclyde, Glasgow, before completing general nurse training in Aberdeen, Scotland. He then worked in neurology, anaesthetics and paediatrics at the Oulu University Central Hospital in Finland for a period of 8 years. He obtained a specialist paediatric nursing qualification from Great Ormond Street Hospital in London. In 1999, he took up the position of principal lecturer in children's nursing at the University of Glamorgan and a year later took on the role of field leader (head of division) of family care. He has edited and authored many positions concerning children's nursing. Currently, he is head of division (Family Care), Faculty of Health, Sport and Science, University of Glamorgan, Pontypridd, Wales.

Vicki Rowse, RSCN, RGN, BA (Hons), MA   Vicki Rowse trained as a nurse at Great Ormond Street Hospital for Sick Children (GOS) in 1983. Further education included an MA in health-care leadership and practice (2008) from the University of Reading. Her practice has included nursing surgical neonates at GOS, Mission Hospital nursing in Zambia, 12 years as a community children's nurse and 7 years as a community children's matron – with a complex care and palliative care team in Winchester. Her achievements include being team finalist for the Nursing Times Awards 2007, being shortlisted for the Nora Reece Award for a master's dissertation in 2009, and being the current holder of a Transforming Community Services Award for developing integrated care for children and families. She is currently working as a community children's matron for Winchester and Eastleigh Healthcare NHS Trust.

Dr Linda Shields, PhD, FRCNA   Linda Shields has held the foundation chair in nursing at the University of Limerick in Ireland, followed by the post of professor of nursing at the University of Hull in England. In addition, she is an honorary professor in the Department of Paediatrics and Child Health at the University of Queensland. Her research interests include the care of children in health services, in particular family-centred care; the health of children in developing countries; paediatric perioperative nursing; and the history of nursing and ethical issues surrounding nursing such as the role of nurses in the euthanasia programmes of the Third Reich. Over her academic career, she has maintained a small clinical load in paediatric perioperative nursing and in 2009, published a book in that highly specialised area of practice. Linda Shields is currently professor of paediatric and child health nursing at Curtin University and works for the Child and Adolescent Health Service, Perth, Western Australia.

Dr Joan Simons RGN, RSCN, RHV, BA (Hons) Community Health Studies, PGDE, PGDAHP, DMS, MA Management Studies, Ed D.   Joan Simons' long-time interest in pain stems from her experience in caring for children and young people with burns. The images of these children have remained etched in her memory till today. She moved on from that area of practice with a feeling of inadequacy in relation to how something as fundamental as pain was dealt with. She believes that the field of pain management has moved on considerably in the last 20 years but realises that comprehensive evidence-based pain management practice has yet to be achieved. Auditing pain management has the potential to increase the profile of children's pain. Currently, she is assistant head in the Department of Health and Social Care, Faculty of Health and Social Care at the Open University, Milton Keynes.

Martin Smith, RN (Level 2), RSCN, BSc (Hons)   Martin Smith qualified as a paediatric nurse in 1998 from the University of Bradford, obtaining a BSc (Hons) in specialist practice as a school nurse in 2002 and further qualifications in palliative care for children and their families from Oxford Brookes University. Her practice has included general paediatric nursing at Frimley Park Hospital, and ENT and day surgery. From 2003 to 2007, he worked as the community children's palliative care coordinator. His interests include paediatric epilepsy care, teaching practice and service development through clinical governance and innovation. His achievements include being team finalist for the Nursing Times Awards 2007. Currently, he works as a community children's nurse and clinical governance specialist for Winchester and Eastleigh Healthcare NHS Trust – both at the Royal Hampshire County Hospital, Winchester.

Amanda Williamson, RGN, RM, LLB, LLM (Family Law and Policy), PGDipHE   Amanda Williamson was previously a lecturer, specialising in neonates at the University of East Anglia. She undertook her master's degree in family law and policy which considered ethical issues in relation to children and medical treatment. She is currently the nurse manager of the Neonatal Intensive Care Unit at the Norfolk Norwich University NHS Hospital Foundation Trust.

Foreword

It is a privilege to write the foreword to this crucially important text, which brings together many different philosophical aspects and ethical issues in children's nursing practice. Children, young people and their families are more aware of their rights than ever before. Indeed, children and young people are seen as active citizens in today's society, with junior citizenship featuring as a core component within school curricula. Today, children themselves wish to be actively involved in decision-making concerning their own care and treatment. It is vital that nurses are appropriately prepared to address the many different issues and scenarios that will increasingly face them in their day-to-day practice.

The text will provide students and practitioners with an understanding of the key principles and the legal framework underpinning children and young people's ethics as they apply to rights. The issues covered will provide insight and rationale to underpin practitioners' decision-making in everyday clinical practice.

The book covers different developmental ages across childhood, as well as settings of care and particular clinical conditions which entail specific issues and challenges for practitioners. The text is divided into four parts: Part I predominately focuses on historical and theoretical perspectives; Part II highlights issues across the age spectrum from neonatal to adolescents; Part III deals with key areas including hospitalisation, treatment processes and the withdrawal of interventions; while Part IV covers overarching aspects such as research and spirituality.

The breadth of topics and areas covered will undoubtedly increase awareness of the ethical, moral and legal issues facing children's nurses of the future. Congratulations to all the chapter authors and the editors who have created a textbook that will, I am sure, be a standard reference for all child health nursing students at both undergraduate and postgraduate levels.

Fiona Smith
Adviser in Children
and Young People's Nursing
Royal College of Nursing

Preface

The gestation of this book has taken almost 20 years, since no sooner had the book *Ethics in Paediatric Nursing* reached the bookshops in 1989 that the long-awaited United Nations Convention of the Rights of the Child (UNCRC) was published and given to the children of the world for their countries to ratify, while in the UK, the Children's Act 1989 was confirmed as law. The care of children was about to change dramatically, as was the education of children's nurses and health-care personnel working with them.

The last 20 years have been an exceptionally active period of change, challenge and concern for health-care workers and those engaged in promoting and safeguarding the well-being of children, and in particular for children's nurses. Ancient and venerable schools of nurses that were flourishing 20 years ago have disappeared and in their place departments of nursing within universities have sprung up all over the UK. With this change in the location of education came also massive changes in the quality of children's nurses' education and with that a need for the humanities, philosophy and ethics, as pertains to the care of children and young people, to be embedded in the new curricula. Even as we write, schools of nursing in the UK are again busily preparing themselves for another major educational revolution, as they adapt their nursing programmes to accommodate the educational

requirements of a children and young person's nurse to be educated to degree level. This new degree-level graduate nurse will need to look more broadly and more intensely at the nature of the work he or she will be undertaking; this book is intended to help in that enormous moral and professional endeavour.

This new edited book on ethical and philosophical aspects of nursing children and young people is intended to reflect some of the contemporary issues encountered while working with children and young people in the twenty-first century and is intended to provoke the reader to consider the place and contribution of the humanities, moral philosophy and ethical discourse in the practice of paediatric nursing.

This book, however, would never have come to fruition were it not for the dedicated and committed hard work of the many contributors of chapters to the project and the tireless help and support of all our families and friends who patiently put up with us as we wrote the chapters and prepared the manuscript for publication over the past 18 months. Thanks are also due to Sue Burr, OBE, the past paediatric nurse adviser at the Royal College of Nursing, for her ongoing support of the project and to Fiona Smith, current adviser in children and young people's nursing at the Royal College of Nursing. Many thanks are also due to Alexandra McGregor, our supportive nursing editor at Wiley/Blackwell publishers. Finally, many thanks to the children who were so keen to inform us of their thoughts and concerns about children's nurses and whose insightful statements have enriched this book.

Thank you once again to all those who have helped this project see the light of day. May it now help illuminate and inform our practice.

Dr Gosia M. Brykcznśka & Dr Joan Simons

Acknowledgements

The editors and chapter authors of this book wish to express their gratitude to the following institutions, publishing houses and authors for granting permission to quote and reproduce poems, photographs, diagrams and texts.

The Royal College of Paediatrics and Child Health (RCPCH) for reproducing a summary of the six principles of ethical conduct in medical research involving children, from RCPCH (2000) Guidelines for the ethical conduct of medical research involving children. *Archives of Disease of Childhood*, **82**, 177–182.

The RCPCH for permission to reproduce the summary of the guidelines for the withdrawal and withholding of treatment from sick children (RCPCH (2004) *Withholding or Withdrawing Life Sustaining Treatment in Children*. RCPCH, London).

UNICEF for permission to reproduce the *Summary of the Convention of the Rights of a Child* (1989). The full version of the UNCRC is available on the UNICEF web site: www.unicef.org.uk/crc.

The International Council of Nurses (ICN), Geneva, for permission to reproduce the summary of *ICN Ethics Code* (2006). The full version of the code is available from the web site: www.icn.ch/ethics.htm.

Great Ormond Street Hospital for Sick Children (GOS), London, for making available a photograph of the GOS chapel.

Rita Pfund for permission to reproduce the poem *Our Little Brother* and for allowing the use of the accompanying photograph.

Rita Pfund for permission to reproduce Figure 20.5 from Pfund, R. (2006) *Palliative Care Nursing of Children and Young People*. Radcliffe Publishing, Oxford (reproduced here with the permission of the copyright holder).

The Journal of Advanced Nursing for giving permission to use the diagram of Guidelines for Spiritual Assessment for Families, in Tanyi, R. (2006) Spirituality and family nursing. *Journal of Advanced Nursing*, **53** (3), 287–294.

Palgrave Macmillan Publishers for permission to reproduce the diagram of Fowler, J. et al. (1991) Stages of faith development in Walker, S. (2005) *Culturally Competent Therapy*. Palgrave/Macmillan, Basingstoke.

Penguin Publications for reproducing the complete poem *Who's Who* (p. 48) by Benjamin Zephaniah in *Talking Turkey's* (1995).

Professor Stephan Millett and Dr Alan Tapper, Centre for Applied Ethics, and Dr David Wall, School of Nursing and Midwifery, Curtin University, for their help and advice about preparation for Chapter 12 by Dr Linda Shields.

Last but most significantly, the editors of this book would like to warmly thank the children and young people whose views about care we have included in this book: Sam Llanwarne, Georgina Llanwarne, Max Llanwarne, Lorna Elwin, Clodagh Simons and Sorcha Simons.

Part I

The Philosophical Foundations of Caring for Children and Young People

What do you think makes a good nurse?

Someone who talks to you and not just your Mum.   (Girl 10yrs)

A good nurse is when they do what they are told and be nice and gentle.   (Boy 8yrs)

Comforting, kind and caring, a nice warming smile.   (Girl 11yrs)

A nurse that is nice and talks to you, one that informs you of what's going on and one that is calm.   (Girl 14yrs)

Someone who is nice to their patients.   (Girl 11yrs)

1 Histories and Philosophies of Childhood

Gosia M. Brykczyńska

Introduction

Is this a holy thing to see
In a rich and fruitful land,
Babes reduced to misery,
Fed with cold and usurious hand?
William Blake (1757–1827, in Warwick 2000 p.71)

These words of the poet Blake were written almost 200 years ago but as this book is going to print, the British public are reeling once again from the disclosed information concerning the family life of baby Peter Connelly, better known to the public as Baby P. As increasingly more information is being made available about the case of Baby P, what is emerging is the extent of the entrenched relentless repetitiveness of generational abuse and neglect and the social fragility and personal inadequacies of the adults concerned. As Andrew Anthony wrote in his investigative report for *The Sunday Observer*:

The savagery was the culmination of generations of abuse and dysfunction, a dreadful violation that was far from inevitable but that had none the less been incubating for decades. The scene of the crime itself seemed to contain all the potent symbols and sordid realities of the feckless, desensitised version of contemporary life.

(Anthony 2009)

At the same time as details of Baby P's life were being put into the public domain, we were being informed about the systematic abuse carried out over 30 years ago by the carers of children in the Haut de la Garenne children's home on the island of Jersey (Byers 2008), while in April 2009 the death of an 11-year-old schoolgirl, Shano Khan, following physical punishment from her primary school teacher sent shockwaves across the Indian subcontinent (BBC News 2009). Meanwhile in the USA, a young woman who was kidnapped as a child has turned up after many years with a tale of confinement, abuse and brainwashing (Moore 2009). No wonder contemporary parents feel justified in saying that they will never let their child out of their sight, stating, I will not let my children ever play or be alone. Finally, a 14-year-old girl in Holland is attempting to be the youngest yachtswoman to circumnavigate the globe. She is contesting the verdict of the courts that she is too young for such feats and should be attending school instead (Watson 2009).

Ethical and Philosophical Aspects of Nursing Children, First Edition. Edited by Gosia M. Brykczyńska and Joan Simons.
© 2011 Blackwell Publishing Ltd. Published 2011 by Blackwell Publishing Ltd.

The question to ask is whether childhood was ever any different for children; that is, were children treated differently in the past? Indeed what did past generations think about children and youngsters? Are our present-day concerns about the quality of life, as experienced by the children of Great Britain and around the world, overly excessive and verging on sentimentality and overprotectiveness? Finally, and most crucially, does the way that we think about childhood influence the way we interact with children – a major concern for all those who work with children (Postman 1982; Druin 1996; Mayall 2002; Jenks 2005; Darbyshire 2007; Towner 2008; Layard & Dunn 2009). This chapter will attempt to address some of these issues giving a general outline of the history of childhood in Europe while acknowledging some of the more prevalent theories, philosophies and models of childhood, and how these may affect our approach to the care of children and young people.

SECTION ONE

Historians' craft or how historians put together the evidence

> …Winds of summer fields
> Recollect the way,
> Instinct picking up the key
> Dropped by memory.
> Emily Dickenson
> (1830–86, in Brinnin 1960)

Most contemporary scholars of the history of childhood are quick to distance themselves from the work of Philip Ariès (1962) and his assertion that the notion of childhood is a modern invention, and from his assertion that historically children were either not considered in the greater scheme of things or that when they were noted, they were taken advantage of and often abused. It would appear that social, cultural and religious practices of adults conspired to create an image of childhood which, to the twenty-first century observer, looked as if the children permanently lived in suboptimal conditions, were socially disregarded and most certainly were not included in the familial affairs of adults. Adults did not seem to be concerned with

the fate (or even the existence) of children. However, contemporary research undertaken by historians of childhood and family life tends to disagree with this extremely bleak picture (Shahar 1990; Cunningham 1995; Hanawalt 1995; Alexandre-Bidon & Lett 2000; Orme 2003, 2006). True, for very many people – if not the majority of people at times – life was hard and brutal. Additionally, life expectancy was low, especially for women, and many children died at birth or prematurely from hunger and infectious diseases. But this harshness of life was shared by everyone (Shahar 1990). It was not specific to children and when life was a bit more bearable there are plenty of evidences that children led a most interesting and varied life (Opie & Opie 1959; Keville-Davies 1991; Kiste 2003; HICD 2006; Orme 2006). There is also plenty of evidence that there was an accepted and well-understood concept of childhood from antiquity up to the present times – even if for most of recorded history the beneficial aspects of childhood, as we know them today, were limited to the ruling classes and the better off children in society. Rebecca Krug (2002) states that by the late Middle Ages there were three Latin definitions relating to that time of life measured from birth to adulthood, namely – *infantia* for infancy; *pueritia* for childhood and *adolescentia* for adolescence. Hardly evidence for an absence of a concept!

To the delight of historians of childhood, various individuals, and by no means all of them famous and wealthy, have managed over the course of the centuries to write down for posterity memories of their own childhood experiences (Holliday 1995; Gold 1997; Fox & Abraham-Podietz 1999; HICD 2006 among many). Many writers in the course of their narratives mention various aspects concerning childhood or the life of children. Hidden away among texts and letters about other matters, they have commented on issues pertinent to our understanding of the lives of children. From the richness of these documents, diaries, novels and tracts, an image emerges of the life of children and the nature of childhood as experienced by children in the distant and near past (Zimler & Sekulović 2008). What is also clear is that while for many children, as for many adults, life was indeed extremely hard, disease was rife and food was scarce, there was not necessarily as much widespread, wanton and vacuous violence and hatred directed specifically *at children* as some commentators would have had us believe (Aries 1962). Of course violence directed at children has unfortunately always existed, and it may have been more prevalent or even more accepted as an inevitable social phenomenon in the past (Hanawalt 1976; Rahikainen 2004); however, it is crucial to remember, as already noted, that violence directed at children still exists today (Amnesty International British Section 1995).

In the process of describing the nature of childhood from the past it is therefore necessary to be careful to avoid unqualified generalisations. The very combination of grinding poverty, lack of parental education and the obligatory and culturally condoned invisible labour of most working women conspired against most of the urban and rural poor in all but preventing them from demonstrating appropriate familial affection and concern for the welfare of their children (Shahar 1990; Cunningham 1991). Unfortunately, almost all of the conditions that were once suffered by European children are still tolerated by some children somewhere around the world today.

Just as in cases of war, where it is accepted wisdom that histories of battles are recorded by the victors, so the vast majority of descriptions of childhood and its events are written by those who have survived into adulthood. The maturation process from childhood to adulthood involves, however, some necessary selectivity of remembered and recallable facts, a phenomenon which Matthews (1994) calls childhood amnesia, and which Catriona Kelly (2007), in her excellent account of the life of Russian children in the waning years of Imperial Russia and through the unbelievably harsh years of the Soviet system, considers as selective 'evocations of the "boxes" or "envelopes" in which children lived' (Kelly 2007:13). No doubt we do tend to predominantly remember the best and the worst of our childhood experiences – and it is often because of such subconscious selectivity of facts, which overly highlights and emphasises certain events, that we unwittingly in the process skew all our remaining memories. The concern here is not for the well-documented psychological trauma following an unpleasant event – the recollection of which is pushed back deep into the subconscious, resulting in various

degrees of mental distress – but, as Matthews (1994) and Kelly (2007) so eloquently point out, the simple and natural growing-up amnesia that is necessary if humans are to function as well-adapted adults. Shahar (1990:5) also observes that: '…As for the writing of adults it is well known that they have difficulties in reliving some of their childhood experiences on the conscious level', since they inevitably describe experiences 'through the filter of selective memory'.

Meanwhile, adults writing about their own childhood often apologise to their readers for sounding boring or sentimental, as Heywood (2001) observes in his study of the history of childhood. Philip Larkin (1922–85) articulated this feeling succinctly in the poem *Coming* adding that he saw his own childhood as 'a forgotten boredom'. Fortunately, historians do not rely solely on what has been written and spoken – such as autobiographies, biographies, novels, school textbooks, medical records and physicians' accounts, judgements handed down in court cases, the legal system itself, parish council and foundling home accounts and such others – to create an image of childhood past (Keville-Davies 1991). To the historian of childhood, childcare professionals and subsequent generations of casual readers, everything from the past is of potentially of great interest and sometimes descriptions of the most simple aspects of daily life seem to later generations of readers to be exotic and worthy of comment (Keville-Davies 1991).

In the recent past, dedicated historical linguists have even managed to retrieve from encroaching oblivion, children's playground lore and language by studying the oral traditions of children's games, which included children's rhymes and children's slang. Researchers began to describe and record the existence of these children's games and their accompanying doggerels, many of which were on the verge of being lost to present generations of scholars and future generations of children (Opie & Opie 1959). The celebrated work of the Opie's in the UK is part of this long scholarly tradition, both in Europe and in the USA, of documenting and recording children's songs and games and is part of the rich and growing scholarly body of knowledge concerning the welfare and social life of children. The little song that the children in Lydney, UK, composed in the 1950s to the tune of *Frère*

Jacques speaks more to us about the children's attitude to school meals at the time, than any lengthy dissertation on the nature of children's diets:

> What's for dinner? What's for dinner?
> Irish spew, Irish spew,
> Soppy semolina, soppy semolina,
> No thank you, no thank you.
> (Opie & Opie 1959:162)

Historians and antiquarians also look at and collect ancient domestic artefacts such as children's furniture, for example, high chairs or cradles, toys and children' s books, clothes, books on advice to parents, etc. They also examine depictions of children in portraits and paintings, on carvings and on ornaments or as illustrations in ancient manuscripts and in historical books and primers intended for children's use (Shahar 1990; Keville-Davies 1991). Together with archaeologists and anthropologists, historians attempt to reconstruct ancient dwellings, and they study the layouts of ancient homes and children's institutions (including foundling hospitals and institutions for orphans and workhouses) to judge and evaluate the nature of the space put aside for children's use. Many ancient artefacts can be seen today in general museums, from Egyptian dolls in the British Museum to Roman sandals in the London Museum. There are also museums dedicated to childhood, such as the rightfully acclaimed Museum of Childhood in London's East End and the Foundling Hospital Museum in Coram Fields, which stands near Great Ormond Street Hospital for Children in central London built at the insistence of nineteenth-century philanthropists and social reformers. Additionally, a trip today to a stately home or a reconstructed Anglo-Saxon village or medieval castle would not be complete without a glimpse of the ancient child's world. This multi-pronged and inter-disciplinary approach to assessing the life of children from the past has enabled scholars of childhood to recreate ever-more accurately the social history of family life and paint detailed pictures of forgotten childhoods (Keville-Davies 1991; Cunningham 1995).

It is only fairly recently, however, that we have begun to ask children themselves about their lives and their childhood experiences, and started to listen to what children have to say (Mayall 2002; Alderson 2008; Layard & Dunn 2009). It is only recently that we have begun to value what children have to say, as evidenced by adults taking seriously the Sixth article of the United Nations Convention on the Rights of the Child (UNCRC), and to listen to the child's own tale be it for legal or for social purposes. This legal obligation can sometimes be difficult to sensitively put into practice, as evidenced by the potential trauma that a 4-year-old witness had to undergo at the Old Bailey (Criminal) Court in London while giving testimony against her abuser (Bennett & Fresco 2009). As Katherine Bennett comments in a fairly comprehensive (American) overview of the use of CCTV in American courtrooms for cases involving young children:

> … protecting the rights of accused persons while guarding against the potential of the criminal justice system to do harm to the child victims of crime continues to be a balancing act.
> (Bennett 2003:268)

We urgently need to find more sensitive and appropriate ways to listen to what children have to say – since for too long we have assumed they were incapable of objectivity or of reliably recognising the difference between truth and fantasy, and we considered them to be fickle-minded – if not upon occasion being spiteful towards their adult carers (Alderson 2008). This was certainly the problem in the past when children's accusations against their carers were not taken seriously enough, as in the notorious case of the Haut de la Garenne children's home on the island of Jersey (Byers 2008). All too often children were simply not listened to or believed (Hallett & Prout 2003; Archard 2004; Leeson 2007).

Children of course can comment most reliably and creatively about many aspects of their lives and fortunately not only about the desperate or criminal aspects of some of their experiences. The Iowa Historical Society together with the University of Iowa have recently launched the *Historic Iowa Children's Diaries Project* (HICD 2006), where they have made available to the public a digitalised collection of diaries written 150 years ago by children and youngsters in rural Iowa. This opportunity to look into the mindset of children of American pioneers is an excellent example of folk history being presented in such a way that it can enlighten and inform subsequent generations of children and adults. Children today are actively encouraged by their teachers and carers to have their say and to express themselves which today is more likely to be via the computer than in the form of diary entries; nonetheless, this gives them a platform to state what they are experiencing for all who have the inclination to hear them or read what they have to say. Professional historians are also aware that the voice of children needs to be heard, and it is therefore heartening that Beryl Rawson, in her excellent and exhaustive account of the lives of children in ancient Rome, states that she was actively searching for evidence of ancient reports written by children themselves concerning their childhood experiences (Rawson 2003). She says that unfortunately none have come down to us, but at least she highlights that crucial distinction in perspectives – the difference between narratives delivered by children about their childhood experiences as it is happening and narratives generated by adults concerning children.

Finally, it needs to be emphasised, that there is not one history of childhood, but many histories of childhood. Apart from obvious differences between any set of individual children's life-experiences, there are other overarching societal and cultural differences which separate children's lives even when they are living at the same time and in the same country, creating experiences of parallel childhoods which often could not be more disparate. Historians and anthropologists have looked at children's lives from all perspectives ranging from the childhoods of aristocratic and noble children, such as John Van Der Kiste's work on *Children at Court* (2003) to Cunningham (1991) who specifically looked at the lives of poor children in Europe. Meanwhile Kelly (2007) looked at the more recent past commenting on the daily life of children in the former Soviet Union, and Laurel Holliday (1995) looked at the recent past when editing the wartime diaries of Central European children from the 1940s. Cultural anthropologists such as Margaret Mead (1901–78) have looked at the lives of children in as far-flung places such as Papua New Guinea while trying all the time to compare the lives of children from different cultures – an endeavour which is necessary to undertake even today, especially with the number of issues arising out of the complexities of our multi-ethnic and multicultural societies. Thus, historically as well as in present times, children, alongside their parents, inhabited various and richly diverse socio-economic worlds – and sometimes even crossed over from one to the other – as did the present-day children involved in the production of the recent Indian film *Slumdog Millionaire*. But for those of us involved in children's nursing it is the fact that these various worlds coexisted at all and that the children of the past have left us legacies of their various worlds, or 'boxes' and 'envelopes' as Kelly (2007) refers to them, which is of prime interest.

SECTION TWO

A review of European childhoods from antiquity to the present

> … See the pictures on the walls,
> Heroes, fights and festivals;
> And in the corner find the toys
> Of the old Egyptian boys.
> Robert Louis Stevenson
> (1850–94, Stevenson 2000a)

As noted, there are almost no extant records from antiquity of what children thought about their own childhood, but there is evidence that from the very earliest of times, once civilisation started to shape family life, this sociobiological institution became important in confirming the stabilisation of society itself and in promoting and transmitting the dominant cultural values of society (Segalen 1986; Clayton 2001). It was also important very early in the history of family life for families to be able to account for themselves and their members, as families needed to know who was a member and who was not a member, and this pivotal distinction had many societal and legal implications – as indeed it still does today. Historically (and in some cultures, even till this day), the sheer number of words for the various levels of consanguinity and kinship acknowledged and recognised within a family was quite astounding, reflecting the importance given to wide-ranging social ties among members of an extended family. In ancient Rome, a child once born had to be formally accepted into the family and the patriarch of the family or father had to decide immediately after birth whether the child would be brought up as *his* son or daughter, or perhaps (for a variety of reasons) left to be brought up outside the family or even abandoned (Marys 1993; Corbier 2001; Rawson 2003). Once the child was formally incorporated into the family, however, family and societal values needed to be transmitted to the child, and the child needed to be taught a skill or trade or some method of survival. There is some debate about the actual extent and widespread use of this *acceptance* ritual in ancient Rome but it does illustrate the significance, at least for some families, of Roman family law and the importance of legal and social obligations towards those children acknowledged as your own (Dixon 1990; Rawson 1991, 2003).

In ancient Roman society, according to contemporary historians, there clearly was a concept of childhood, and there was recognition of the needs and concerns for the education of children, and a large section of Roman law was concerned with children and their hereditary rights (Rawson 1991). Although not too much funeral art represents children, where this does occur it is most beautifully and tenderly represented (Dixon 1990; Rawson 2003:18). Additionally, from the careful reading of Greek and Latin literature, a picture emerges of children who enjoyed playing games, although the teacher-philosophers Plato and Aristotle would have liked to curtail some of the playtime of children and have them study more. There is even evidence of a toymaking industry present in ancient Rome (Rawson 2003:19).

This childhood world in late antiquity was present and real for the children of city dwellers, the Greek and later Roman elite, and children of the relatively well to do. But the ancient world also practised the institution of slavery, and poor peasants (both free and enslaved) worked the land for their master, while free labourers and tradesmen supported the infrastructure of the state – and for all of them life could be hard. Women would have looked after small children, but with the high mortality rate associated with childbirth, this meant that many children were orphaned, and an orphaned child's fate was uncertain at best (Dixon 1990; Rawson 2003). There is some recent research on the art of mothering and the lives of women in ancient Rome and some interesting insights into the early life of newborns (Dixon 1990;

Rawson 2003). For children without families, however, the usual fate was being sold into slavery or being left to a life of prostitution or begging. In many ways, not much has changed in this respect over the centuries. There was (and still is) a huge economic divide between the life of the rich and well off and the life of the poor and infirm – a distinction not just relevant to developing countries. In the ancient pagan world of antiquity, a concept of *societal* responsibility for the welfare of these orphaned children and their families, should they fall on hard times, was all but unknown (Rawson 2003). Within the concept of an extended family adoptions of children and taking-in of impoverished relatives did occur, but this was more likely to be the case in the more affluent sectors of society. In Europe, it was the acceptance of Christianity as the state religion by the Roman Emperor Constantine in the fourth century AD which heralded the start of a church- and state-sanctioned provision of a safety net for the poorest and most destitute of society – but even this activity did not stop some the worst aspects of child neglect and cruelty.

The advent of Christianity meant that all children (in the eyes of God) were seen as important and deserving of our respect, not only the children of the well to do. The writings of some of the early Fathers of the Church shed some light on what educated early Europeans of late antiquity thought about children and how they formulated a theology of childhood, family life and marriage. We have some interesting insights therefore about family life and children in late antiquity from the writings of St Augustine (354–430). Augustine initially considered the child to be an innocent, but he modified his tone substantially when he reflected on his own rather adventurous youth and childhood (Chadwick 1986). In his famous autobiography, writing about infancy in general terms he observed:

> He was not old enough to talk, but whenever he saw his foster-brother at the breast, he would grow pale with envy. This much is common knowledge. Mothers and nurses say that they can work such things out of the system by one means or another, but surely it cannot be called innocence …

(Augustine 1961:28)

Augustine, prior to his conversion to Christianity, had a son, Adeodatus, and he was amazingly faithful to him over 14 years and to his concubine even though under Roman law this was not a necessity. Augustine in his autobiography describes his childhood and the life of children, generally, accurately and often quite tenderly, but when he describes, as above, scenes from the nursery it is as a fifth-century-male, uninformed as we are today of infant and child psychology (Chadwick 1986). As a result, to Augustine even an infant's tantrums were an indication of the non-innocence of children, something that seemed contradictory to the spiritual idea of the 'innate innocence of children'. Augustine proceeds to describe in his autobiography several discrete stages of child development, commenting on all of these and many aspects of his own childhood, such as the often-quoted reference to playing games and unfair punishments:

> … But we loved to play, and punishments were imposed on us by those who were engaged in adult games. For the amusement of adults is called business. But when boys play such games they are punished by adults, and no one feels sorry either for the children or for the adults …
>
> (Augustine 1961:30)

Augustine, the Bishop of Hippo, was busy fighting the Pelagian heresy and, as a result of his renewed thinking about baptism and especially infant baptism, concluded that all humans including newborns are burdened with sin, and only baptism can remove the burden of this sin and ensure their eternal life (Chadwick 1986). Augustine believed that when children are naughty or bad, they are showing sinful tendencies, and it is the original sin of Adam which accounts for these tendencies. He also believed that it is only the child's physical immaturity which can be considered innocent, for a newborn child's soul has the same burden and tendency to evil as that of any un-baptised adult (Stortz 2001). The effects of such thinking, in regards to infants and small children has led many Christian educationalists (down the centuries) to see in the misdemeanours and youthful errors of many young children resurgences of these evil tendencies, which, in turn, they feel need to be curtailed often by harsh punishment. Although Augustine had himself been physically punished

as a young boy, his comments and recollection of the events do not seem to inform future generations of educationalists and parents to be more moderate and refraining:

> … Though I was small my devotion was great when I begged you not to let me be beaten at school … our parents scoffed at the torments which we boys suffered at the hands of our masters. For we feared the whip as much as others fear the rack, and we no less than they, begged you to preserve us from it.
>
> (Augustine 1961:30)

As Martha Stortz notes, Augustine's influence on the understanding of children in theology '… formed and informed, transformed and deformed Christian attitudes towards children' (Stortz 2001:79). The cumulative effect of his writings, even allowing for the context of his times, was that subsequent pastoral teaching concerning children was effectively overly condemning of human nature and prone to advocating punishments (often physical punishments) as a mechanism to correct the natural exuberance and behaviours of children. Moreover, as a pastor he was aware of the marital problems of many members of his diocese in Northern Africa, and although he was aware of the practice of infanticide and abandonment of infants, he did not condemn the parents too harshly. Some of his more angry outbursts were reserved, however, for condemning the consequences of human nature and sexual activity, stating in a tract, *De peccatorum meritis*, that, 'the very root of sin lies in carnal generation' (Chadwick 1986:113).

Early medieval (Christian) thinking about children as represented by the writings of Thomas Aquinas (1225–74) acknowledged that loving a child and acceptance of a child was something natural to humans – and being part of our nature, was therefore a good thing. Additionally, Aquinas saw a difference between simply nature-generated concern for one's children and genuine care for children that also involves volition and intellectual reflection. Aquinas thought that care of children continued all through a child's life which had the effect of binding families together for life and promoting mutual responsibilities. Following Artistotelian arguments, Aquinas assumed that well-adjusted parents would care for their children and would strive to protect them against assaults from outsiders, thus having complete control over the child. However, as Traina (2001) points out in her review of Aquinas's approach to children, Aquinas considered respect and love towards one's parents to take precedence over love and concern for one's children on the basis that your parents have already given you life and love and protection – for which you need to be grateful and owe them respect in keeping with the third commandment – while your children are as yet an unknown entity and quite likely to die anyway (Traina 2001:121)!

Regardless of the actual longevity of children's lives, Aquinas certainly realised that loving one's children was a strong primal emotion and part of our basic nature, and he knew that whether or not our parents were still alive, and in need of care, we would certainly not stint love and affection on our children. Accordingly, apart from the provision of spiritual care, he considered the main tasks of parenthood to be the provision of material welfare for one's children and providing for their education (Traina 2001:121). Moreover, Aquinas's recommendation that parents educate their children was not just a pious wish, for he as many others put much emphasis on education and the need for knowledge and scholarship to underpin moral and social decision-making (Copleston 1955).

There is increasing historical evidence that post-antiquity Europe had an unbroken tradition of basic schools designed to teach children to read and write (Cunningham 1995; Orme 2006). There is documentation that these schools existed in ancient Greece, and we know that both Plato and Aristotle were involved in forms of teaching. Schools functioned throughout the Roman period and various artefacts that were used by Roman schoolboys are now displayed in museums. Schools that were attached to royal courts and cathedrals also existed until recent times. Moreover, contrary to the public myth, not all medieval schools were attached to monasteries, and many schools in cities were run by lay masters of varying intellectual abilities as noted by Orme (2006). Medieval schools were run predominantly for boys, since girls, if the parents chose to educate them, were educated at home, or sometimes even in a nunnery, though this was discouraged (Shahar 1990; Cunningham 1995; Meale 1996; Orme 2006). It was not till several centuries later that the state in England and other European countries saw it fit to educate all children – including girls – from every economic background. Even this endeavour was considered a controversial move at the time, and it took the vision and effort of many social reformers, parliamentarians and even philosophers – such as John Stuart Mill (1806–73) – to bring the notion of universal education for children to fruition.

Aquinas himself as a boy had been sent by his parents to be educated by the Benedictines at the Abbey of Monte Cassino, and as a young man he had studied at the universities of Naples, Paris and Cologne spending most of his time as a Dominican friar engaged in scholarly activities (Copelston 1955). His childhood was comfortable and his education for the times was one of the best. In keeping with the prevailing thinking at the time, however, Aquinas also saw a distinction in the needs and requirements between boys and girls, and he completely justified parental preferences for boys over girls. There is evidence that right through the Middle Ages girls tended to be abandoned at birth more often than boys, that they were weaned earlier in favour of boys, that they were denied the educational opportunities which was offered to boys – even among the relatively well-off families – and in order to be married (or enter a convent) they required a dowry. Some parents may have even felt blessed to have had daughters, but even these so-called open-minded parents did not want too many of them! Above all, medieval society reflected a rigid hierarchy, and as Traina (2001), observes,

> Nearly everyone spent a significant portion or even all of life under the power of others: nuns under abbesses; slaves under masters; peasants under nobles. Yet unlike adults, who normally both submitted to and exerted control, children were always at the bottom of the heap.
>
> (Traina 2001:126)

Aquinas was aware of this well-structured social hierarchy, but without advocating immediate social change or reform he insisted instead that parents should take their familial responsibilities towards their children seriously (Copelston 1955).

Fascinating as this review of medieval thinking about children may be, it is not Aquinas's thinking on family obligations that had the most lasting effect on European society's attitudes towards children but his religious ideas that helped formulate a medieval theology concerning the child's soul and spirituality. For Aquinas, as for Aristotle, the child was essentially an incomplete and immature adult, lacking in full wisdom and virtue, but the child did have all the necessary potential to become a mature and wise person and an honest virtuous citizen who would ultimately, if he or she led a good life, share in the Sonship of God – a Pauline theological concept which to the contemporary reader, as Traina observes, was articulated unfortunately in a 'troublingly gendered' format (Traina 2001:128). She continues that it was precisely Aquinas's recognition of the child's developmental capacities, however, even allowing for their presentation in a medieval theological context, which makes his theories about the nature of children acceptable to educationalists even today. Finally, it is important to note that the reason why one is looking at the life of children through the prism of religion is that for much of this period the majority of people who would have written and commented on the world around them were men of the clergy or monks and nuns, who have left us the bulk of documentation concerning children's lives.

Meanwhile, as already noted medieval children could be married off very early and sent to monasteries and obliged to work from a very early age. They were also given enormous responsibilities at an early age, such as running huge monasteries, defending their kingdoms in battle and ruling city states (Orme 1984; Heywood 2001; Woosnam-Savage 2008). There are of course many instances of adults acting as regents to boy-kings and rulers, but there are also cases of very young people who were simply burdened with the affairs of adults and who even found themselves on the battlefields (Orme 1984; Woosnam-Savage 2008). For children of noblemen, preparing for knighthood and warfare was a major undertaking and some youths undoubtedly looked forward to their lives as knights. Training for the role, however, included the wearing of (heavy) armour and learning all the martial arts necessary to be effective in combat, such as the skill of being able to jump 'on and off horses while armed and even while holding a naked sword' (Orme 1984:188). As Robert Woosnam-Savage (2008) curator of Leeds Royal Armouries observes:

The play and practice was for the battlefield and not just the 'playground'. Even in death some children could not escape the association of the sword. Children, presumably of royal birth, could be buried with swords as the finding in 1957 of the grave of a Frankish youth of about six years of age under Cologne Cathedral showed.

At the other end of the social spectrum were the children of peasants and poor city dwellers who were also sometimes pressed into warfare and who would probably have gone to the battlefield without any training whatsoever (Woosnam-Savage 2008). These young people were also expected, however, to help their parents financially at a trade or skill, or work the land and thereby contribute to the household economy. It would appear from the many records available across all of Europe that children and young people were forced into early social maturation and they took up their place in society much earlier than children do today (Cunningham 1995; Heywood 2001). As already noted, a young girl recently requested her school to give her permission to be absent for over a year in order to be able to undertake a solo trip around the world in a boat (Watson 2009). This case brings into sharp focus yet again the ongoing debate about when childhood begins and when it finishes and what are the obligations of adults and society towards children (Hanawalt 1992; Mayall 2002; Alderson 2008). See also Chapter 9 in this book for a review of current thinking surrounding the notion of adolescence and its relevance for healthcare workers.

Somewhat later, the comfortably well-off children of the English chancellor and Renaissance man of letters Thomas More (1478–1535) were being lovingly educated and cared for in a manner which we would consider to be a privilege even today (Bridgett 1892; Kenny 1983)! More enjoyed his family life and provided his children, including his daughters, with the highest standards of education of the day which consisted of Latin and Greek, logic, philosophy, astronomy and mathematics (Kenny 1983:18). In a letter to one of his daughter's tutors, More says that he wishes them to be well educated in letters and virtue because 'erudition in women is a new thing and a reproach to the idleness of men' (Kenny 1983:18). More's eldest daughter Margaret wrote letters to her father in such excellent Latin that her writings won praise even from Erasmus of Rotterdam (1466–1536), the great advocate of Renaissance humanism, who was a good friend of More (Kenny 1983:19). More strove to educate his daughters with humour and paternal concern, ever solicitous that they should not only be well behaved, genteel and lead virtuous lives but also be capable of sound reasoning and logic. As More commented in a letter to his daughters in 1522:

> How can a subject be wanting when you write to me, since I am glad to hear of your studies or of your games, and you will please me most if, when there is nothing to write about, you write about that nothing at great length. Nothing can be easier for you, since you are girls, loquacious by nature, who have always a world to say about nothing at all. One thing, however, I admonish you, whether you write serious matters or the merest trifles, it is my wish that you write everything diligently and thoughtfully. [Letter of Thomas More to his children, 1522]
>
> Bridgett (1892:133–134)

More, was quite open with his affection towards his children, as observed in his letter (in Latin) to his daughter:

> You ask, my dear Margaret, for money with too much bashfulness and timidity, since you are asking from a father who is eager to give, and since you have written to me a letter such that I would not only repay each line of it with a golden philippine, as Alexander did the verses of Cherilos, but, if my means were as great as my desire, I would reward each syllable with two gold ounces. [Letter of Thomas More to his daughter Margaret, 1520]
>
> Bridgett (1892:135)

Well might we wonder how common was this type of family life and interaction with children. As already noted, More himself was well aware that the extent of the formal education which he gave his daughters at that time was still a novel undertaking. However, we do know that throughout the Middle Ages some girls were educated and were therefore literate, since nuns (at least) in mon-asteries were expected to read scripture and devotional prayers, and many women have left for posterity their letters and papers not to mention poems and ballads and religious tracts which they wrote *themselves*, that is, were not dictated to clerks or chaplains (Wilson 1984). More recent scholarship in this area has confirmed this supposition and historians of medieval literacy even go further suggesting that women read not only for their own immediate needs and pleasure but also wrote texts which helped them in managing their homes and estates (Marchand 1984; Williard 1984; Boffey 1996; Meale 1996; Krug 2002). What is new in the More household is the extent of education he provided for his daughters – an undertaking noted by other scholars of the day such as Bishop Cuthbert Tunstall (1474–1559) who dedicated his textbook on arithmetic (*On the Art of Calculation*) to More's children (Kenny 1983:18)!

Meanwhile, children of peasants, labourers, merchants, and artisans, as well as professionals – such as lawyers and physicians – also experienced a childhood, but that childhood, especially in the context of rural poverty, did not extend much beyond the seventh or eighth year of a child's life. After that time, the child was increasingly expected to financially help out its parents and contribute in some form to the family economy (Cunningham 1995; Heywood 2001).

Needless to say, in an agrarian economy there tended to be more work in the summer than in the winter and there were longer working hours in the summer; but the work had its own pastoral rhythm, which some historians in the past have tended to romanticise. Seamus Heaney (the Irish Nobel Prize-winning poet) writing in the 1930s could well have been articulating the sentiments of countless rural children from previous centuries when he wrote about a father working the fields with a horse-plough while a child followed him in the furrows. The poem written from a child's perspective observes accurately the bond between the child and the parent, the child dreaming of following literally and figuratively in its father's footsteps, since the child muses, 'All I ever did was follow, In his broad shadow around the farm' (Heaney 2000).

Katrina Honeyman, however, reflecting contemporary research notes, that '...the romantic view, which juxtaposes the harshness of factory life with a pre-industrial golden-age, is a minority position' (Honeyman 2007:175). Work on the land could be as dangerous and hard for a youngster as work on medieval construction sites – such as building city walls and cathedrals and latterly in factories – but on the whole, rural work lent itself to a slower pace of living and certainly small children could be better supervised by their family, as Heaney's poem implies. From various reports in chronicles and diaries and even paintings, we can surmise that much of this agrarian-based rhythm of work, involving rural children's contribution to the family purse, changed very little over the centuries up to the advent of the Industrial Revolution. As Honeyman (2007) states concerning the debate surrounding child labour in the eighteenth century:

> That children should work was hardly the question. The nature of work conducted by children was hotly contested … Until the later eighteenth century, however, the consensus was that children should be productive for both economic and moral reasons.
>
> (Honeyman 2007:3)

The Industrial Revolution, therefore, did not throw children into paid work or even work outside the home, as that was already familiar practice, but it did change the nature of the work that children did (Horrell & Humphries 1995; Honeyman 2007). For the first time children were deliberately commercially *exploited* on a large scale. They worked inhumane hours from an incredibly young age, in unhealthy environments, for ridiculously low pay or, as in the case of parish poor children, for no pay at all, but in return for some food and clothing and, with some luck, a learnt trade or skill (Cunningham 1995; Honeyman 2007).

Towards the end of the eighteenth century and at the beginning of the nineteenth century as the new steam-propelled technology to produce cloth in a fast and inexpensive way was being introduced by entrepreneurs and businessmen, the exploitation of children (and women) who were hired to work in these cotton and silk mills began (Cunningham 1995; Honeyman 2007). Initially, mill owners sought to utilise existing adult labour from the surrounding areas, which explains why the mills tended to be located in or near towns and cities. But as the adult labour force from the surrounding areas dried up, ever-younger children of the existing labour force were also utilised and encouraged to find employment in the mills. As noted, these children were paid a pittance. There is quite a lively scholarly debate as to the actual economic and social significance of the labour of these children and the monies paid to them, and its effect on their family life (Horrell & Humphries 1995; Rahikainen 2004; Honeyman 2007). That the mill owners grew incredibly rich from the cheap labour of their workforce is well documented, but did parents send children to work in the mills because they brought in much-needed cash to augment the meagre family budget – even though we know it was a tiny contribution to the overall family income – or did the parents actually strive to have more children and thereby increase their potential earners so that the extra children could bring in extra cash? Finally, did the parents actually have a choice about how and where and when their children worked?

In 1843, the Victorian poet, Thomas Hood, sent anonymously to *The Punch* the ballad *The Song of the Shirt*, in which he described the timed labour of seamstresses.

> … With fingers weary and worn,
> With eyelids heavy and red,
> A woman sat in unwomanly rags,
> Plying her needle and thread …

The woman had little choice about her work and only dreamed about going out into the country – of having a break just for 1 h. Most parents sent their children into the mills and to the mines in order to bring in extra money. No doubt the parents were taken in by the sales pitch of the supervisors and mill owners, but their own working lives in the mills were not necessarily that much better off either (Cunningham 1995). Exploitation of children in factories and mills was occurring not only in Great Britain but also in the USA and other major industrialising countries of Europe. In Rhode Island, on the East coast of America, Samuel Slater opened his first textile mill and the majority of his first employees were children between the ages of 7 and 12. By 1830, 55% of all the millworkers on Rhode Island were children (Buhle *et al.* 1983)!

There were two groups of children exploited in the factories and mines. One group consisted of children who had families and who were paid wages, however small; and the other group consisted of children who were orphans and came from the poor houses. In eighteenth-century Britain, poor, abandoned and orphaned children were the responsibility of parish councils. As more agrarian families were becoming impoverished and moving to the cities and as more children were being abandoned, the finances of the parishes which looked after these children in special homes and workhouses were also increasingly being stretched. Rather than have the children become a long-term burden to the parish it was thought more appropriate to teach the children a trade or skill and give them the opportunity of becoming an apprentice. Sending children to be apprenticed to learn a trade was nothing new of course – this was common practice. It was considered a good economic solution for the children and also a sound moral approach as laziness was considered by society to be a great social wrong. It is not surprising, then, given this moralising approach to the welfare of the children, that there were a fair number of nonconformist entrepreneurs at this time who genuinely considered the work of the children in the mills and factories as good for the children themselves and as helping in building character.

Soon after the articulation of this theory of moral labour, there was the wholesale deportation of poor parish children from their workhouses in small towns and rural areas to the textile mills and mines. These children were not paid wages, and any money from the transaction went to the parishes from which they came. Initially, some of the mill owners were not aware of the conditions under which the children had to work, but this soon changed. It is to the merit of some of the Evangelical and Quaker nonconformist reformers that they were among the first to protest about the working conditions for children in the mills and agitated for reform and change. As early as 1802, the Factory Act was designed in England to stop this exploitation of the pauper-apprentice work system, but the law was only aimed at improving the life of children

from the workhouses who had no parents and therefore were the legal concern and responsibility of society. Meanwhile, children who had parents were not included in the recommendations and continued to work in the factories and mills (Bowditch & Ramsland 1968).

Joshua Drake from Dundee, a father who had a daughter working in the mills, stated to the Sadler Committee in 1832, which was set up to look into the working conditions in the mills, that he himself had worked in the mills since he was 5. In the summer he worked from four in the morning till ten or eleven at night – or 'as long as we could stand on our feet' (Bowditch & Ramsland 1968:86). Corporal punishment was frequently meted out to the children and they (especially the children from the parish workhouses) often tried to escape from the mills but were forcefully brought back and severely punished. He noted:

> There was a boy taken and tied upon another man's back, and they flogged him round the place … If the law could do anything for it, I would have them punished by law as for assault, where assault leaves a visible mark…
> (Bowditch & Ramsland 1968:82)

In 1833, a royal commission established by the government recommended that children aged over 11 be allowed to work a maximum of 12 h per day, but that younger children should work less hours and that those under 9 years of age were no longer permitted to work at all. But this too was just a recommendation, and not all factories followed suit immediately and, most crucially, it only applied to the textile industry. There were very many industries that were not included in the various subsequent factory acts, most notably the work of chimney sweeps whose fate was immortalised by the writers and social activists Charles Dickens and Charles Kingsley in their works of fiction. Only after much further lobbying, the 1847 Factory Act limited the working hours for adults and children to 10 h daily.

Meanwhile, in 1842 the Ashley Mines (Royal) Commission was set up to look into the welfare of workers, especially children, in the coal pits and mines. A 10-year-old boy Alexander Gray, who worked a pump, was interviewed and he stated to the Commission:

I pump out the water in the under bottom of the pit to keep the men's room (coal face) dry. I am obliged to pump fast or the water would cover me. I had to run away a few weeks ago as the water came up so fast that I could not pump at all. The water frequently covers my legs. I have been two years at the pump. I am paid 10d a day. No holiday but the Sabbath. I go down at three, sometimes five in the morning, and come up at six or seven at night.

To the same commission, 18-year-old Ann Eggley who worked in a coal mine since she was 7 stated:

I am sure I don't know how to spell my name … the work is too hard for me … father said – it was both a shame and disgrace for girls to work as we do.

(Bowditch & Ramsland 1968:87)

A 6-year-old girl testified to the committee that she had been down the mines for 6 weeks already and that she carried 'a full 56 lbs. of coal in a wooden bucket. I work with sister Jesse and mother. It is dark the time we go'. We learn from her that she was working down the mines with other members of her family.

Not until the 1860 Mines Regulation and Inspection Act, however, were all females and boys under the age of 12 prohibited from working underground. Interestingly, in order to be able to prove that a young person was of a certain age and therefore could legally work in the mines and factories, young people needed birth certificates. The 1837 Registration Act made it compulsory for all births, marriages and deaths to be registered at a registry office which was a separate document from a church record. Now, younger children who had previously only attended Sunday Schools (most of which taught some basic reading skills not only scripture) because they had been engaged working in mills and factories and mines had time to attend formal schooling during the week.

The first Elementary Education Act was not passed till 1870, however, which was 10 years after the 1860 Mines Regulation Act! This act made basic education obligatory for all 5- to 10-year olds. Slowly, over the years the school leaving age has risen. The school leaving age in Great Britain was only raised to 16 in 1973, although present governments are trying again to increase the obligatory leaving age. It is upon a youngsters 16th birthday that town/parish councils could relinquish their responsibilities towards the young people in their care. This too is slowly changing; councils and professionals working with youngsters are beginning to realise that a 16-year old – especially one who has been in care for most of his or her life and was looked after by local councils and lived in children's homes – is hardly in a position to be capable of being left entirely alone in the world to fend for itself (DCSF 2006; Leeson 2007; RCN 2008). Meanwhile, at 16 a youngster can legally marry and join the army but still may not buy alcohol or cigarettes or vote in national elections. (See Chapter 9 for some of the current ethical issues concerning work with adolescents.) Over the centuries, the lives of children and adolescents have changed a lot in many respects but have changed very little in others.

SECTION THREE

Thinking about childhood – reflecting on children

The contemporary child and youngster in the UK is perceived in several different ways, depending upon which school of thought the observer adheres to (Mayall 2002; Hallett & Prout 2003). Moreover, contemporary society has well-developed and entrenched ideas about the nature of children and young people and, depending upon the social context, changes and adapts its thinking and subsequent child-directed activities (Mayall 2002; Alderson 2008). There are at least three prevalent current images of children, which society readily recognises: the image of the innocent child, the image of the child as a threat to present and future society and the image of the child as a potential contributor to society (Larkin 2000; Mayall 2002; Towner 2008). Philip Darbyshire (2007) in his recent article on the nature of contemporary childhood picks up on some of the concerns and issues embedded in these classifications of contemporary children, adding suggestions as to how to *normalise* their childhood and bring back some joy into their lives.

The image of the child as being innocent is quite prevalent however throughout history, and as we saw with the thinking of Augustine and then Aquinas this image has had much popularity in church circles up to this day (Brueggemann 2008; Towner 2008). But the innocence of the child is not just due to the absolution of original sin following baptism, as Augustine originally suggested, which would have been a rather fragile situation at best. Prepubertal children were considered innocent and pure (of sexual knowledge and activity) and therefore holy, and should they become the unfortunate victims of slaughter and murder (martyrdom) as the Holy Innocents in the Bible story – who fell at the swords of Herod's soldiers – they were much admired and venerated as saints. Devout children who died young were also venerated and often canonised, their cult spreading across medieval Europe as examples of saintly innocents. It was also considered significant that in the New Testament children were portrayed positively and with compassion (Gundry-Volf 2001; Brueggemann 2008).

Medieval society admired and strove to emulate the *innocence* of children and children saints in varying ways, with some practices being rather endearing, for example, the tradition of the Boy Bishop enacted in many parts of Europe (till this day) on the feast of Saint Nicholas. Constructing hagiographies of saintly children shaped in turn the way that society subsequently conceptualised the *good child*. This perspective easily alters into seeing children as potential *victims* of a bad world, and therefore requiring society to have a tighter control over the life of a child so that the child would *not* fall prey to those intent on corrupting its innately good morals or otherwise harming the child/youngster (Darbyshire 2007). Even today, the public often refer to and conceptualise children as being innocent individuals and their innocence becomes all the more true and precious should a child or young person become the victim of a crime such as rape or murder. This is only too evident in how the media portray children who are the victims of various crimes, and goes some way to explain the confusion the public have over children who start to bond with their abusers, as noted in the recent case of Jaycee Lee Dugard (Moore 2009).

The perspective that children are seen as innocent players in the social life of adults contributes to the adult approach which disallows and dismisses the child's attempt to break out of conformity and social expectations of accepted childhood behaviours with the admonition 'that good children do not do behave like that', demonstrating a lack of understanding of even normal children's behaviour (Mayall 2002; Hallett & Prout 2003). The perspective that children are innately innocent can also, as a consequence, potentially demonise adults, since if the child is innocent and pure (and can do no wrong), the adult must be at fault. The compromise position that children might at any one time be somewhere on a scale between being totally socially and morally innocent, as the newborn child, and demonstrating the conniving awareness of a savvy adolescent is usually forgotten or overlooked. As children mature so does their awareness of the world around them and the formalisations of their interactions with the world; this is a long process (Mayall 2002). Very young children can (technically) operate computer chat sites, but this does not mean that they are socially ready or even aware of some of the potential consequences of their actions (Mitchell *et al.* 2003).

Children can also be seen as threats. The unruly child can be seen as a threat to society – to the established order. Since children are often unaware of societal norms and potentially ill adapted to living in our society, they need to be acculturated into its ways and norms. This is most commonly done through parents explaining societal values to children and through schools imparting moral education. Schools were founded as much to transmit to children prevailing societal and cultural values and norms as teach children how to read and write. Most parents still want schools to transmit certain moral values to children, but some parents who disagree with the prevailing norms and values expressed in contemporary schools want their children to be educated at home. The present rise of children being educated at home in Europe and the USA – assuming it is not just a middle-class passing fad – is an interesting social statement concerning the level of disquiet some parents have expressed concerning contemporary schooling. More importantly and worryingly, it reflects a serious level of non-sharing of prevalent societal values and a subsequent lack of social cohesion.

Children are seen as threats because they often demonstrate counterculture behaviours and some adults can feel threatened and rendered helpless by their actions. Youth workers comment, however, that most young people are totally unaware of the extent to which many adults are intimidated by them – a complete mismatch of perspectives. The contemporary poet, Gareth Owen, in his poem *All the Sad Young Men*, echoes concerns that had been raised by the child rights campaigner Janusz Korczak (Efron 2008). Abused and misunderstood young boys tend to grow up to be themselves abusing and *still* misunderstood adults (Owen:1995:17).

There are of course a lot of troubled children, and children who in their disrupted lives act out and often damage or destroy much that they come into contact with (see Chapters 9 and 10). Whether there are currently more emotionally disturbed children and whether the antisocial behaviour of some of them is worse than in the past is the work of child psychologists, sociologists, children's lawyers and the juvenile justice system to assess (Bradshaw & Mayhew 2005). Suffice to say here that such emotionally disturbed and socially disruptive children do exist, and that they too need to be seen as children and young people first – in need of expert help – and only as social offenders later, however unacceptable their actions. The UK justice system was reprimanded by children's rights lawyers when the two youngsters who killed Jamie Bulger were not treated as juveniles by the UK legal system. There is nothing new in the phenomenon of children killing children, but every time it occurs it is an indication of societal, familial or emotional problems. Children can also appear as threats to each other, for example, the current fashion among some youngsters of carrying knives and increasingly being prepared to use the knives against other young people, with all-too-often fatal consequences. Even more prevalent are cases of youngsters bullying and harassing other children, including cyber harassment. Children are not only increasingly being targeted by adults but also by other youngsters on the computer and they find themselves threatened and vulnerable. Mitchell *et al.* (2003) sums it up succinctly stating:

…threatening and offensive behaviours have been directed on the Internet to youths, including threats to assault or harm them, their friends, or their property and efforts to embarrass or humiliate them. Once again, the concern of parents and other officials is that the anonymity of the Internet may make it a fertile territory for such behaviours.

(Mitchell *et al.* 2003:9)

Finally, children can be perceived as potentials, that is, potential adults and basically not representing much in themselves at the present time but considered to be of great worth as future adults and future contributors to society. Thinking of children as *potentials* is the preferred conceptualisation of children by governments and states – children are the future tax-paying citizens of the nation and are necessary to continue the many long-term plans of society, such as work and pay for the future state pensions of the retired. This pragmatic conceptualisation of children need not completely negate the present worth of a child, but it has had some interesting consequences in terms of how some adults have approached children in the past and continue to approach them to the present day. By regarding the child as representing a future adult, there is an implicit understanding of the developmental aspects of childhood, but it also represents a conceptualisation of children where the child's current childhood concerns can be easily overlooked as being transient and therefore lacking in social and economic weighting. Since children are only children for a short period in their lives, society is sometimes ambivalent as to whether it is worth investing in and promoting this transient phase of young people's lives.

All too often one hears statement such as 'children's concerns are not weighty and important like those of adults', 'they will grow out of their concerns', 'they will forget their pains'. This had been the situation in the late 1800s in regards to the need to build specific children's hospitals and children's wards in general hospitals in order to accommodate the large number of sick children. It then became an ethical and medical issue to convince hospital governors, paediatricians and children's nurses that these sick children needed their parents around them if they were to be well cared for and to thrive. Unfortunately, there is no room here for a review of the history of children's nursing and the history of children's health-care provision; it is a fascinating and separate chapter in the social history of childhood (Hutchinson 1999; Bradley 2001; Kelsey 2002).

The Victorian poet R.L. Stevenson (1850–94) portrays an idyllic picture of the sick child convalescing in bed:

> When I was sick and lay a-bed,
> I had two pillows at my head,
> And all my toys beside me lay
> To keep me happy all the day …
>
> (Stevenson 2000b)

This is not that dissimilar a picture to the one drawn for us by children in British hospitals in the early 1900s (BJN 2007), but these rosy pictures of convalescing youngsters were unfortunately not the whole story. Most children were inadequately cared for by staff who were ill equipped to care for them, and at some point in the nineteenth century up to the middle of the twentieth century, it was even considered appropriate in hospital circles to keep hospitalised children separated from their families. Attempts were made, however, to improve the health of children and reduce infant mortality, and much effort was put into improving the quality of life of children both in Europe and in North America and Australia (Warsh & Strong-Boag 2005). At the present time, children have their own designated hospitals and qualified professionals who work with them, and most importantly they are not separated from their families. Indeed, they go to hospital only when their care and treatment is not possible in their home, and then they go accompanied by their parents or familiar carers.

Meanwhile, orphaned and poor children in the early 1900s were sent thousands of miles away to what was considered a better life and future for them, such as the famous railway children in the USA, or the children sent from the UK to Australia – all done with little regard to the emotional impact on the child (Holt 1992). When children themselves are asked about their needs and requirements for a good childhood, they often mention the presence of a reasonably harmonious family life, attendance

at school and a lack of grinding poverty. This seems to suffice. A young girl during World War II, pondered in her diary about her schooling, even though there was a war going on'… I wondered what will happen to our school, but Mama said that when a country is fighting for its survival, there is no time for schooling' (Holliday 1995:3). It is rare, that children and youngsters should mention specifics such as brand name toys or games, types of clothing or even the absence of disease, as vital prerequisites for a good childhood. Obviously, the response depends on the age of the child or young person, their educational and social background, personal experiences with the health-care and educational system and, most significantly, the actual year when the question is posed, that is, the political and sociocultural context in which the question is posed. When children were recently asked in the UK what for them constituted a good childhood, a 9-year-old girl in the first instance did note the absence of wars …

> I think the things that stop children and young people from having a good life are: wars, unkind people, parents that argue and split up, not having parents, not having enough food and water and not being able to live feeling safe.
>
> (Layard & Dunn 2009)

Children are traumatised by the presence of violence, whether between nations or among family members, and would, if they only could, avoid being confronted with the results of this violence. Currently, the presence of child soldiers in parts of Africa and Asia is a distressing phenomenon – and one that NGOs and aid agencies are attempting to address. Unfortunately though, as we have noted in this chapter, children down the ages have been caught up in the affairs and wars of adults and more often than not have fallen victim to the horrors of these adult conflicts (Amnesty International British Section 1995).

Conclusion

It has taken an awful lot of political and social campaigning over many decades, and taken the efforts of many scholars, child psychologists, paediatricians, children's nurses and concerned individuals to reach the point where we are today, where children are respected as individuals for what they are, with rights and privileges conferred on them precisely because they are children and young people living in the present; not in some distant future state and time.

In this chapter, I have reviewed the histories and philosophies of childhood and demonstrated how the daily lives of children have changed over the centuries. It is clear that many aspects of children's lives have changed for the better, but that unfortunately other aspects have changed little – for at least some children. Moreover, the quality of life for all children depends heavily on adults understanding the nature of childhood and the needs of children if they are to flourish and develop in an optimal fashion.

Some social reformers working for the welfare of children have even sacrificed the joys of having their own children in order to care for and promote the interests of other people's children, such as the legendary Polish paediatrician and child psychologist, Henry Goldszmit (pen name Janusz Korczak) (Veerman 1992; Efron 2008). Concerning the dedication of Korczak for his orphaned children, Veerman (1992) notes:

Korczak served the child and his rights as no one else in history did. Not only did he formulate ideas about the rights of the child, but he put them into practice for more than thirty years.
(Veerman 1992:93)

While reviewing the history of childhood for this book, the enduring image of the good doctor Korczak has stayed with me. Like him I dream of a world in which children's nurses and healthcare workers will stay committed to furthering the welfare of the child and never grow complacent for there is always so much more that can be done for the children and young people we work with. But this work will be more efficacious and rewarding if we do not lose sight in our endeavours of the essential nature of the child and do not neglect the needs of the small child present within each of us. As Korczak noted, it is important to:

...know yourself before you attempt to know children...first and foremost you must realize that you too, are a child whom you must first get to know...
(Korczak 2007)

References

Alderson, P. (2008) *Young Children's Rights – Exploring Beliefs, Principles and Practice*, 2nd edn. Jessica Kingsley, London.

Alexandre-Bidon, D. & Lett, D. (2000) *Children in the Middle-Ages*. University of Notre Dame Press, Notre Dame, Indiana.

Amnesty International British Section (1995) *Childhood Stolen – Grave Human Rights Violations Against Children*. Amnesty International British Section, London.

Anthony, A. (2009) Baby P: Born into a nightmare of abuse, violence and despair, he never stood a chance. *The Observer*, 16 August 2009.

Archard, D. (2004) *Children – Rights and Childhood*. Routledge, London.

Ariès, P. (1962) *Centuries of Childhood*. Vintage Books, New York.

Augustine, St (1961) *Confessions*. Penguin Classics, London.

BBC News (2009) Delhi girl left in sun to die. *BBC News Channel*, 14.06 GMT, 17 April 2009. http://news.bbc.co.uk/I/hi/world/south_asia/804238.stm

Bennett, K.J. (2003) Legal and social issues surrounding closed-circuit television testimony of child victims and witnesses. In: *The Victimization of Children: Emerging Issues* (eds J.L. Mullings, J. Margquart & D. Hartley), pp. 233–271. The Haworth Maltreatment & Trauma Press, Binghamton, New York.

Bennett, R. & Fresco, A. (2009) Trail ordeal of girl, 4. *The Saturday Times*, 2 May 2009, p. 1.

BJN (*British Journal of Nursing – Professional Issues*) (2007) Experiences of children in hospital: BJN 100 years ago. *British Journal of Nursing*, **16** (12), 748.

Blake, W. (2000) Holy Thursday (II). In: *The Nations Favourite Poems of Childhood* (ed. A. Warwick), p. 71. BBC Worldwide Ltd, London.

Boffey, J. (1996) Women authors and women's literacy in fourteenth and fifteenth century England. In: *Women and Literature in Britain, 1150–1500* (ed. C.M. Meale), pp. 159–282. Cambridge University Press, Cambridge.

Bowditch, J. & Ramsland, C. (eds) (1968) *Voices of the Industrial Revolution – Selected Readings*, 6th edn. University of Michigan Press, Ann Arbor, Michigan.

Bradley, S. (2001) Suffer the little children – The influence of nurses and parents in the evolution of open visiting in children's wards 1940–1970. *International History of Nursing Journal*, **6** (2), 44–51.

Bradshaw, J. & Mayhew, E. (2005) *The Well-Being of Children in the UK*. Save the Children & The University of York, London.

Bridgett, T.E. (1892) *Life and Writings of Sir Thomas More*, pp. 133–134. Burns & Oates, London.

Brinnin, J.M. (ed.) (1960) *Emily Dickinson*, No. 104, p. 108. Dell Publishers, New York.

Brueggemann, W. (2008) Vulnerable children, divine passion, and human obligation. In: *The Child in the Bible* (eds M.J. Bunge, T.E. Fretheim & B.R. Gaventa), pp. 399–422. William B. Eerdmans Publishing Company, Grand Rapids, Michigan.

Buhle, P., Molloy, S. & Sansbury, G. (eds) (1983) *A History of Rhode Island Working People*. Regine Printing Co., Providence, Rhode Island.

Byers, D. (2008) Remains of five children found at Haut de la Garenne Jersey former children's home. *Times Online*, 31 July 2008. www.timesonline.co.uk/tol/news/uk/crime/article 4434012.ece

Chadwick, H. (1986) *Augustine (Past Masters Series)*. Oxford University Press, Oxford.

Clayton, P.A. (2001) *Family Life in Ancient Egypt*. Hodder Wayland, London.

Copleston, F.C. (1955) *Aquinas: An Introduction to the Life and Work of the Great Medieval Thinker*. Penguin Books, London.

Corbier, M. (2001) Child exposure and abandonment. In: *Childhood, Class and Kin in the Roman World* (ed. S. Dixon), pp. 52–73. Routledge, London.

Cunningham, H. (1991) *The Children of the Poor: Representations of Childhood Since the Seventeenth Century*. Oxford University Press, Oxford.

Cunningham, H. (1995) *Children and Childhood in Western Society Since 1500*. Pearson Education Ltd, Harlow, Essex.

Darbyshire, P. (2007) 'Childhood': Are reports of its death greatly exaggerated? *Journal of Child Health Care*, **11** (2), 85–97.

DCSF (2006) *Care Matters: Transforming Lives of Children and Young People in Care*. Department for Children, Schools and Families, London.

Dixon, S. (1990) *The Roman Mother*. Routledge, London.

Druin, A. (1996) A place called childhood. *Interactions*, **3** (1), 17–22.

Efron, S.E. (2008) Moral education between hope and hopelessness: The legacy of Janusz Korczak. *Curriculum Inquiry*, **38** (1), 39–62.

Fox, A.L. & Abraham-Podietz, E. (1999) *Ten Thousand Children: True Stories Told by Children Who Escaped the Holocaust on the Kindertransport*. Behrman House, Inc, West Orange, New Jersey.

Gold, A.L. (1997) *Reflections of a Childhood Friend – Memories of Anne Frank*. Scholastic Inc, New York.

Gundry-Volf, J.M. (2001) The least and the greatest: Children in the New Testament. In: *The Child in Christian Thought* (ed. M.J. Bunge), pp. 29–61. William B. Eerdmans Publishing Company, Grand Rapids, Michigan.

Hallett, C. & Prout, A. (eds) (2003) *Hearing the Voices of Children – Social Policy for a New Century*. RoutledgeFalmer, London.

Hanawalt, B.A. (1976) Violent death in fourteenth and fifteenth century England. *Comparative Studies in Society and History*, **18** (3), 297–320.

Hanawalt, B.A. (1992) Historical descriptions and prescriptions for adolescence. *Journal of Family History: Studies in Family, Kinship and Demography*, **17** (4), 341–351.

Hanawalt, B.A. (1995) *Growing Up in Medieval London: The Experience of Childhood in History*. Oxford University Press, Oxford.

Heaney, S. (2000) Follower. In: *The Nations Favourite Poems of Childhood* (ed. A. Warwick), p. 139. BBC Worldwide Ltd, London.

Heywood, C. (2001) *A History of Childhood*. Polity Press, Cambridge.

Historic Iowa Children's Diaries Digital Collection (HICD) (2006) *The University of Iowa Libraries Digital Library Services*. digital.lib.uiowa.edu/diaries

Holliday, L. (ed.) (1995) *Children's Wartime Diaries*. Simon & Schuster/Pocket Books, New York.

Holt, M.I. (1992) *The Orphan Trains: Placing Out in America*. University of Nebraska Press, Lincoln, Nebraska.

Honeyman, K. (2007) *Child Workers in England 1780–1820*. Ashgate Publishing, Aldershot.

Horrell, S. & Humphries, J. (1995) The exploitation of little children: Child labour and the family economy in the Industrial Revolution. *Explorations in Economic History*, **32** (4), 485–516.

Hutchinson, K. (1999) Restored to life, and power, and thought. *International History of Nursing Journal*, **4** (3), 36–39.

Jenks, C. (2005) *Childhood*, 2nd edn. Routledge, London.

Jerrold, W. (ed.) (2004) *The Complete Poetical Works of Thomas Hood*. Kessinger Publishing Company, Whitefish, Montana.

Kelly, C. (2007) *Children's World – Growing Up in Russia 1890–1991*. Yale University Press, New Haven, Connecticut.

Kelsey, A. (2002) Health care for all children: The beginning of school nursing 1904–1908. *International History of Nursing Journal*, **7** (1), 4–11.

Kenny, A. (1983) *Thomas More (Past Masters Series)*. Oxford University Press, Oxford.

Keville-Davies, S. (1991) *Yesterday's Children: The Antiques and History of Childcare*. Antiques Collectors' Club, Woodbridge.

Kiste, J.V.D. (2003) *Childhood at Court*. The History Press Ltd/Sutton Publishing, Thrupp/Stoud.

Korczak, J. (2007) *Loving Every Child* (ed. S. Joseph). Algonquin Books/Workman Publishing, Chapel Hill, North Carolina.

Krug, R. (2002) *Reading Families: Women's Literate Practice in Late Medieval England*. Cornell University Press, Ithaca, New York.

Larkin, P. (2000) Coming. In: *The Nations Favourite Poems of Childhood* (ed. A. Warwick), p. 165. BBC Worldwide Ltd, London.

Larkin, M. (2009) *Vulnerable Groups in Health and Social Care*. Sage Publications Ltd, London.

Layard, R. & Dunn, J. (2009) *A Good Childhood – Searching for Values in a Competitive Age*. The Children's Society/Penguin Books, London.

Leeson, C. (2007) My life in care: Experiences of non-participation in decision-making processes. *Child and Social Work*, **12** (3), 268–277.

Marchand, J. (1984) The Frankish Mother: Dhuoda. In: *Medieval Women Writers* (ed. K.M. Wilson), pp. 1–29. The University of Georgia Press, Athens, Georgia.

Marys, S. (1993) Infanticide in Roman Britain. *Antiquity*, **67** (257), 883–888.

Matthews, G.B. (1994) *The Philosophy of Childhood*. Harvard University Press, Cambridge, Massachusetts.

Mayall, B. (2002) *Towards a Sociology for Childhood – Thinking from Children's Lives*. Open University Press, Maidenhead.

Meale, C.M. (1996) "…alle the bokes that I have of latyn, englisch, and frensch": Laywomen and their books in late medieval England. In: *Women and Literature in Britain, 1150–1500* (ed. C.M. Meale), 2nd edn. pp. 128–159. Cambridge University Press, Cambridge.

Mitchell, K.J., Finkelhor, D. & Wolak, J. (2003) Victimization of youths on the internet. In: *The Victimization of Children – Emerging Issues* (eds J.L. Mullings, J.W. Marquart & D.J. Hartley), pp. 1–41. The Haworth Maltreatment & Trauma Press, Binghamton, New York.

Moore, M. (2009) Jaycee Lee Dugard walks into police station 18 years after disappearance. *Daily Telegraph on-line* (Telegraph.co.uk), published 9.17 pm 27 August 2009 on www.telegraph.co.uk/news/worldnews/northamerica/usa/6101545.

Opie, I. & Opie, P. (1959) *The Lore and Language of Schoolchildren*. Oxford University Press, Oxford.

Orme, N. (1984) *From Childhood to Chivalry – The Education of the English Kings and Aristocracy 1066–1530*. Methuen Press, London.

Orme, N. (2003) *Medieval Children*. Yale University Press, London.

Orme, N. (2006) *Medieval Schools – From Roman Britain to Renaissance England*. Yale University Press, New Haven, Connecticut.

Owen, G. (1995) All the sad young men. In: *The Fox on the Roundabout and Other Poems*, pp. 16–18. CollinsChildren'sBooks, London.

Postman, N. (1982) *The Disappearance of Childhood – How TV is Changing Children's Lives*. W. H. Allen & Co., London.

Rahikainen, M. (2004) *Centuries of Child Labour: European Experiences from the Seventeenth to the Twentieth Century*. Ashgate Publishing, Aldershot.

Rawson, B. (ed.) (1991) Adult-child relationship in Roman society. In: *Marriage, Divorce, and Children in Ancient Rome*, pp. 1–7. Clarendon Paperback/Oxford University Press, Oxford.

Rawson, B. (2003) *Children and Childhood in Roman Italy*. Oxford University Press, Oxford.

RCN (2008) *Adolescence: Boundaries, Connections and Dilemmas*. Royal College of Nursing, London.

Segalen, M. (1986) *Historical Anthropology of the Family*. Cambridge University Press, Cambridge.

Shahar, S. (1990) *Childhood in the Middle Ages*. Routledge Publishing, London.

Stevenson, R.L. (2000a) Children. In: *The Nations Favourite Poems of Childhood* (ed. A. Warwick), p. 108. BBC Worldwide Ltd, London.

Stevenson, R.L. (2000b) The land of counterpane. In: *The Nations Favourite Poems of Childhood* (ed. A. Warwick), p. 109. BBC Worldwide Ltd, London.

Stortz, M.E. (2001) Where or when was your servant innocent? Augustine on childhood. In: *The Child in Christian Thought* (ed. M.J. Bunge), pp. 78–102. William B. Eerdmans Publishing Company, Grand Rapids, Michigan.

Towner, S.W. (2008) Children and the image of God. In: *The Child in the Bible* (eds M.J. Bunge, T.E. Frentheim & B.R. Gaventa), pp. 307–322. William B. Eerdmans Publishing Company, Grand Rapids, Michigan.

Traina, C.L.H. (2001) A person in the making: Thomas Aquinas on children and childhood. In: *The Child in Christian Thought* (ed. M.J. Bunge), pp. 103–133. William B. Eerdmans Publishing Company, Grand Rapids, Michigan.

Veerman, P.E. (1992) Janusz Korczak and the rights of the child to respect. In: *The Rights of the Child and the Changing Image of Childhood*, Chapter VII, pp. 93–112. Martinus Nijhoff Publishers, Dordrecht.

Warsh, C.K. & Strong-Boag, V. (eds) (2005) *Children's Health Issues in Historical Perspective*. Wilfrid Laurier University Press, Waterloo, Ontario.

Warwick, A. (ed.) (2000) *The Nation's Favourite Poems of Childhood*. BBC Worldwide Ltd, London.

Watson, R. (17 November 2009) Confined to port: Sailor girl not ready for solo voyage round the world, rules court. *Saturday Times*, 31 October 2009, p. 31.

Williard, C.C. (1984) The Franco-Italian Professional Writer: Christine de Pizan. In: *Medieval Women Writers* (ed. K.M. Wilson), pp. 333–263. The University of Georgia Press, Athens, Georgia.

Wilson, K.M. (ed.) (1984) *Medieval Women Writers*. The University of Georgia Press, Athens, Georgia.

Woosnam-Savage, R.C. (2008) "He's armed without that's innocent within." A short note on a newly acquired medieval sword for a child. *Arms and Armour*, **5** (1), 84–95.

Zimler, R. & Sekulović, R. (eds) (2008) *The Children's Hours – Stories of Childhood*. Arcadia Books, London.

2 Theories of Moral Philosophy Applied to Paediatric Nursing

Gosia M. Brykczyńska

Introduction

According to Pat Benner *et al.* (2009) current nurse education is aimed at enabling nursing students to successfully complete three high-end apprenticeships in order that they may become competent registered nurses. These apprenticeships are as follows: a cognitive apprenticeship – facilitated through the theoretical and scholastic rigour of academia, a skilled know-how of clinical practice apprenticeship – ensured through appropriate clinical placements with suitable mentors as practical guides and the preparation for ethical comportment apprenticeship – delivered through the philosophical and professional components of the nurse education course. In their thought-provoking book, they report on their findings from a large review of nurse education, recommending a major refocusing of some of the sacrosanct subjects and ideas currently taught within nurse education programmes. They see the need for facilitating the moral discourse of nurses in order to enable the growth of what they refer to as moral comportment. Transmitting professional and socially appropriate nursing values and ethos has always been a challenge for nurse educators, and perhaps the best place to start is to consider the nature of nursing moral vocabulary and to examine some underlying theories which shape nurses' moral debates – something also noted and recommended in Davis & Fowler (2006) chapter on teaching nursing ethics.

Moral concerns have always been with us. For as long as humanity has been reflecting on its activities and expressing concern over the moral choices which it has had to face, philosophers have been around to help articulate ethical arguments (Stumpf & Fieser 2003; Fowler & Tschudin 2006). In varying degrees and in different ways, almost all cultures which have been studied, and certainly all those cultures which possess a written record of their history, have expressed awareness of and appreciation for philosophy and in particular moral philosophy. Different cultures have relied on different philosophical traditions to inform their moral debate, and this richness in plurality of approaches in regarding the world and human activities should not be glossed over, for there are as many world views as there are cultures and, therefore, there are many philosophical traditions.

For the purposes of this book, however, only a review of the main ways of moral reasoning as expounded by moral philosophers in the European tradition will be considered. Since modern nursing, as a recognisable separate profession allied to medicine, is considered to be a product of European social and religious culture, examining European ways of moral reasoning which have underpinned and shaped the profession seems most fitting and useful (Fowler 2006; Fowler & Tschudin 2006). In this book devoted to the myriad concerns and issues surrounding the morality and philosophy of paediatric nursing, a short review of the most commonly encountered ethical theories should be of some help. Although most nurses undertake some sessions in health-care ethics during the course of their professional education, this is often of a very cursory nature. Therefore, to help the reader who may be unfamiliar with some aspects of these theories and to re-familiarise others with their content, this chapter will explain the basic tenets of some of these philosophies.

Deontology – non-consequentialism

Among the several theories of moral philosophy relevant to health-care workers, non-consequentialism, or theories of deontology, assumes special significance. All so-called professional codes of conduct, such as the Nursing and Midwifery Council (NMC) professional code of conduct which is binding for all UK-registered nurses, the General Medical Council (GMC) code of conduct which binds physicians, the Medical Research Council (MRC) code for researchers and so on, are based on ethical principles embedded in the moral theories of deontology. Deontology, from the Greek word *deon* meaning duty/law, is the moral theory which states that our moral conduct should be guided by more than just concern for good or optimal consequences of our actions; it should be additionally based on universally recognisable rules and regulations, which it is *our duty* to obey. Our moral conduct should be guided by some absolute principles which explain the duties which we need to adhere to and respect. Obviously, we need to take into account some aspects of the consequences of our actions – not to do so would be at best short-sighted and at worst dangerous – but the main moral motivation for our actions should not be concern for the resulting production of good over evil but doing that which we ought to

do because it is the right thing to do and it is our duty to do it. That is, we should conduct ourselves in such an ethical manner as to reflect in our behaviours and motivation other more universal principles of conduct than just concern for the consequences of our actions.

If I only buy my train ticket when I know that inspectors are likely to board my train, I am behaving morally on those occasions, but the rationale for my moral behaviour leaves something to be desired. Deontologists would require me to always buy my train ticket regardless of whether there is a ticket inspector around, on the basis that not buying a ticket could not be made into a universal moral law binding on everyone at all times and, additionally, that not paying for my train tickets is not an intrinsically good action since it is a form of stealing. The philosopher who is best known for articulating this moral theory is the East Prussian philosopher Immanuel Kant (1724–1804). (See Scruton (1982) or Stumpf & Fieser (2003) for more details on his life and work.)

Immanuel Kant, writing during the eighteenth century, wanted to prove to his contemporaries that it was possible to justify moral actions without recourse to a theological or religious discourse. While he himself was a devout Christian, he was concerned that secularist writers and thinkers (especially after the French Revolution of 1789) would weaken secular arguments for moral behaviour in refuting Christian-based moral theology. He believed that morality was not only possible without reference to religion and theology, but, given the intellectual climate of his times, quite essential. He therefore set out to articulate what today is considered the basis of deontological reasoning present in much of our social and civic thinking (Scruton 1982). Much of his writings take for granted that the moral agent would be a thinking, reflective person of goodwill. This assumption is in fact common to many philosophers of various persuasions, and needs to be fully appreciated if the theories these philosophers articulate are to be properly evaluated.

Kant believed that every person was governed by a universal moral law, or, as he put it, a *supreme moral law*. This idea was a result of his belief that each individual has an intrinsic value – that people are important and special by the very virtue of being human beings; that they are in fact ends unto themselves as opposed to some means to an end, just as a small fish may be considered food for a larger fish in the natural order of the food chain. The small fish has little intrinsic value in itself. It has value only because it is part of the food chain, part of nature. For Kant, people were important in themselves (they respected themselves and looked after themselves), and these same rational beings likewise respected and treated other individuals with care.

To explain this theory in practical terms, he articulated the so-called categorical imperatives – or maxims. These imperatives were to direct and inform the moral agent along specific lines of arguments and judgements. We will list in the following the three most comprehensive maxims.

Categorical imperative I

To act only on the maxim through which you can and at the same time will that it should become universal law.

This is sometimes called the principle of universality, or, the golden rule – *Do unto others as you would have them do unto you*. Kant explained that if you wanted to lie – because you considered it was not in someone's best interest to be privy to the truth – could you at the same time desire and indeed will (which is an even stronger requirement) that everyone always do exactly the same? Indeed, would you really want everyone to behave like that – even towards you should you be at the receiving end of such moral reasoning sometime in the future? In her seminal work on lying, the applied philosopher Sissela Bok (1978) devoted a whole chapter to the phenomenon of lying in health-care contexts. The chapter raises some interesting points concerning the entrenched aspects of paternalistic lying so prevalent in health-care work and still encountered in paediatric contexts. In a more recent thought-provoking article, de Raeve (2002) has also commented on the ethical issues surrounding aspects of trust and integrity pertaining to nurses and their work.

Categorical imperative II

No person should be treated merely as a means to an end, but always as an end unto themselves.

Kant was in awe of the human person. He thought that the individual was unique, and his appreciation for the intricate biology and spirit of the individual led him to acknowledge that human beings have their own intrinsic worth. He considered that humans represent an intrinsic value in and of themselves and are not to be thought of as merely the playthings of gods (as ancient Greek mythology insinuated) or the property of others (as demonstrated in the possession of serfs in Russia or later the maintenance of slavery in Europe and USA). Kant had lived through the turbulent times of the French Revolution, and the populist slogan of *Liberty, Equality and Fraternity* (to all) were well known to him (Scruton 1982). This thinking leads on to considering that all humans, including children, have some intrinsic basic rights; this theory will be re-examined later in this chapter and in other chapters of this book.

The maxim 'never to treat a person solely as a means to an end' resonates today whenever the bioethical issues surrounding certain in vitro fertilisation cases are publicised, where parents attempt to conceive a child with a particular set of genetic characteristics in order to obtain organs and tissue from this newly generated offspring thereby helping cure a sibling from a terminal illness. Not only is the newly conceived child brought into existence primarily for reasons other than its own intrinsic worth and value but there is also the possibility that other potential children (embryos) were discarded in the process only because they did not have the sought-after characteristics. It is hard not to quote Kant's maxim in such cases however much we may want to sympathise with the parents.

This maxim is also relevant for children's nurses in the way that they treat the children in their care – as important and significant individuals meriting professional attention and concern in the present moment and not for what they will or might become some day, that is, *future* adults and potential contributors to the social good. This is a sentiment most relevant to the work of paediatric nurses as some young patients unfortunately will never grow up and develop into mature adults. Some children only have the *now* in which to be themselves. Some of these ethical issues will be explored further in subsequent chapters of this book.

Categorical imperative III

Finally, Kant thought that in determining the merits of a particular action we should consider whether it would be possible to impose upon other independent and valued moral agents the universisable moral act in question. He put it thus:

> The agent must always act as if he were a king creating a universal law for his kingdom of ends in themselves.

The effect of such thinking together with the other imperatives is that when we consider our moral actions, we should be capable of following general, universal moral principles, which we are personally satisfied to follow and indeed desire that everyone else follow, in order to demonstrate respect towards others and the duty we owe to others – people like us are also valued members of humanity. Therefore, I will never lie, cheat, steal, break my promises, etc. It is this aspect of his thinking which underpins our codes of professional conduct.

In 1979, the applied philosophers Tom L. Beauchamp and James F. Childress wrote their first textbook on the *Principles of Biomedical Ethics*, a classic text which has since been translated into many languages and has had numerous imprints and editions. Their four biomedical principles of non-maleficence, beneficence, justice and autonomy encapsulated in an easily understood framework the necessary moral imperatives required in health-care practice. These principles were derived from an understanding of deontology and were applied to the issues and concerns of health-care workers. Steven Edwards (2006:66) justifies this principle-based approach to ethical nursing, stating that nurses find the principles relatively easy to understand and to apply in their working environments, since the principles already reflect 'compatibility with professional nursing practice'. The principles, however, are general and, in practice, can and do sometimes contradict each other; some philosophers consider the principles to lack the capacity for attention to detailed particularities of practice. Nonetheless, for the first time a textbook on medical ethics captured the imagination of health-care workers around the world on a truly amazing scale.

Possibly, the biggest problem, however, for twenty-first century health-care workers and those involved with the care of children is that while most members of society may find Kantian deontology rather hard to accept (and understand), it does form the basis of most of our professional codes of conduct and public legislation which also governs our publicly sanctioned nursing activities. There is therefore the inescapable and inbuilt potential for conflict of moral perspectives – the deontological imperatives of duty and universality of moral conduct (according to Kantian philosophy) which is required of health-care professionals as explained in the writings of Beauchamp & Childress (2008) and Edwards (2006) versus a tendency to think and react along the lines of more utilitarian pragmatism which is the prevailing (and potentially less morally demanding) form of ethical reasoning undertaken by the rest of society. We will now look at the theory of utilitarianism.

Utilitarianism – consequentialism

Utilitarianism is that form of ethical reasoning which is primarily concerned with the end result of our moral actions. When deciding upon a particular moral activity, consideration is given to the quantity of beneficence and public welfare that will be increased and generated due to my actions, rather than the intentions I might have had in undertaking a particular action or even for the consideration of some higher principles, for '…Utility, or the Greatest Happiness Principle, holds that actions are right in proportion as they tend to promote happiness, wrong as they tend to produce pain …' (Mill 1998:55).

The greatest exponent of this form of ethical reasoning was the English philosopher John Stuart Mill (1806–73), who was as colourful and interesting a public figure during his lifetime as Immanuel Kant was a retiring and a relatively unknown pedantic academic. (For an account of JS Mill's life and works see Stumpf & Fieser 2003.) While both were later considered giants of philosophical discourse, it was JS Mill who captured the public imagination, giving a reasoned voice to concepts of modern democracy which are felt and indeed integrated into contemporary political life even today. Based on the work of his mentor, the reformist and writer Jeremy Bentham (1748–1832), JS Mill stated what seemed intuitively right and natural to many people, namely, that what we desire most from life is happiness and contentment and that most of our actions (directly or indirectly) are geared towards attaining and promoting happiness. Therefore this natural inclination cannot help but be morally acceptable; as he noted '... men do desire happiness; and however imperfect may be their own practice, they desire and commend all conduct in others towards themselves, by which they think their happiness is promoted' (Mill 1998:74). Mill went even further and stated that we should actually strive to bring about happiness by opting for those moral decisions that promote happiness and refrain from those activities that decrease the overall amount of happiness.

Needless to say, such a moral theory is extremely attractive, and it would appear that so long as it can be demonstrated that our moral activities promote our happiness, our moral obligations towards society are resolved. However, Mill was not so naive, and the true happiness which he had in mind was a happiness for the public good; as he noted, people do '... desire to be in unity with [] fellow creatures, which is already a powerful principle in human nature, and happily one of those which tend to become stronger, even without express inculcation, from the influences of advancing civilization' (Mill 1998:77). He couched his theory of utilitarianism with so many caveats and clauses that ultimately the moral integrity of the utilitarian was as impressive as that of the serious deontologist from Königsberg. For Mill, a moral act was considered good if it promoted the happiness and well-being of the majority of the people. Inbuilt into this theory, however, was a conscious recognition that some individuals might lose out and that the wishes of a minority of individuals may well be overruled or disregarded for the greater good of the whole community. This particular aspect of his social and political philosophy has come to be understood as the basis of our modern democratic system of government. It also forms the heart of Mill's ethical theory on utilitarianism.

Mill wrote his classic essay *On Utilitarianism* in order to explain to the public the principle of utility and to defend the ideas of his mentor, the reformer Jeremy Bentham. In the process, however, he came to articulate his own interpretation of the moral philosophy of utilitarianism, which ultimately differed quite substantially from Bentham's original

ideas. Mill acknowledged the difference between different types of happiness putting far greater emphasis on the quality of happiness generated as opposed the amount of happiness; as he stated, 'It would be absurd that [-] the estimation of pleasures should be supposed to depend on quantity alone' (Mill 1998:57). The main thrust of utilitarianism, whether it is focused on ethical rules or actions, was to separate the motivation for the action from the deed itself and to separate the person from the act, that is, it is not the person's volition which determines whether an act is morally good or bad but the positive and good consequences of that action, which is the promotion of happiness. Because of this emphasis, Mill acknowledged that much thought would need to go into our moral actions and that we would need to attempt to sensibly predict the consequences of our actions and choose wisely our ethical acts. Underlying much of this thinking was Mill's belief that the public should be educated and well schooled in order to be capable of making these appropriate decisions concerning their true happiness!

True to such assertions, Mill was himself a great social reformer, lobbying for universal education for all citizens and standing for parliament on a reforming platform. He married the suffragette Harriet Taylor (1807–58) with whom he wrote many pamphlets and books and was close friends with many Victorian poets and writers, in particular Coleridge (1772–1834) and Wordsworth (1770–1850). He retired early to the south of France due to ill health. Many critics thought that his attitudes as expressed in his treaties *On Utilitarianism* published in 1863 were somewhat paternalistic and that his theory of utilitarianism contained several basic fallacies and lacked intellectual rigour and coherence. But Mill at least acknowledged that in order to make a reasoned ethical decision one ought to have a modicum of knowledge and information, that is, a basic education. In conclusion, utilitarianism rejects personal bias and moral intuition, thereby avoiding the problems noted with plurality of principles that deontology engenders and with it the frequent clashes of these principles and the resultant difficulties in ethical decision-making.

Accordingly, it could be argued that the shortened working hours for health-care workers legislated by the European Union is a utilitarian solution to individual preferences (and work practices). Overall, more goodwill be accomplished if patients are treated by rested and healthy carers than if they are looked after by dangerously exhausted staff. Thus, even if we personally wanted to and were prepared to work extra hours in the day or week, this approach might not be in the long-term interest of our patients and the majority of other health-care staff. In such a case, we should be prepared to put aside our personal preferences (which we may well have convinced ourselves promotes our personal happiness and good) and accept those decisions which promote the common good for the majority of health-care staff and patients. It is another deliberation entirely whether shortening the working hours of health-care workers may not, in the short term, deprive patients access to sufficient numbers of qualified health-care professionals until more staff can be educated. In the meantime, this policy may cause exhaustion for the existing staff.

Rights theories

During the late seventeenth and eighteenth centuries, other philosophers and reformers were debating about human rights. For European observers of the late-eighteenth-century political and social scene, it was clear that society was polarised between the haves and the have-nots, and that even hard-won political and legal assurances of security and safety were beginning to be eroded and count for very little. A king could still force you to take up arms, a *Seigneur* could still set arbitrary demands on your time and labour, and a far-flung ruler could demand from you import taxes – and in all of this there was very little recourse to the law. Indeed, the law was the enforcer of many of these top-down decisions that affected the majority of citizens. While this situation was not necessarily that different from previous centuries, it was the increase of a literate and mobile middle-class town population, sandwiched between people of immense wealth on the one side and peasants and labourers of the land on the other, which led to the airing and subsequently writing of commentaries on the injustices of the situation (Stumpf & Fieser 2003). It is almost inevitable that unrest and grumblings would become manifest by the late eighteenth cen-

tury. Add to this the clamouring for independence from colonials in the Americas, an increase in Christian sectarianism which meant that many Europeans were leaving the familiar territories of Europe to escape religious persecution and starting up new lives in the new lands, and a series of bad economic decisions by potentates resulting in poverty and famine in Europe and the result was chaos and revolution. This was the socio-economic and political context for the formation of a group of insightful statesmen and thinkers who started commenting and reflecting on the social injustices of the situation. The result of this debate was some fairly lofty writings and declarations concerning the welfare and entitlements of ordinary people in respect to their person (Stumpf & Fieser 2003).

An understanding of the need for articulating human rights and the acknowledgement of the existence of human rights – or entitlements – had been commented upon by several earlier philosophers and writers, such as the English philosophers Thomas Hobbes (1588–1679) and John Locke (1632–1704). But it was the later writers of the enlightenment however, such as the Frenchman Jean Jacques Rousseau (1712–78) and the early American thinkers and politicians such as Thomas Jefferson (1743–1826) and Benjamin Franklin (1706–90), who contributed most to the subsequent debate on human and political rights (Waldron 1984; Stumpf & Fieser 2003).

Not all commentators, however, were that enamoured by the concepts as they were presented by these philosophers. Jeremy Bentham thought that the writings represented just a collection of lofty ideals and empty words not amounting to much – or, as he put it, they were no more than 'nonsense on stilts'. But the idea that human beings (precisely because they are humans) may have inherent rights caught the social if not political and philosophical imagination; as Austin states '... The central assumption of the rights paradigm is that every person can make certain claims based solely on their humanness' (Austin 2003:105). Most of these early rights, however, as presented to the public of the late eighteenth and early nineteenth centuries were socio-political in nature and concerned such areas of life as the right to own property, to bear arms, to profess a particular religion free from interference and the right to life. In these basic rights, we can see the influence of the early colonial

American thinkers who were also trying at this time to justify their move towards independence (Austin 2003). These early declarations of human rights did not, of course, include giving women the right to vote, or even acknowledging women's independent status; women were still *owned* by their husbands and had no civic presence. Neither were the rights of slaves or serfs included, or their fate and existence seriously debated; nonetheless it was a major step forward in acknowledging that people (i.e. individuals other than the aristocracy or landed gentry) have some basic rights vis-à-vis a potentate or ruler and that a legitimate state could not allow these rights of its citizens to be violated.

Slowly these early basic rights became incorporated into the laws of various countries and over the next two centuries these rights were elaborated upon to incorporate significantly more than just socio-political entitlements of the public (Waldron 1984; Austin 2003). Increasingly, these human rights had more to do with requisites for basic human existence and happiness and less to do with the early preoccupation with socio-political oppression. Today, most governments around the world subscribe to the Universal Declaration of Human Rights (UN 1948) and within Europe, *The Charter of Fundamental Rights of the European Union* (2000). Additionally, as health-care professionals working with children, there are many aspects of the 1989 United Nations Convention of the Rights of the Child (UNCRC) which are not only binding on professional workers in regards to the care and welfare of children but which provide the non-disputed legal context in which health-care services to children and their families must be delivered (UN 1989; Alderson 2008). See Chapter 3 for an elaboration of children's rights in regards to health-care provision.

As with all moral theories, there are some issues with rights-based approaches to moral interaction (Waldron 1984; Austin 2003). Probably the most obvious is that citizens need to understand what is actually meant by their human rights, and they need to know what rights they themselves are entitled to, this point being brought out quite forcefully in the implementation of the UNCRC (Alderson 2008). They also need to know what are their corresponding obligations or duties in respect to these rights (Austin 2003). For example, a child has the right to a free and universal education sup-

plied by the state, but society agrees in return to pay taxes to the state which will facilitate the funding of state-provided universal education. There are many such matched societal rights and duties, and people are becoming more aware of their rights but less cognizant of their corresponding responsibilities or obligations. Sometimes, however, reciprocity in terms of responsibilities and obligations concerning rights is too diffuse for a simple 'matching game' (Waldron 1984; Austin 2003). Finally, in measure, as governments become more affluent and can afford to spend more of its citizens' taxes on social programmes and the implementation of human rights, that which is considered to be a basic entitlement also changes.

Whereas all *basic* human rights are by definition also basic human needs and quite often are also clearly articulated by individuals as basic human wants, not all human wants are also basic human needs. For example, wanting something very much does not automatically make that want a basic human need which is essential for my survival and the promotion of my welfare. This confusion between rights, needs and wants is partly to blame for an ever-increasing perception by the public that human rights theories are generally ineffectual in promoting moral awareness and that they are lacking in philosophical rigour with the inevitable resultant diminution of societal support. There is much fine-tuning that still needs to be done before the majority of the population recognises and appreciates the subtleties of rights theories and their implementation in daily life (Stumpf & Fieser 2003). There are many examples of conflicting rights, yet most of the time what is really being discussed and put to the test are not basic human subsistence rights – which for the most part are not disputed – but particular human wants which do not necessarily reflect vital human needs. Fortunately, there are still many activists who do strive to promote human rights, especially children's rights, such as the sociologist and children's rights campaigner Priscilla Alderson (2008).

In the interwar period in Poland, Henryk Goldszmit (1877–1942), a young and enthusiastic paediatrician who could have easily made for himself a full-time career as a children's writer, started to talk out about the specific need for the articulation of children's rights. These were novel concepts in Europe during the 1920s and 1930s, but Henryk

Goldszmit – or Janusz Korczak as he was better known from his *nom de plume* – was undoubtedly an exceptional person (Lewowicki 1994; Lifton 1997).

Working with children in pre-war Poland, Korczak the writer, paediatrician and educationalist saw that children were essentially disenfranchised. They lacked the respect and dignity which they deserved. They were citizens without a voice and without the basic rights accorded to adults. Korczak started therefore to write about children's rights – such as the right to their own name, to having a secret, to professing a faith, to an education, to make mistakes, even to die prematurely, but above all to be nurtured with love and affection (Joseph 1999). Today, we recognise these sentiments in regards to the care of children wherever they may be and they are deservedly well reflected in the UNCRC. But this was by no mere happenstance; it was precisely the celebrations connected with the centenary of Janusz Korczak's birth that prompted the Polish government to celebrate 1978 as the Year of Korczak and to encourage the UN to incorporate his thinking into the celebrations by the UN of 1979 as the UN Year of the Child. Seeing the need to revise and update the post-war UN Declaration of Children's Rights of 1959, which had no force of law and was only at best a recommendation, the Poles requested UNICEF to form a working party to re-draft this document. Ten years later, the working party put out the UNCRC for ratification and as of today 192 countries around the world have signed the convention and have agreed to be bound by its legislation. The UNCRC elaborates on three main areas of children's rights: provision rights such as for education and the best possible and appropriate health care; protection rights such as freedom from abuse, early labour, being robbed of their culture and faith; and finally participation rights in their welfare, care and social activities (Veerman 1992; Freeman 1997).

Like with the United Nations Declaration of Human Rights (UNDHR), also known as the Universal Declaration of Human Rights, this convention is only as good as the commitment of countries and their governments to adhere to the legislation (which they themselves have signed up to). Unfortunately, we still have politically unstable areas of the world where children are forced to serve in armies as child soldiers. There are parts of the world where poverty is still so entrenched that children are forced to be part of the workforce at the expense of their own basic education. There are countries where children are still tried in adult courts and can be subject to capital punishment and there are parts of the world where children can be taken away forcefully from their parents for ideological and political reasons (Amnesty International 1995; Alderson 2008). There is therefore no place for complacency and much work still needs to be done before most (if not all) children in the world can be assured of their basic rights. At least now, unlike in the past, children themselves can bring their grievances to courts of human rights and argue their case. No longer must their cause be brought to court by an adult – which is always one more barrier to overcome and can potentially mean that adults will not perceive the necessity or urgency of the case in the same way that children do. If children are angry or upset enough over a violation of their rights, they can take their grievance to a court of human rights. In the United Kingdom, there is also a children's commissioner whose task it is to look out for the promotion of children's rights (Freeman 1997; Alderson 2008).

We can see from this review of deontology, utilitarianism and principle-based ethics that there are several different ways of moral reasoning. There is also, however, regardless of individual preferences, the ever-present requirement, particularly for members of professions working with vulnerable people such as children and their families, to be a person of goodwill, indeed to be a good person. Concentrating on *being* a morally good person (as opposed just *doing* the correct acts) can itself result in acquiring a particular world view – a particular way of appreciating the world around us – and in being a particular type of person (Brykczynska 1992b). This emphasis in moral philosophy on *who* we are as opposed to what it is that we do is known as virtue ethics.

Virtue ethics

It is generally accepted that the first recognised person to articulate this philosophical approach in Europe was the ancient Greek philosopher and educationalist, Aristotle (384–322 BC). Aristotle was concerned with the education of young Greeks, and so well known was his approach to the development and schooling of youngsters that Philip II of Macedon asked him to educate his son Alexander the Great (356–323 BC). In his writings, Aristotle commented on many things, from the natural world around him to various aspects of Greek literature and politics. He also put much thought into determining how to go about becoming a good person, that is, how to become a good citizen (Barnes 1982; Stumpf & Fieser 2003).

For Aristotle, as for many Greeks at that time, it was important that the well-educated man of the state reflect certain characteristics and values. The statesman (and also warrior) needed to reflect certain esteemed values in their lives. Aristotle listed these personal values (or virtues) and elaborated upon them in his classic work *The Nichomachean Ethics*. He considered that the statesman and warrior needed to be a good citizen and therefore would need to be trustworthy, magnanimous, honest, courageous and so on. He recognised that these virtues would need to be worked upon if they were to become second nature to the individual. Aristotle assumed that in time the committed person would indeed become trustworthy, honest, courageous, etc. The more these virtues were practised, the more likely they were to become habit and normal behaviour. Of all the virtues that contributed to the make-up of the good person, Aristotle thought that wisdom, especially practical wisdom, was the most important, commenting '... that there is no virtue without wisdom' (Aristotle 1962:171).

It is important, of course, to understand what Aristotle had in mind by advocating practical wisdom. As he stated: 'Virtue or excellence is not only a characteristic which is guided by right reason, but also a characteristic which is united with right reason; and right reason in moral matters is practical wisdom' (Aristotle 1962:172). He further noted, practical wisdom is '... concerned with human affairs and with matters about which deliberation is possible' (Aristotle 1962:157). It cannot be overemphasised just how important Aristotle's work on the nature and promotion of virtues subsequently became and just how far-reaching his influence on the discourse of philosophy for following generations of scholars including health-care workers (de Raeve 2006a).

It is often stated that Aristotle's work on virtue ethics was recovered from obscurity by the medieval scholar and saint Thomas Aquinas (1225–74), who re-articulated and re-formulated Aristotle's theory of virtue ethics for a Christian medieval readership in his major work *Summa Theologica*. The works of Aquinas were themselves in turn re-examined and re-interpreted for a contemporary readership by recent European writers and philosophers such as Martin Heidegger (1889–1976), who has profoundly influenced contemporary notions of phenomenology and ontology. Today, there is again a renewed scholarly interest in the philosophy of virtue ethics following a seminal article on the subject by the analytical philosopher Elizabeth Anscombe in 1958 (Anscombe 1958). Currently a virtue-based approach to moral philosophy is reflected in the work of several ethicists such as Michael Slote (1992, 2007), Joan Porter (1990), Alistair MacIntyre (2007) and Virginia Held (2006) among many, and in the thinking of health-care professionals such as Brykczynska (1995), Darling-Smith (1993), Scott (2003) and de Raeve (2006a), reflecting perhaps the frustrations with and inadequacies of the other main ethical perspectives – something also noted by Driver (2001) who cautions however not to completely abandon consequentialist theories of morality in the move towards appreciating virtue ethics.

During recent wars and conflicts, all manner of human behaviour has been recorded, and the most affected by the horrors of war are those living in the deprived and poorest areas of the globe; moreover war affects women and children disproportionately. There has been – perhaps inevitably – during this time more evidence of violence, cruelty and selfishness than heroism or compassion. But there were also some uplifting and rather public examples of virtuous behaviour during these times, such as the rescuing of Jewish children from Central Europe via the Kinder-transport and arranging for them to be cared for in England (Fox & Abraham-Podietz 1999). Most virtuous behaviour, however, is not acted out on such a public stage (Wuthnow 1991), but where there are examples of public altruism and heroic virtuous behaviour, there is also (usually) sincere appreciation and recognition by the public (Wuthnow 1991). In the heart of the city of London, there is a unique monument to *everyday* heroes. Tucked away in Postman's Square, in the shadow of the ancient hospital of St Bartholomew, are plaques on a wall which commemorate unsung heroes who have paid with their lives for acts of altruism and courage. Interestingly, some of these acts were committed by children. Acts of altruism and courage are not the sole prerogative of adults or professionals.

Of course, virtue ethics as an approach to moral development and education has been around since the times of Aristotle, and is shared in various formats by many different cultures, but its modern re-emergence, and some would say dominance, among some public workers and health-care professionals is most probably due, as noted, to a level of dissatisfaction with the efficacy of the other main moral theories (Murdoch 1970; de Raeve 2006a). But some scholars, philosophers and health-care professionals question the extent of the value and level of interest surrounding the popularity among health-care professionals of virtue ethics. Louise de Raeve (2006b) has written a good explanation of this critique by philosophers, while other nurses have questioned the uncritical acceptance of virtue ethics – most notably Peter Allmark (1998). These writers are sceptical of the so-called moral benefits which this philosophical approach is supposed to engender, since they argue that the approach neither offers a key to solving moral dilemmas nor offers a philosophical interpretation of prevailing moral quandaries – the two most common instances for health-care workers when they are in need of a philosophical guide. They argue that Aristotle's approach offers little comfort in times of moral distress. Additionally, moral philosophers tend to distinguish between notions of *virtue ethics* and *virtue theories*; meanwhile, of concern to educationalists is the vexing question of whether virtue can realistically be taught – which was the subject of a fascinating lecture series (Darling-Smith 1993) and something de Raeve (2006c) also elaborates upon. Virtues certainly are better taught by example, the use of reflection and the humanities than in a traditional lecture format.

What is still relevant today, however, is the importance and emphasis on cultivating the virtues and especially the virtue of practical wisdom – or moral comportment (Roach 1995, 2002; de Raeve 2006a; Benner *et al*. 2009). The virtue-ethics approach to being a good person, together with a judicious employment and understanding of other moral theories in resolving moral dilemmas and quandaries, seems to be well reflected in current nursing

ethics literature and accounts for the current emphasis by educators in encouraging the next generation of professionals to take more personal responsibility for who they are and more responsibility for the professional and personal decisions which they make (Brykczynska 1995; Scott 2003; de Raeve 2006a,c). This approach is increasingly being reflected in the thinking of the NMC about the nature of the contemporary nurse (NMC 2008).

Caring and nursing ethics

As more women began to study and comment upon moral theories, they noted that in most instances the theories were written from a gendered perspective (Larrabee 1993; Liaschenko & Peter 2003; Noddings 2003). Just as female historians have noted that male historians (especially in the past) have often omitted the perspectives of the vanquished, the downtrodden and the insignificant small folk, such as trades-people, children or women, so theories of philosophy appear to have been written for a primarily male readership, concerning for the most part matters of interest to men, such as politics and justice and social decision-making. This is not to say that women were not interested in matters of governance or social justice or rights theories, and the last 70 years have been testimony to the ever-expanding scope of their philosophical interests and scholarship. Indeed, there has been a steady flow of eminent female philosophers (in recent times) concerned with a variety of socio-cultural and political issues such as Mary Warnock (1992), Mary Midgley (2005) and Virginia Held (1984, 2008). But they also wrote on aspects of compassion, empathy and caring, for example, Virginia Held's (2006) recent book on caring ethics, Bowen's (1997) book on gender sensitive ethics and Helen Oppenheimer's (2003) book on approaches to ethics, as well as the health-care ethicists Simon Roach (1997, 2002) and Verna Tschudin (2003) among others, who alongside such philosophers as Gaylin (1976) and Mayeroff (1971) and more recently Stan van Hooft (1995) present another interpretation of virtue-based professional caring ethics (Brykczynska 1992a, 1997; Davis & Fowler 2006; Gastmans 2006).

At the present time, female scholars are re-shaping our thinking and understanding of many traditional moral approaches, for example, the work of Noddings (2003), Virginia Held (2006) and Bowen (1997). The Gilligan-Kohlberg debate of the 1970s which spurred interest in feminist ethics, in turn gave credence to those professionals concerned with caring ethics (Roach 1997, 2002). These predominantly female philosophers argue that since half of all human activity is represented by the activities of women, and since women spend much of their time creating, facilitating and fostering relationships, this womanly activity of creating and facilitating interrelationships also needs to be represented in the interests of moral philosophers (Bowen 1997). As Liaschenko & Peter (2003:33) note 'What makes feminist ethics feminist is the study of moral theorising with respect to gender'. Moreover, the caring that modern women engage in covers not only the domestic area but also a large part of the public sector. It is not surprising therefore that the area of feminist ethics which struck a cord with health-care and public sector professionals was the literature on caring and caring ethics. The nursing literature on caring ethics reflects therefore the rise of enthusiasm surrounding the topic (Brykczynska 1997; Liaschenko & Peter 2003). Some moral philosophers are cautious, however, and analyse the philosophical nature of caring and the limitations of caring ethics in significant depth, thereby significantly contributing to the scholarship on the subject (van Hooft 1995, 2003; Held 2006).

As Pam Smith's important work on nurses' labour noted, the caring work of nurses is emotionally draining, yet this necessary activity needs to be continued *but* with greater support and public acknowledgement (Smith 1992). Nurses spend much of their time caring for others and the moral distress, quandaries and issues which they face, although sometimes addressed by major moral theories, for the most part go unrecognised and unappreciated. Much of a nurse's time is spent addressing patients' pain and suffering and that can become stressful, but analysing the concepts of pain and suffering can be helpful (Brykczynska 1992b; Carnevale 2009). However, it is relational aspects of the work of nurses that is found to be most difficult to cope with. How nurses weave in and out of relationships, how they form these relationships and how and why they set professional boundaries seems to be a fundamental aspect of nursing which is well articulated in the profes-

sional caring literature as well as illustrated by Duncan Randall in this book.

As with virtue ethics, it is a matter of debate whether we consider caring ethics to be a major moral theory in the same way as deontology or utilitarianism and therefore to be considered as a useful guide to moral decision-making on par with other philosophical theories. As shown, no one philosophical theory answers all criticisms and as de Raeve (2006b) notes, both Martha Nussbaum and Alistair MacIntyre – two philosophers writing from a neo-Aristotelian perspective – are cautious if not sceptical of the benefits that virtue ethics can bring to the debate. Meanwhile writings on caring ethics never aspired to be textbook guides to moral conduct. In its present format caring ethics owes some of its ideas to the writings of Aristotle and virtue ethics but it does not intend to be a *prescription* for health-care morality; it does, however, offer insights into a rationale for being a particular kind of health-care professional – one in possession of wisdom and compassion; or as Stan van Hooft (2003:11) eloquently states:' … the caring person feels caringly, thinks caringly, and thereby acts virtuously. Caring conceived in this way is neither merely an interpersonal emotion nor just a professional practice; it is the very ethical life of nursing'.

Conclusion

Pat Benner *et al.* (2009) in their recent study recommend bringing everyday nursing ethical concerns to be the centre of nursing education and they urge nurse educators to focus more on the everyday practices of ethics, as experienced by health-care professionals. They recommend that nurses recognise the basic humanity of their patients, strive to preserve their patient's dignity, have the courage and wisdom to know how and when to respond to substandard practices, know how to be an effective patient advocate without being patronising and robbing the patient of self-determination, be professionally competent and, finally, learn the interpersonal skills of empathy and compassion based on listening to the patient, all without abrasive intrusion into the patient's personal space. This is not that dissimilar to the recommendations from the contributors to Anne Davis' (Davis *et al.* 2006) co-edited recent book aimed at nurse educators, or the position of van Hooft (2003). As Roach (1995:8) commented 'The caring paradigm is, in itself, a source of power'. It is, as she notes, in the very patient–nurse relationship 'exposed in the relational reality'. The contributors to this book have attempted to show precisely how this all-encompassing, interrelational, moral comportment demonstrated in caring ways of being, may be – and upon occasion should be – expressed in a paediatric nursing context and how it is the most powerful asset that nurses bring to their work.

References

Alderson, P. (2008) *Young Children's Rights – Exploring Beliefs, Principles and Practice*, 2nd edn. Jessica Kingsley Publishers, London.

Allmark, P. (1998) Is caring a virtue? *Journal of Advanced Nursing*, **28**, 466–472.

Amnesty International (1995) *Childhood Stolen – Grave Human Rights Violations Against Children*. Amnesty International British Section, London.

Anscombe, G.E. (1958) Modern moral philosophy. *Journal of the Royal Institute of Philosophy*, **33** (124), 1–19.

Aristotle (1962) *Nicomachean Ethics* (translated with notes by Martin Ostwald). Bobbs-Merrill Educational Publishing, Indianapolis.

Austin, W. (2003) Using the human rights paradigm in health ethics: The problems and the possibilities. In: *Approaches to Ethics – Nursing Beyond Boundaries* (ed. V. Tschudin), pp. 105–114. Butterworth-Heinemann, Edinburgh.

Barnes, J. (1982) *Aristotle* (Past Masters Series). Oxford University Press, Oxford.

Beauchamp, T.L. & Childress, J.F. (2008) *Principles of Biomedical Ethics*, 6th edn. Oxford University Press, New York.

Benner, P.E., Tanner, C.A. & Chesla, C.A. (2009) *Expertise in Nursing Practice: Caring, Clinical Judgement and Ethics*, 2nd edn. Springer, New York.

Bok, S. (1978) *Lying – Moral Choice in Public and Private Life*. Vintage Books/Random House, New York.

Bowen, P. (1997) *Caring: Gender Sensitive Ethics*. Routledge, London.

Brykczynska, G. (1992a) Caring – A dying art? In: *Nursing – The Challenge to Change* (eds M. Jolley & G. Brykczynska), pp. 1–45. Edward Arnold, London.

Brykczynska, G. (1992b) Caring – Some philosophical and spiritual reflections. In: *Nursing – The Challenge to Change* (eds M. Jolley & G. Brykczynska), pp. 225–262. Edward Arnold, London.

Brykczynska, G. (1995) Reflective practice: An analysis of nursing wisdom. In: *Nursing: Beyond Tradition and Conflict* (eds M. Jolley & G. Brykczynska), pp. 9–28. Mosby, London.

Brykczynska, G. (ed.) (1997) A brief overview of the epistemology of caring. In: *Caring: The Compassion and Wisdom of Nursing*, pp. 1–10. Edward Arnold Publishers Ltd, London.

Carnevale, F.A. (2009) A conceptual and moral analysis of suffering. *Nursing Ethics*, **16** (2), 173–183.

Charter of Fundamental Rights of the European Union (2000) Available on the EU websites: www.eucharter.org and www.europarl.europa.eu/charter

Darling-Smith, B. (ed.) (1993) *Can Virtue be Taught?* University of Notre Dame Press, Notre Dame, Indiana.

Davis, A.J. & Fowler, M. (2006) Caring and caring ethics depicted in selected literature: What we know and what we need to know. In: *Essentials of Teaching and Learning in Nursing Ethics – Perspectives and Methods* (eds A.J. Davis, V. Tschudin & L. de Raeve), pp. 165–179. Churchill Livingstone/Elsevier, Edinburgh.

Davis, A.J., Tschudin, V. & de Raeve, L. (2006) *Essentials of Teaching and Learning in Nursing Ethics*. Churchill Livingstone, Edinburgh.

Driver, J. (2001) *Uneasy Virtue*. Cambridge University Press, Cambridge.

Edwards, S. (2006) A principle-based approach to nursing ethics. In: *Essentials of Teaching and Learning in Nursing Ethics – Perspectives and Methods* (eds A.J. Davis, V. Tschudin & L. de Raeve), pp. 55–65. Churchill Livingstone/Elsevier, Edinburgh.

Fowler, M. (2006) Social ethics, the profession and society. In: *Essentials of Teaching and Learning in Nursing Ethics – Perspectives and Methods* (eds A.J. Davis, V. Tschudin & L. de Raeve), pp. 27–36. Churchill Livingstone/Elsevier, Edinburgh.

Fowler, M. & Tschudin, V. (2006) Ethics in nursing: An historical perspective. In: *Essentials of Teaching and Learning in Nursing Ethics* (eds A. Davis, V. Tschudin & L. de Raeve), pp. 13–26. Churchill Livingstone, Edinburgh.

Fox, A.L. & Abraham-Podietz, E. (1999) *Ten Thousand Children*. Behrman House, Inc., West Orange.

Freeman, M.D.A. (1997) *The Moral Status of Children: Essays on the Rights of the Child*. Martin Nijhoff Publishers, Boston.

Gastmans, C. (2006) The care perspective in healthcare ethics. In: *Essentials of Teaching and Learning in Nursing Ethics – Perspectives and Methods* (eds A. Davis, V. Tschudin & L. de Raeve), pp. 135–148. Churchill Livingstone/Elsevier, Edinburgh.

Gaylin, W. (1976) *Caring*. Knopf Publishers, New York.

Held, V. (1984) *Rights and Goods – Justifying Social Action*. University of Chicago Press, Chicago.

Held, V. (2006) *The Ethics of Care: Personal, Political and Global*. Oxford University Press, Oxford.

Held, V. (2008) *How Terrorism is Wrong*. Oxford University Press, New York.

van Hooft, S. (1995) *Caring: An Essay in the Philosophy of Ethics*. University Press of Colorado, Denver.

van Hooft, S. (2003) Caring and ethics in nursing. In: *Approaches to Ethics – Nursing Beyond Boundaries* (ed. V. Tschudin), pp. 1–13. Butterworth/Heinemann, Edinburgh.

Joseph, S. (1999) *A Voice for the Child: The Inspirational Words of Janusz Korczak*. Collins Publishers, London.

Larrabee, M.J. (1993) Gender and moral development: A challenge for feminist theory. In: *An Ethic of Care: Feminist and Interdisciplinary Perspectives* (ed. M.J. Larrabee), pp. 3–19. Routledge, Chapman and Hall, London.

Lewowicki, T. (1994) Janusz Korczak 1878–1942. *Prospects: The Quarterly Review of Comparative Education*, **XXIV** (1/2), 37–48.

Liaschenko, J. & Peter, E. (2003) Feminist ethics. In: *Approaches to Ethics – Nursing Beyond Boundaries* (ed. V. Tschudin), pp. 33–43. Butterworth/Heinemann, Edinburgh.

Lifton, B.J. (1997) *The King of Children – The Life and Death of Janusz Korczak*. St Martin's Griffith, New York.

MacIntyre, A. (2007) *After Virtue – A Study in Moral Theory*, 3rd edn. University of Notre Dame Press, Notre Dame, Indiana.

Mayeroff, M. (1971) *On Caring*. Harper & Row, New York.

Midgley, M. (2005) *The Essential Mary Midgley*. Routledge, Abingdon, Oxon.

Mill, J.S. (1998) *Utilitarianism* (Oxford Philosophical Texts) (ed. R. Crisp). Oxford University Press, Oxford.

Murdoch, I. (1970) *The Sovereignty of Good*. Routledge & Kegan Paul, London.

NMC (2008) *The Code: Standards of Conduct, Performance and Ethics for Nurses and Midwives*. Nursing and Midwifery Council, London.

Noddings, N. (2003) *Caring: A Feminine Approach to Ethics and Moral Education*, 2nd edn. University of California Press, Berkeley.

Oppenheimer, H. (2003) Mattering. In: *Approaches to Ethics – Beyond Nursing Boundaries* (ed. V. Tschudin), pp. 73–82. Butterworth/Heinemann, Edinburgh.

Porter, J. (1990) *The Recovery of Virtue*. SPCK Publishing, London.

de Raeve, L. (2002) Trust and trustworthiness in nurse-patient relationships. *Nursing Philosophy*, **3**, 152–162.

de Raeve, L. (2006a) Virtue ethics. In: *Approaches to Ethics – Nursing Beyond Boundaries* (ed. V. Tschudin), pp. 109–122. Butterworth/Heinemann, Edinburgh.

de Raeve, L. (2006b) A critique of virtue ethics. In: *Approaches to Ethics – Nursing Beyond Boundaries* (ed. V. Tschudin), pp. 109–122. Butterworth/Heinemann, Edinburgh.

de Raeve, L. (2006c) Teaching virtue ethics. In: *Approaches to Ethics – Nursing Beyond Boundaries* (ed. V. Tschudin), pp. 123–134. Butterworth/Heinemann, Edinburgh.

Roach, S.M. (1995) A dominant paradigm of the modern world. In: *Power, Politics and Public Policy: A Matter of Caring* (ed. A. Boykin), pp. 3–10. National League for Nursing, New York.

Roach, S.M. (ed.) (1997) *Caring from the Heart: The Convergence of Caring and Spirituality*. Paulist Press, Mahwah, New Jersey.

Roach, S.M. (2002) *Caring, the Human Mode of Being: A Blueprint for the Health Professions*, 2nd revised edn. Canadian Healthcare Association Press, Ottawa.

Scott, P.A. (2003) Virtue, nursing and the moral domain of practice. In: *Approaches to Ethics – Nursing Beyond Boundaries* (ed. V. Tschudin), pp. 25–32. Butterworth-Heinemann, Edinburgh.

Scruton, R. (1982) *Kant*. Oxford University Press, Oxford.

Slote, M. (1992) *From Morality to Virtues*. Oxford University Press, New York.

Slote, M. (2007) *The Ethics of Care and Empathy*. Routledge, London.

Smith, P. (1992) *The Emotional Labour of Nursing – How Nurses Care*. Macmillan Press Ltd, Houndsmills, Basingstoke.

Stumpf, S.E. & Fieser, J. (2003) *Socrates to Sartre and Beyond – A History of Philosophy*. McGraw Hill Publications, New York.

Tschudin, V. (2003) Narrative ethics. In: *Approaches to Ethics – Nursing Beyond Boundaries* (ed. V. Tschudin), pp. 61–72. Butterworth/Heinemann, Edinburgh.

UN (1948) *Universal Declaration of Human Rights*. United Nations, New York. Full version also available on the UN website: www.un.org

UN (1989) *Convention of the Rights of a Child (UNCRC)*. UNICEF, Geneva. Full version also available on the UNICEF website: www.unicef.org

Veerman, P. (1992) *The Rights of the Child and the Changing Image of Childhood*. Martinus Nijhoff Publishers, Boston.

Waldron, J. (1984) *Theories of Rights (Oxford Readings in Philosophy)*. Oxford University Press, Oxford.

Warnock, M. (1992) *The Uses of Philosophy*. Blackwell Publishers, Oxford.

Wuthnow, R. (1991) *Acts of Compassion – Caring for Others and Helping Ourselves*. Princeton University Press, Princeton, New Jersey.

Suggested further readings

Baron, M.W., Pettit, P. & Slote, M. (1997) *Three Methods of Ethics*. Blackwell Publishers, Oxford.

MacIntyre, A. (1998) *A Short History of Ethics*, 2nd edn. Routledge, London.

Reed, J. & Ground, I. (1997) *Philosophy for Nursing*. Edward Arnold, London.

3 A Review of Children's Rights as Applied to Paediatric Nursing

Jim Richardson

Introduction

Only 30 years ago, few people would have felt that a whole chapter on the rights of the child would have been necessary in any book. At that time the child's rights were generally not considered in detail. Parents had rights, school teachers had rights but children did not necessarily have explicit rights.

This situation has changed radically in that more and more people, organisations and policies are focused on developing and ensuring the rights of the child and young person. This atmosphere is dynamic and exciting and new progress in this area is made continually. The Royal College of Paediatrics and Child Health held a conference which took stock of achievements in children's health rights on the 20th anniversary of the United Nations Convention on the Rights of the Child (UNCRC). Coincidentally, this was also the 50th anniversary of the influential 1959 Platt Report.

This chapter will determine what the child's rights are and will use the UNCRC (UN 1989) as an organising framework for exploring these. An assessment will be made of practical implications of children's rights in service provision in child health nursing care.

One area which causes consternation when discussing issues related to children and young people is how precisely should a child be defined. Historically, our understanding of what a child is has evolved considerably. Traces of this can be seen in some confused areas of the law. A young person may marry at 16 or learn to drive at 17 so might be assumed then to have made the transition to adulthood.

However, the age of criminal responsibility in England, Wales and Northern Ireland is 10 years – and in Scotland this is as low as 8. What then does this reflect in terms of the distinction between childhood and adulthood? It would seem to suggest that children as young as 9–10 must have the ability to be responsible for their actions in committing a crime. Other societies place this age of taking responsibility much later at around 16.

The UNCRC (United Nations 1989) recognises as a child anyone under the age of 18. This will always be a debatable issue but recognises that children and young people who continue in full-time education until their late teens remain in a partially dependent position and, therefore, have specific vulnerabilities. Increasingly, public policy uses 18 as the distinguishing point between young adulthood and full adulthood. From the point of view of

Ethical and Philosophical Aspects of Nursing Children, First Edition. Edited by Gosia M. Brykczyńska and Joan Simons.
© 2011 Blackwell Publishing Ltd. Published 2011 by Blackwell Publishing Ltd.

public services, the modern tendency is to offer a choice of adult or child services to young people around 16–18 years of age. This is also the case when young people are offered the choice of being cared for on a children's ward or on an adult ward.

The rights that are accorded to children through international agreements such as the UNCRC can be seen as a set of entitlements that the child can reasonably be expected to either be provided with or protected from. This is an important distinction and the terms positive and negative rights are well established. A positive right is something that a child should be given such as a name or a nationality (*UNCRC Article 7*), while a negative right is something that a child should be able to expect to be shielded from such as protection from violence, abuse or exploitation (*UNCRC Article 19*) (see Appendix II).

One factor which has been used in the past in determining what rights one is entitled to is the ability to respond to rights by being able to discharge corresponding responsibilities. This ability is the hallmark of an autonomous, competent individual. Children, during their maturation, are developing their ability to be autonomous especially as they move nearer to young adulthood. This is quite an extended process and is highly dependent on the characteristics of each individual person. We are all different in terms of the rate of our maturation and, particularly in the middle school years, in the stability of that achievement.

Ethical principles

Ensuring the rights enlisted in the UNCRC indicate provision of the rights outlined by Beauchamp & Childress (2008), which can be summarised as follows.

Autonomy

This is the right of the mature individual to determine what happens to them. The autonomous individual understands the implications of choices and has the right to make those choices. This is the basis of independent informed consent to medical or nursing treatment (GMC 2007). Adults are assumed to be competent to make autonomous

choices unless some factors limit this competence. Children and young people are increasingly seen as progressively gaining the ability to exercise competence and autonomy as they mature. This assumes the child as *becoming* competent and this should be recognised in facilitating the child's participation in decision-making. This is a challenging area in the practice of children's and young people's nursing.

Beneficence

This is *doing good*. This is an attractive concept and one which health professionals will recognise. However, it is not always easy to define what *good* is in terms of the impulses for an action and also in terms of the potential result of that action. The UNCRC is helpful in providing, within its articles, a series of concrete provisions which, if assured, will help to ensure that good is done and through this the child enjoys a benefit.

Non-maleficence

This is the twin of doing good and means avoiding harm. Again, *harm* is an elusive concept and while it might be easy to understand in concrete terms, it may be rather more difficult to grasp in its more abstract forms. It is easy to understand that an intravenous infusion must be carefully monitored to avoid physical harm in the form of extravasation which might cause blood vessel and soft tissue damage and inflammation/infection in the form of phlebitis. Also, the risk of over- or under-dosage of fluid or medications is a risk. It is rather more challenging to grasp the harmful impact of, for example, failing to respect culturally determined customs and values. This can have a very harmful effect on the child who is absorbing and accommodating the cultural norms of their family and community, but this process is still incomplete.

Respect

This is the recognition and acknowledgement that all other people, including children and young people, have the right to be treated with dignity.

This means all the conventionally understood things such as treating others with courtesy and kindness. Of course, in the content of health care with all the attendant decisions and pressures this can be something of a challenge to maintain. However, a realisation that treating someone badly, and, it could be argued, especially a child or young a person, is positively damaging is crucial. The old axiom 'do unto others as you would have them do unto you' has often been cited as a yardstick for respect.

Justice

Justice is treating someone fairly. It consists, among other things, of equity – that is, treating everyone in the same way. Again, recent history has lessons to teach. In the past, when paediatric cardiac surgical services were scarce, babies with Down's syndrome who had associated congenital cardiac defects were often not offered surgical treatment, while babies with a cardiac defect who did not have Down's syndrome were offered such care. Today this would be unacceptable because of our sense of equity; of all human values, that of all human life having equal worth is crucial, and society would not now tolerate such discrimination. However, there are new sources of inequity, such as when new and expensive forms of therapy may be made available to some patients when local decision-makers decide to fund them. Others may be denied these treatments because they are not identified as priorities for funding in the locality where they happen to live. This is the so-called *post-code lottery* against which great progress is being made through the work of agencies such as the National Institute for Health and Clinical Excellence.

Another area which children's and young people's nurses will encounter inequality is in the phenomenon of child poverty (UNICEF Innocenti Research Centre 2007). Inequalities exist in any society and are often concentrated in areas of relative deprivation where there is significant unemployment, poor housing, restricted resources and overstretched, compromised public services. These circumstances can be expected to have a large negative impact on the well-being of families and most importantly on growing children and young

people. Poverty is self-perpetuating and has proven to be a cycle which is difficult to break. A number of initiatives and policies aim to alleviate childhood poverty with the long-term objective of ensuring that children have their basic needs satisfied and have the best possible chance to achieve their optimal potential. These policy directions aim to reduce inequality and assure that all children are respected and treated with dignity.

In order to secure justice, it is important that truth-telling is maintained as an important value. This is another aspect of respect. It is not difficult to understand how truthfulness in working with children and young people is important in establishing mutual trust in a therapeutic relationship. However, it may be difficult in all circumstances for nurses to maintain the pure idea of truthfulness. Sometimes children will need to have the full truth of their situation, particularly in severe, acute or life-limiting illness, delivered to them in manageable *packets* of information in a format which they can accept and manage. Sometimes parents will not want their child to receive the full truth, particularly if that truth is difficult and distressing.

This will always be a challenging situation and one with which the children's nurse needs to work on systematically. Over time, families can often be helped to move gradually to talking about their difficulties, but they usually need considerable help to do so. However, when they achieve this there is considerable benefit for all family members in being able to be open and communicative about the challenges they face in coping with a child's serious health issue. The UNCRC gives clear guidance in this area (*Article 18*).

In terms of truth-telling, children's nurses sometimes face difficulties when a child or young person discloses something to them but asks that they tell no one else. This disclosure may relate to the child being badly treated and the child may feel uncomfortable or afraid of the consequences of their disclosure. A guiding principle which will be helpful here is that of non-maleficence, or avoiding harm; if the child is at risk of suffering harm then the nurse must judiciously share this information to ensure that the child is safeguarded (GMC 2009). Of course, this sharing of information would happen only within established guidelines and with senior, responsible professionals who are in a position to ensure that the child is protected with a minimum of necessary disruption to the child's family and life while ensuring confidentiality as far as is possible and practicable (DCSF 2008).

Concepts of childhood

Within modern society, how we view children and young people has changed considerably in a short time and continues to do so. We are moving from a position where the child is seen as dependent and others, parents or primary carers, must make decisions on their behalf to ensure their safety and well-being. Health professionals, including children's nurses, were also inclined to be rather paternalistic in terms of feeling that, on the basis of their professional knowledge, skills and expertise, they knew best and only had to give instructions to secure compliance and achieve improvements (Charles-Edwards 2003). Within this orientation it was not always felt important to give the child full information about their situation. In recent years, we have been moving steadily away from this approach, as our sense of what a child is and what that child's rights are changes. We are now appreciating more fully each child's, and family's, unique ability to participate in decision-making and planning in relation to the child's medical and nursing care. It is obvious that we all differ in terms of our abilities, our responses to difficult situations and our beliefs and past experiences. Therefore, how this engagement happens must be tailored to suit the people involved. Our increasing willingness to work in this fashion marks a quantum leap from simply nursing a child on the basis of what we as professionals believe to be the priorities and the necessary nursing actions. Nonetheless, all tendencies to tokenism must be avoided in this respect.

These changes are occurring with the growing realisation of the abilities of children and young people as they move along the continuum between dependence and independence. Of course, this is a rather fluid transition as being faced by stressful and distressing situations in strange environments can cause the child to move again towards greater dependence on parents. Parents in their turn can find themselves experiencing distress and helplessness and will, in this context, experience great need for information, support and guidance.

Our growing appreciation of how the child and young person is indeed capable of participating, with the help of parents and skilled nurses, in their own care and in exercising choice about how that care happens is mirrored in the wider changes in society (Franklin & Sloper 2005; Whitty-Rogers *et al.* 2009).

The UNCRC has had a great impact on policy development in the UK. In every sector of public services children are more and more being seen as participants rather than passive, dependent recipients of these services; such as in school councils in primary and secondary schools, helping to prepare support plans with family social workers, participating in decision-making in family courts. The list could go on and on. It may be useful to consider what is driving these developments. The UNCRC itself is influencing policies and the way in which services are delivered. The Welsh Assembly Government has derived seven core aims from the Convention.

The seven core aims ensure that *all* children

(1) Have a flying start in life;
(2) Have a comprehensive range of education and learning opportunities;
(3) Enjoy the best possible health and freedom from abuse, victimisation and exploitation;
(4) Have access to play, leisure, sporting and cultural activities;
(5) Are listened to, treated with respect and have their race and cultural identity recognised;
(6) Have a safe home and community which supports physical and emotional well-being;
(7) Are not disadvantaged by poverty.

These core aims are used as a checklist to ensure that all new policies will have a positive impact on child citizens.

The introduction of children's commissioners in each of the UK's home nations has been an important innovation. The English children's commissioner, Professor Al Aynsley Green, has done fundamentally important work in his Office's *11 Million Project*, which has been promoting awareness among children and young people, as well as the adult population, of the rights guaranteed in the UNCRC. The first Welsh children's commissioner, the late Peter Clarke, consulted widely with children in Wales about what they thought could be done to improve their daily lives. It is perhaps not surprising that the priorities they drew up included improving toilet facilities in schools and free access to drinking water during the school day. Mr Clarke was mocked in some sections of the media for the campaign he instituted to secure these basic provisions. He, however, courageously and doggedly lobbied to ensure that decent toilet facilities and drinking water were made available to all Welsh school children. On closer examination, it can be seen clearly that this helps to ensure children's comfort, health and well-being and, crucially, dignity.

The work of the commissioners has led to further developments in children's participation since their work is always informed by children's views. Mechanisms for consultation were set up using new electronic media and representative workshops. Children and young people were facilitated in responding to policy proposals and making sure that their views reached policy-makers. Also, these mechanisms ensured that children's and young people's priorities were made known to legislators.

This has led naturally to the establishment of youth parliaments where young people are able to debate and contribute their views to the wider political process. As a consequence, we are beginning to see children and young people as citizens, active citizens, in entirely new ways.

All of the Commissioners have focused strongly on promoting a wide awareness of the UNCRC as a clear and helpful statement of children's rights (UKCC 2008). The UNCRC is a helpful tool for children's and young people's nurses in their everyday work. It may be helpful to consider in more detail how the UNCRC came about and how it is organised. The UNCRC was accepted by the United Nations in 1989 but actually had two predecessors in 1924 and 1959 (Milne 2008). It is notable that both of these early versions were produced in the aftermath of a World War, in the context of which human rights, generally, and children's rights, especially, had been widely ignored. The impetus for producing the 1989 UNCRC was provided by Poland at a time when that country was on the point of democratising (see Chapter 2). The UNCRC was ratified by the UK in 1991 and is a live document in that the UK reports regularly on progress in implementing the rights contained in the docu-

ment via the United Nations Committee on the Rights of the Child. The last report was submitted in 2007.

The UKCRC document is easily accessible (website: www.unicef.org) and exists in a number of formats and versions for different audiences. The 54 articles in the definitive document contain a good deal of detail but simplified versions strive to present a clear, succinct statement of rights. There are wallchart versions which are useful for display in child care areas such as community clinics, children's wards and school nurses' offices (www.cewc-cymru.org.uk). This is helpful in raising awareness among the professionals as well as the children, young people and families using their services.

The four children's commissioners in the UK have also done a good deal of work in disseminating the Convention and its message as widely as possible. In this way they seek to achieve a high degree of awareness of children's rights among the public at large. This heightened awareness should lead to consideration of children's rights being stimulated and lead to these being promoted generally. The Scottish children's commissioner has produced two sets of cartoons, one for children and one for teenagers, illustrating each of the UNCRC's articles (www.sccyp.org.uk). These show in a colourful and entertaining way the core message of each of the articles. These have proven to be very useful in all sorts of educational settings including children's and young people's nursing education.

The UKCRC was conceived of as consisting of a number of articles each addressing a right. It has become customary to divide these up into three groupings or classifications: protection, provision and participation. This can be illustrated by examining some of the Charter's articles in more detail.

Protection

This category encompasses a number of rights which protect the child from harm including that which would have a negative impact on the child's development or opportunities. Articles in this category explicitly deal with any form of exploitation which might have a damaging effect on the child.

Article 9. This article ensures that children's right not to be separated from their parents is respected. This right is absolute unless, of course, the parents mistreat their child. The thinking behind this article will be immediately familiar to any children's nurse who has worked in the area of child protection. The paramount requirement is to ensure that the child is not harmed in any way while preserving the integrity of the family as far as is possible. This is a fine balance and action must be based on a calculation of potential risk. Positive professional support and guidance may have a beneficial outcome in terms of keeping the family together. However, some parents will persist in placing their own needs before those of their children and on occasion the child may need to be moved to a safer, more nurturing environment.

Article 9 also makes provision for the situation in which the child's parents are separated. It makes it clear that in such circumstances the child has the right to maintain contact with both parents. This is a contentious issue in Britain today as criticism has been levelled at the Family Courts on the basis that more could be done to ensure this right. Again, this right would only be applicable in situations where contact did not carry the risk of harm.

Article 11. Under the terms of this article, children should not be removed from the country illegally (UKBA 2008). This is of significance for children's nurses, for example, in situations where a child may be taken out of the country so that culturally determined practices which are illegal in this country can be performed. One example of this is female genital mutilation. This is an age-old practice which is valued by some communities but which has enormous and severely damaging effects both physically and psychologically.

Provision

Article 22 stipulates that when a child comes into the country as a refugee they should have the same rights as children born in that country. There is good evidence that this is not always the case (Crawley 2009). There are clear risks that these children may be exposed to poverty, underprovided for in the education system and subject to discrimination. It is important that children's nurses ensure that the spirit of this right is pro-

tected in the health services (Carnevale *et al.* 2009). This will often involve special measures such as the assured provision of professional interpreters and ensuring that culturally sensitive and safe care is delivered. This is an area where children's nurses can be politically active in lobbying to protect the rights enshrined in *Article 22.*

A right to an education is stipulated in *Article 28.* In the working environment of the children's and young people's nurse this is an important consideration. Under 5s education, especially playwork, has generally been inconsistently available although its value is well established in promoting early learning and fostering readiness for *formal* post-5 education. This is all the more important for children with enduring or chronic health needs. In some areas, in a difficult economic climate, there has been a contraction in the provision of such services both in the primary and secondary healthcare sectors. Here, again, is an arena where children's nurses might act as *activists* to help assure this right.

Participation

The third 'P' category of articles address facets of children's and young people's participation. This is perhaps the area where most progress has been achieved in the UK over recent years.

Article 13 lays down that children and young people have right to receive, and to share, information with the proviso that this information is not harmful to the child or to others. This is closely linked to the requirements of *Article 12* which states that children have a right to say what they want to happen when adults are making decisions which affect the child. It goes on to reinforce the principle that the child's opinions should always be taken into account. Taken together, these two articles form the basis for the child's having a greater opportunity to have a say in decisions in relation to their health care. Children's nurses have slowly been becoming accustomed to this being a fundamental aspect of their everyday work. As with most of these rights, further progress is required in making this reality, but real, clearly visible steps forward have already been taken. As before, if the child's understanding of the situation is immature and any objection they might have about a proposed procedure or treatment might lead to their suffering tangible harm, then their objection can be overridden. However, there are ways and means of achieving this and the child still needs to be treated kindly, gently and with respect. Also, of course, allowing the child a degree of choice in the small matters of what is happening to them can help them to maintain a sense of a degree of control.

Subtle shifts in the way language is used indicate the direction of development. In the past when the child had to be held still for the performance of important, and often unpleasant, clinical procedures, this was termed *restraint*. Nowadays we have policies to help guide us in the proper use of *therapeutic holding*. Another area where great strides forward can be seen is that of advocacy. Where advocacy occurs a particular set of skills is used by an adult to facilitate the child in having their voice heard (DoH 2002; NYAS 2009).

All in all, these principles underpinning the UNCRC could be argued to form a fourth 'P' – that of promotion. The Charter can be seen to be aiming to foster a more positive image of children, their capabilities and childhood generally. This has the potential to achieve a shift for the better in society's reactions to and expectations of children and young people. It might be said that we are at the start of a long road in this respect!

Perhaps the most important article from the viewpoint of the children's nurse is *Article 42*. This article calls for all government authorities to make the Charter known to all parents and children (Mitchell 2005). This is where we, as children's nurses and public servants, have a responsibility to disseminate information on the rights enshrined within the Charter to parents, children and young people and to make sure that they are understood. Only then can children and families lay claim to the rights to which they are entitled.

Conclusion

In a relatively short space of time, children's rights in society have developed into a sophisticated and comprehensive framework underpinned by the UNCRC. This development is a process rather than an event and despite considerable progress, more is required (CRDU 2003). Children's nurses should be at the forefront of not only integrating every aspect of the Charter into their daily work but also in fostering further development in this important social change.

References

Beauchamp, T.L. & Childress, J.F. (2008) *Principles of Biomedical Ethics*. Oxford University Press, Oxford.

Carnevale, F., Vissandjee, B., Nyland, A. & Vinet-Bonin, A. (2009) Ethical considerations in cross-linguistic nursing. *Nursing Ethics*, **16**, 813–826.

Charles-Edwards, I. (2003) Power and control over children and young people. *Primary Health Care*, **13** (8), 43–49.

Crawley, H. (2009) *The Situation of Children in Immigrant Families in the United Kingdom (Innocenti Working Paper)*. UNICEF, Florence.

CRDU (2003) *The United Nations Convention on the Rights of the Child*. Children's Rights Development Unit, London.

DCSF (2008) *Information Sharing: Guidance for Practitioners and Managers*. Department for Children, Schools and Families, London.

DoH (2002) *National Standards for the Provision of Children's Advocacy Services*. Department of Health, London.

Franklin, A. & Sloper, C. (2005) Listening and responding? Children's participation in health care within England. *International Journal of Children's Rights*, **13**, 11–29.

GMC (2007) *0–18 Years: Guidance for all Doctors*. General Medical Council: London.

GMC (2009) *Confidentiality*. General Medical Council: London.

Milne, B. (2008) From chattels to citizens? In: *Children and Citizenship* (eds A. Invernizzi & J. Williams). Sage, London.

Mitchell, R.C. (2005) Postmodern reflections on the UNCRC: Towards utilising Article 42 as an international compliance indicator. *International Journal of Children's Rights*, **13** (3), 315–331.

NYAS (2009) *Making Choices*. National Youth Advocacy Service, Cardiff.

UKBA (2008) *UK Border Agency Code of Practice for Keeping Children Safe from Harm*. UK Border Agency, London.

UKCC (2008) *UK Children's Commissioners' Report to the UN Committee on the Rights of the Child*. UK Children's Commissioners, London.

UN (1989) *UN Convention on the Rights of a Child*. United Nations, Geneva.

UNICEF Innocenti Research Centre (2007) *Child Poverty in Perspective: An Overview of Child Well-being in Rich Countries*. UNICEF: Florence.

Whitty-Rogers, J., Alex, M., McDonald, C. & Austin, W. (2009) Working with children in end-of-life decision making. *Nursing Ethics*, **16** (6), 743–758.

Suggested further readings

Alderson, P. (2008) *Young Children's Rights: Exploring Beliefs, Principles and Practice*, 2nd edn. Jessica Kingsley Publishers, London.

CRDU (2003) *The United Nations Convention on the Rights of the Child*. Children's Rights Development Unit, London.

Invernizzi, A. & Williams, J. (2008) *Children and Citizenship*. Sage, London.

Part II

Ethical Aspects of the Continuum of Care

My Nurse

When I go to hospital
My nurse would treat me well,
She'd know just how to cure me
With medicine and pills

When I went to A&E
My nurse was standing by
She never took her eyes off me
And helped me not to cry

When I go to hospital
My nurse is always there,
To help me and to cure me
And give me lots of care.

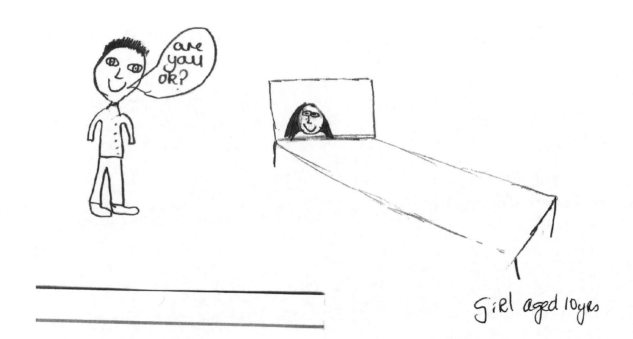

girl aged 10yrs

4 Beginning of Life: Ethical Issues in Neonatology Nursing

Amanda Williamson and Julie Mullett

The time came to make the agonising decision to turn off Mason's life support, to allow our son to rest in peace in heaven.

(Amanda Mason's Mum 2009; East Anglia's Children's Hospices Annual Review 2008–09)

Introduction

Since the 1960s, developments in neonatal medicine have meant that more babies are surviving at younger and younger gestations (Nuffield Council of Bioethics, NCOB 2004). The neonatal intensive care unit (NICU) has become a highly specialist and technical environment. Medical and nursing staff have become highly skilled in supporting sick babies and prolonging life. However, not all babies will survive; some will survive with severe disabilities, and the cost of such medical advances may mean that very difficult ethical decisions have to be made by parents and staff caring for these babies. The decisions may include whether or not to commence resuscitation on a baby at the edge of viability (24 weeks gestation) or who has a life-threatening congenital abnormality and whether or not to continue treatment on a baby who is thought to have a life-limiting disorder or a significant risk of

disability so that it may not necessarily be in the best interests of the child to provide active treatment.

This chapter will explore the ethical aspects of decisions that may have to be made in relation to neonatal care. Although organisations such as the NCOB (2004), the British Association of Perinatal Medicine (BAPM) (Wilkinson *et al.* 2008) and the Royal College of Paediatrics and Child Health (RCPCH) (RCPCH 2004) may provide guidance to practitioners, the ethical decisions made must reflect a number of complex interactions and considerations. One decision that is correct for one family may not be correct for another.

It is important to remember that at the heart of any decision made, the *best interest* of the baby must remain paramount (*The Children Act* 1989 s1; NCOB 2004; RCPCH 2004).

How should ethical decisions be made in a NICU?

Ethical decisions made in a NICU often raise significant emotions. The ethical decisions made in a neonatal setting are particularly unique; they may be decisions made on the edge of viability where the long-term outcome is uncertain or may

Ethical and Philosophical Aspects of Nursing Children, First Edition. Edited by Gosia M. Brykczyńska and Joan Simons.
© 2011 Blackwell Publishing Ltd. Published 2011 by Blackwell Publishing Ltd.

be decisions of withdrawing treatment because the treatment is thought to be *intolerable* for the baby and the risk of long-term disability or morbidity is uncertain. Babies in NICUs are reliant on their family and those caring for them to be their advocate and decide what is in their *best interest*. Parents find themselves in a position where they are asked to make difficult decisions that they had probably never perceived of at the start of their pregnancy about a child they have had little or minimal time to get to know. Parents are reliant on staff caring for their child to guide them though a difficult and painful process. This raises the question as to how ethical decisions should be made in a NICU and who is best placed to make that decision.

Baumann-Holzle *et al.* (2005) identify a number of ways that the decision could be made:

- Unilaterally by the head of the neonatal unit
- By following strict rules and guidelines
- By an ethics committee or ethical consultants
- By parents
- By doctors and nurses working and caring for the infant

This list will form the structure of this chapter. However, it should be noted that complex decisions made in relation to neonatal care may also be made by the legal system; for example, in Re A (Children) (Conjoined Twins: Surgical Separation) (2000) a decision was made by the Court of Appeal to separate conjoined twins against the wishes of their parents. This was a very complex case in which the separation of the twins meant that one twin (Mary) was certain to die as she was reliant on her sibling (Jodie) to circulate oxygenated blood for both of them. If the twins were not separated, doctors estimated that they would both die within 6 months. Medical staff wanted to separate the twins to give Jodie a good chance of survival. However the parents did not feel able to give their consent to separate the twins.

Unilateral decision making

The danger of unilateral decision making is not only that it is susceptible to that person's own interpretation of the situation, their own life experiences, but that it is also open to bias. It is also a significant responsibility for an individual to undertake. However, due to the very complex nature of ethical decisions that must be made within the NICU setting, unilateral decision making is not recommended (Baumann-Holzle *et al.* 2004).

Rules and guidelines

Guidelines and ethical frameworks have been developed by the NCOB (2004), RCPCH (2004) and BAPM (Wilkinson *et al.* 2008) to guide health-care professionals towards making appropriate ethical decisions in relation to neonatal care. The legal system may also provide rules for health-care professionals to follow. The problem with any rule is that each baby and their family are unique and a rule that may be appropriate for one family may not be appropriate for another. All guidance must acknowledge the need for cases to be judged on an individual basis.

BAPM (Wilkinson *et al.* 2008) developed a framework to help guide clinicians who make decisions about the management of babies born extremely prematurely at less than 26 weeks gestation.

Key features of the framework include:

- Ensuring that accurate clinical information is available to professionals to enable appropriate decisions to be made.
- The best estimation of gestational age should rely not only on scanning information but also in conjunction with the parents.
- Discussions with parents should include information about the expected outcome based upon local and national data.
- Any decision made should be individualised and should be led by senior staff of all disciplines.

Summary of framework

- If the gestational age is certain and is less than 23 + 0 weeks gestation, it is recommended in the best interests of the child for resuscitation not to be carried out.

- If the gestational age is certain at 23 + 0–23 + 6 and the fetal heart is heard during labour, BAPM recommend that an experienced professional in resuscitation should attend the birth. It is in the best interests of the baby not to start resuscitation, particularly if the parents request resuscitation not to be commenced. If bag and mask inflation is commenced, the response of the heart rate will be critical in any further decisions to be made.
- If the gestational age is certain at 24 + 0–24 + 6, resuscitation should be commenced unless parents and staff believe that the baby's chance of survival will be severely compromised. Again the response of the baby's heart rate in response to resuscitation will be able to aid decision making further. If the baby appears more immature than expected deciding not to commence resuscitation may be considered in their best interests.
- If the gestational age is 25 + 0 weeks or more, BAPM say that it is appropriate to resuscitate these babies. This was based on the evidence from the EPICure 2 Perinatal Group (2008) which found that survival at that gestation since 1995 had increased from 54% to 67% but that morbidity had not changed.

The RCPCH (2004) identify five circumstances in which withholding or withdrawal of treatment may be justified. These include the brain dead child, the permanent vegetative state, the no-chance situation, the no-purpose situation and the unbearable situation. For neonates, perhaps the most significant may be the no-purpose situation and unbearable situation. The no-purpose situation identifies circumstances in which the child may survive if treatment is given but that this treatment may not be in the child's best interest. The unbearable situation occurs when the family feel that continuing treatment is more than can be borne and the family wish to withdraw treatment or for the child to receive no further treatment (RCPCH 2004). Despite such unbearable situations arising, the NCOB (2004) unreservedly rejected any idea of active ending of neonatal life even if that life was seen to be intolerable.

Although the RCPCH and BAPM give guidance, in practice it is still the responsibility of the individual practitioner, trust and neonatal network to interpret and implement the guidance. This chapter will explore later how individuals' own experiences and beliefs may influence their own decision making. However, guidance helps practitioners and families to make decisions that are individual and appropriate for each baby.

Legal guidance may also be used to aid decision making. Dewar (1998:467) notes that 'Family law engages the passions as no other part of our legal system does: and it is the hallmark passion that must exceed rationality'.

The Abortion Act (1967) allows termination of pregnancy up until 24 weeks of completed pregnancy. However decisions are also made at a similar gestation depending upon a child's *best interest* under the Children Act 1989. This may present health-care professionals with a complex ethical consideration where on the one hand they are being asked to terminate a fetus that in another circumstance they would be asked to treat. McCullough & Chervenak (1994) claim that neonatal practice in the United Kingdom is based on the premise that when a fetus becomes viable, it acquires the status of a person. However, this is not the case legally. According to St George's Healthcare NHS Trust v S (1998, 2FLR 728) 'a pregnant woman was entitled, as an adult of sound mind, to refuse medical treatment, even if her own life and that of the unborn child depended upon some treatment'. In this case, a woman refused life-saving treatment for herself and her unborn baby, as she wished her baby to be born naturally. However, medical staff made an application under section 2 of the Mental Health Act 1983 and a Caesarean section was carried out against her wishes. The woman applied to the court for a review of the decision. This means that a fetus does not obtain any rights until it has an independent existence from its mother. The NCOB (2004) identifies that the value that a person puts on the life of a fetus or a newborn infant is an important consideration when making decisions about critical care. It regards the moment of birth as the significant threshold in potential viability. The rights a baby gains at birth include rights under the *Human Rights Act* (1998) and (although not legally binding) rights under the United Nations Convention on Rights of the Child (UNCRC) (UN 1989) which would be considered by the court in any child cases. The NCOB (2004) agrees with the legal position and says that although it may be *morally* wrong for a woman to act in a way which is harming her future child, it would be wrong to force a woman to have medical or surgical interventions to benefit a fetus.

The Children Act (1989) may offer guidance as to who can make decisions as in Section 3 (1) it introduces the concept of parental responsibility. It states parental responsibility is 'all the rights, duties, powers and responsibilities which by law a parent has in relation to the child and his property'. The mother automatically gains parental responsibility. The father gains responsibility automatically if the parents are married. If parents are unmarried, the father automatically gains parental responsibility if he is named on the birth certificate (*The Adoption and Children Act* 2002). This could be problematic for staff in NICUs if the baby has not had its birth registered and the mother may be too ill to give consent or estranged from her partner. If the father is not on the birth certificate then he must apply for a court order to gain parental responsibility. Parents have a legal duty to provide or take steps to provide medical treatment to prevent unnecessary suffering or injury. Only where all persons with parental responsibility exercise a veto will medical treatment be prohibited. There is an ongoing case re Baby RB, where his parents cannot agree on whether to withdraw life support or not on a 1-year-old child who is unable to breathe unaided (*The Times* 2009).

Health-care practitioners have a legal obligation to do 'what is reasonable to safeguard or promote the welfare of the child' (*The Children Act* 1989 s.3 (5)). However this must not go against parents' wishes particularly where there is no consensus. Should they wish to do this they must seek the leave of the court and apply for a Section 8 Specific Issue Order (*The Children Act* 1989 s10 (4)). The court may use its inherent jurisdiction to consent or refuse treatment on behalf of a minor. It is a protective jurisdiction allowing the court to plug legal loopholes in complex cases where there is no statutory provision available. In any decision regarding children, the child's welfare shall be the court's paramount consideration and any order must have a demonstrable benefit for the child (*The Children Act* 1989 s1(1)). The court would take into consideration UNCRC 1989 when making any decision in relation to a child which includes the right to life. The court must ensure that it adheres to the *Human*

Rights Act (1998) in any decision it makes in regard to neonates which includes the right to life without prejudice. A study by Issacs *et al.* (2006) found that it is best if parents and staff can agree on the need for intensive treatment of a neonate. The RCPCH (2004) claim that duty of care and partnerships of care are fundamental principles in the ethical decision-making process involving children.

Role of ethics committees

Clinical ethics committees are now becoming more common in the United Kingdom. The RCPCH (2004) describe the functions of these committees as including discussion, analysis and advising for individual cases. They may provide an opportunity for staff to analyse the appropriate action in difficult and complex ethical cases. However, the problem with ethics committees is that they may seem too distant from the case, and it may be difficult for families to give their thoughts or feel they have had their views appropriately represented to a committee. If the committee is associated to a trust, it may not appear independent and there may be concerns that judgements are not based upon individual outcomes but on the good for all. Parents may not agree with a decision and a good working partnership between parents and staff may be lost. Cuttini *et al.* (2000) found that overall if a hospital had an ethics committee advising on their clinical cases, the probability of ever having withdrawn mechanical ventilation from a neonate increased. This may be because hospitals that have more complex cases are more likely to have an ethics committee. Or it could be that a collective responsibility means that staff feel more able to make decisions that lead to withdrawal of mechanical ventilation.

Partnership decision making

Almost all NICUs in the United Kingdom would claim to offer family-centred care. 'Family centred care is a philosophy of care that helps families whose baby required hospital care to cope with the stress anxiety and altered parenting roles that accompany their baby's condition' (Neonatal.Org 2009:11). There is perhaps no more significant time during neonatal care where the need for true family-centred care is required as when decisions about withholding or withdrawal of treatment are being made.

However, the Parents of Premature Babies Project (POPPY) (POPPY 2009) found that family-centred care within NICUs in the United Kingdom was variable with some units offering much better level of support for families than others.

Sudia-Robinson & Freeman (2000) identify that it is parents who are ultimately responsible for their babies' medical care and that parents often want to be active participants in decisions regarding their babies' care. They identify that parents may have a very wide range of knowledge and understanding of the care their babies may receive. They claim that it is important that parents be actively engaged in any decision-making process. McHaffie et al. (2001) also support this finding. Their study found that the majority of parents wanted to be actively involved in decision making on behalf of their child and did not appear to suffer adverse consequences by doing so. However, they say that the timing of events during the decision-making process and the management of death is critical. If parents were given time to assimilate the reality at each stage of the process, their dissatisfaction was reduced. This is supported by the POPPY Study (2009) which found that parents found it very distressing to be given conflicting advice. The study found that if parents received little bits of information, it allowed them to assimilate the information given before they received more. It is important that parents have accurate and consistent information upon which to make their choices (McHaffie et al. 2001). A paper by a specialist group which discusses withdrawal of mechanical ventilation says that parents must be given time to make any decision and that they 'walk alone in their own shoes' Tobin in Issacs et al. (2006:314). Tobin claims that parents should be allowed a margin of error in their decision making. A very difficult concept for parents may be that 'sometimes being the very, very, best parent does not mean fighting to cure but fighting to do the best you can for your child's quality of life' (Craft & Killen 2007:10).

A study by Hammerman et al. (1997) explored the response of pregnant women towards the treatment of critically ill and/or malformed neonates. They concluded that maternal cultural background and beliefs more profoundly influenced any ethical decision making than a woman's past life experience. Tobin in Issacs et al. (2006) says that parents' religious and other beliefs should be respected by health-care professionals even if the professionals' own beliefs differ from those of the parents. A study by Cuttini et al. (2000) found that doctors with significant religious beliefs did alter their decision making in cases where a decision to commence active treatment for neonates who were at high risk of death or severe disability was involved. Tobin in Issacs et al. (2006) identifies that if parents are to make wise decisions, they must rely on sensible advice from well-informed, experienced and humane health-care professionals. There is always a danger of health-care practitioner bias. A doctor who rated religion as extremely or fairly important was less likely to have withheld intensive care, withdrawn mechanical ventilation or to have administered analgesia to relieve pain (Cuttini et al. 2000). It is not uncommon for nursing staff to note that different decisions in regard to a baby's care may be made according to which consultant is managing the baby that day.

Boyle et al. (2004) claim that although parents in the United Kingdom are involved in the decision-making process as to whether or not resuscitation of a 25-week gestation baby should be undertaken, most centres would ultimately resuscitate babies born at 25 or 24 weeks gestation even if the parents did not wish for that to happen. A study by Janvier & Barrington (2005) found a much higher rate of resuscitation at tertiary centres rather than smaller neonatal centres. They identify that it could be that parents in the tertiary centres requested more resuscitation or it could be an influence of neonatologists' own views and a reflection on the way discussion of treatment was undertaken. This raises the concern that although parents may believe they have given informed consent, they are dependent on the information given to them by staff caring for their babies. Decisions will be almost always made from a position of probabilities not certainties (RCPCH 2004).

Tobin in Issacs et al. (2006) says that it is the responsibility of doctors to truly evaluate the benefits of burdens and treatments on a child and they must resist pressure from parents to do the wrong thing if it is not in the best interests of the child. In Portsmorth NHS Trust v Wyatt (Portsmouth

NHS Trust v (1) Derek Wyatt (2) Charlotte Wyatt (by her guardian CAFCASS) and Southampton NHS Trust (Intervener) 2004, 07/10/2004), where the parents and medical staff disagreed over treatment and medical staff did not want to mechanically ventilate the baby if her condition deteriorated, Justice Hedley said 'Although I believe and find that further invasive and aggressive treatment would be intolerable to Charlotte, I prefer to determine her best interests on the basis of finding what is the best that can be done for her'. The NCOB (2004) states that the concept of *intolerability* described situations in which the continuation of treatment could not be seen to be in the *best interests* of the baby because it would impose an intolerable burden on the baby. Tobin in Issacs *et al.* (2006) says there are two ways in which life-sustaining treatment may be considered not to be in the best interests of the child. These are when treatment does not offer a sufficient therapeutic to the child or when it entails a too great a burden on the child. However, this raises the dilemma as to who decides that the treatment is not therapeutic or is too much of a burden. The RCPCH (2004) try to identify what makes a disability intolerable. The term *intolerable* could mean 'that which cannot be borne' or 'that which people should not be asked to bear' (RCPCH 2004:25). However, people's own views on what is intolerable may vary according to their own life experiences and judgements. If intensive treatment does not provide a benefit for the baby, treatment may be legally and ethically withdrawn even if the parents disagree (Issacs *et al.* 2006).

The NCOB (2004) says that economic considerations must not be the only consideration in maximising health benefits; equity and justice should be significant considerations in the decision-making process. Staff should be aware of but not driven by the resource implications of their decisions; their decisions should be clinically led (NCOB 2004, para 13). Issacs *et al.* (2006) suggest that pressure on intensive care beds is not a valid reason to withdraw or withhold ventilation of a neonate. However, Zupancic *et al.* (2000) claims that resuscitation and intensive treatment of very premature children with a high chance of long-term disability or death may not be financially justifiable in a public health-care system. The NCOB (2004, para 26) identifies very clearly that no person involved in intensive care treatment of neonates should feel pressurised to allow babies to die because of the risk of a disability.

The problem for health-care professionals is that they always commence from a position of uncertainty. There will always be children who survived despite withdrawal of treatment. The RCPCH (2004) say that this does not mean that the decision to withdraw or withhold treatment was then necessarily wrong.

Neonatal nursing staff

Neonatal staff are trained to undertake interventions that prolong life (Williamson *et al.* 2009); this means that staff may feel internal conflict and a sense of failure when a decision to withdraw treatment is made. Yam *et al.* (2001) found that nursing staff on NICUs often felt angry about the dilemma of providing both curative and palliative care. Wynn (2002:122) explores ethics in a neonatal nursing setting; she claims nurses ask the questions 'Is there a person here? How do I know the care I am giving is doing more good than merely sustaining biological life? How do I know if this patient has a future?'

A study by Spence (1998) explored the involvement of neonatal nurses in ethical decisions made and to what extent they saw themselves as advocates for the babies in their care. The study covered nurses working in both NICUs and special care baby units. The study found that nursing staff were more likely to be involved in clinical decisions rather than ethical decisions. She found that nurses had most concern for neonates who had an unclear diagnosis and that neonatal nurses viewed themselves as advocates for the babies in their care. Term babies who had suffered a significant degree of hypoxia appeared to cause neonatal nurses particularly high levels of concern. However, a study by Monterosso *et al.* (2005) found that neonatal nurses actually used their clinical knowledge and experiences to guide ethical decision making. They recommended that a multidisciplinary model for ethical decision making should be used. This means that the perspective of the nursing staff directly involved in the care of the baby may be utilised. The Nursing Midwifery Council (NMC) guidance for nurses states that you should 'make the care of people your first concern, treating them as individuals and respecting their dignity' (NMC 2008:1).

Spence (1998) found that nurses identified knowledge, assertiveness, communication, empathy and experience as essential to enable nurses to act as a baby's advocate. She also identified that nurses must be willing to step into this role and acknowledge the pivotal role that they could play in a decision-making process. Nurses' own experiences may alter their attitudes to an ethical situation. A study by Bellini & Damato (2009) found that nurses with more years of neonatal nursing experience were less supportive of the initiation of aggressive care modalities for patients not for resuscitation. They found that the nurses' level of education do not alter their view. This perhaps highlights the importance of a person's own life experiences, attitudes and beliefs in regard to ethical decision making.

Conclusion

The neonatal nurse must remember to be aware that the decision being made is for a baby and its family, and that their own life experiences should not become prejudicial in any decision-making process. The NMC (2008:1) say 'you must always be able to justify your decisions, and be open and honest, act with integrity and uphold the reputation of your profession'.

Neonatal nurses work very closely with the families of babies in their care. This means that they may be able to offer a unique and supportive role to families during any decision-making process; however, it is a role that neonatal nurses must be willing to accept if they are to become true partners in the ethical decision-making partnership.

Reflective scenario

Sarah Jones has just had a Caesarean section for pre-eclampsia toxaemia at 24 weeks gestation. She is currently heavily sedated on the high-dependency unit. Her partner Joe is with their baby (Sam) who is extremely ill on the NICU. Sam has been found to have a congenital abnormality that is incompatible with life.

Questions

Who would be able to make the decision about whether to continue treatment?
How should the decision be made?
What factors may influence the decision-making process?

References

Abortion Act (1967) An Act to amend and clarify the law relating to termination of pregnancy by registered medical practitioners. United Kingdom Parliament.

Amanda Mason's Mum (2009) *East Anglia's Children's Hospice Annual Review 2008–2009*. EACH, www.each.org.uk

Baumann-Holzle, R., Maffezzoni, M. & Bucher, H.U. (2005) A framework for ethical decision making in neonatal intensive care. *Acta Paediatrica*, **94**, 1777–1783.

Bellini, S. & Damato, E.G. (2009) Nurses' knowledge, attitudes/beliefs and care practices concerning do not resuscitate status for hospitalised neonates. *JOGNN*, **38** (2), 195–205.

Boyle, R.J., Salter, R. & Arnander, M. (2004) Ethics of refusing parental requests to withhold or withdraw treatment from their premature baby. *Journal of Medical Ethics*, **30**, 402–405.

Craft, A. & Killen, S. (2007) *Palliative Care Services for Children and Young People in England*. Department of Health, UK.

Cuttini, M., Nadai, M., Kaminski, M., *et al.* (2000) End-of-life decisions in neonatal intensive care: Physicians' self reported practices in seven European countries. *The Lancet*, **355** (17), 2112–2118.

Dewar, J. (1998) The normal chaos of family life. *Modern Law Review*, **61** (4), 467.

EPICure 2 Perinatal Group (2008) Survival and early morbidity of extremely preterm babies in England: Changes since 1995. *Archives of Diseases in Childhood*, **93** (Suppl.), A33–A34.

Hammerman, C., Kornbluth, E., Lavie, O., Zadka, P., Aboulafia, Y. & Eidelman, A. (1997) Decision-making in the critically ill neonate: Cultural background v individual life experiences. *Journal of Medical Ethics*, **23**, 164–169.

Human Rights Act (1998) HMSO, London.

Issacs, D., Kilham, H., Gordon, A., *et al*. (2006) Withdrawal of neonatal mechanical ventilation against parent's wishes. *Journal of Paediatrics and Child Health*, **42**, 311–315.

Janvier, A. & Barrington, K. (2005) The ethics of neonatal resuscitation at the margins of viability: Informed consent and outcomes. *The Journal of Pediatrics*, **147** (5), 579–585.

McCullough, L.B. & Chervenak, F.A. (1994) *Ethics in Obstetrics and Gynecology*. Oxford University Press, Oxford.

McHaffie, H., Lyon, A. & Hume, R. (2001) Deciding on treatment limitation for neonates: The parents' perspective. *European Journal of Pediatrics*, **160**, 339–344.

Monterosso, L., Kristjanson, L., Sly, P., *et al*. (2005) The role of the neonatal intensive care nurse in decision-making: Advocacy, involvement in ethical decisions and communication. *International Journal of Nursing Practice*, **11**, 108–117.

NCOB (2004) *Critical Decisions in Fetal and Neonatal Medicine Ethical Issues*. Nuffield Council on Bioethics, London, http://www.nuffieldbioethics.org

Neonatal.Org (2009) *Neonatal Standards for Stakeholder Comment on: Family Centred Care, Surgery, Transfers, Workforce Data, Governance* at http://www.neonatal.org.uk/standardsquestionaire

NMC (2008) *The Code: Standards of Conduct, Performance and Ethics for Nurses and Midwives*. Nursing and Midwifery Council, London.

POPPY (2009) *Family-centred Care in Neonatal Units: A Summary of Research Results and Recommendations from the POPPY Project*. Parents of Premature babies Project, NCT, London.

Portsmouth NHS Trust v (1) Derek Wyatt (2) Charlotte Wyatt (by her guardian CAFCASS) and Southampton NHS Trust (Intervener), 07/10/2004 (2004) EWWHC 2247 (Fam).

RCPCH (2004) *Withholding or Withdrawing Life Sustaining Treatment in Children: A Framework for Practice*, 2nd edn. Royal College of Paediatrics and Child Health, London.

Re A (Children) (Conjoined Twins: Surgical Separation) (2000) *The All England Law Reports*, **4**, 961–1070.

Spence, K. (1998) Ethical issues for neonatal nurses. *Nursing Ethics*, **5** (3), 206–217.

St George's Healthcare NHS Trust v S (1998) 2FLR 728 'a.

Sudia-Robinson, T. & Freeman, S. (2000) Communication patterns and decision making among parents and health care providers in the neonatal intensive care unit: A case study. *Heart & Lung*, **29**, 143–148.

The Adoption and Children Act (2002) Office of Public Sector Information, London.

The Children Act (1989). HMSO, London.

The Times (2009) 4 November 2009, p. 23.

UN (1989) *United Nations Convention on Rights of the Child*. United Nations, New York.

Wilkinson, A., Ahluwalia, J., Cole, A., *et al*. (2008) British association of the management of babies born extremely preterm at less than 26 weeks gestation. A framework for clinical practice at the time of birth. *Archives of Diseases in Childhood FNN Online*, **94**, 2–5. doi:10.1136/adc.2008.143321.

Williamson, A., Devereux, C. & Shirtliffe, J. (2009) Development of a care pathway for babies being discharged from a level 3 neonatal intensive care unit to a community setting for end-of-life care. *Journal of Neonatal Nursing*, **15** (5), 164–168.

Wynn, F. (2002) Nursing and the concept of life: Towards an ethics of testimony. *Nursing Philosophy*, **3**, 120–132.

Yam, B., Rossiter, J. & Cheung, K. (2001) Caring for dying infants: Experiences of neonatal intensive care nurses in Hong Kong. *Journal of Clinical Nursing*, **10**, 651–659.

Zupancic, J.A., Richardson, D.K., Lee, K. & McCormack, M. (2000) Economic of prematurity in the era of managed care. *Clinical Perinatology*, **27** (2), 483–497.

Suggested further readings

NCOB (2004) *Critical Decisions in Fetal and Neonatal Medicine Ethical Issues*. Nuffield Council on Bioethics, London, http://www.nuffieldbioethics.org

RCPCH (2004) *Withholding or Withdrawing Life Sustaining Treatment in Children: A Framework for Practice*, 2nd edn. Royal College of Paediatrics and Child Health, London.

Wilkinson, A., Ahluwalia, J., Cole, A., *et al*. (2008) The management of babies born extremely preterm at less than 26 weeks gestation. A framework for clinical practice at the time of birth. *Archives of Diseases Childhood FNN Online*, **94**, 2–5. doi:10.1136/adc.2008.143321.

5 Ethical Issues in Caring for Toddlers and School Age Children: Ethical Aspects of the Role and Work of the Health Visitor

Monica Davis

Introduction

This chapter will explore some of the ethical issues in health visiting whilst highlighting a few of the challenges health visitors face on a daily basis. Ethics in nursing has been of great importance because it revolves around moral judgements or putting it simply, about aspects of *right* and *wrong*; therefore, it is about moral behaviour (Hawley 2007). Edwards (1996) uses the terms ethics and morals synonymously and involves analysis of actions which may result in harm or benefit to an individual. Beauchamp & Childress (2001) talk about professional morality, having standards of conduct which are on the whole accepted by professions such as medicine. These include aspects such as informed consent, confidentiality, respecting autonomy and protection from harm and can be applied to nursing.

The ethical issues that will be discussed in this chapter are non-maleficence, beneficence, autonomy, and nurse–patient relationship, specifically veracity. Utilitarianism will also be focused on in relation to immunisation. Many ethical issues emerge when caring for toddlers and school age children, not least because they are so precious but also because parents or carers on the whole want to do the best for their children. This may, however, conflict with what professionals consider as being in the child's best interest; in nursing it could be argued that our moral duty is to all our clients including the children without partiality. Some of the ethical issues are relevant not just for health visitors but also for parents/carers revolving around immunisation concerns, domestic abuse (domestic violence) and of course safeguarding children. These issues will be discussed in this chapter, along with the challenge that increasingly, parents, health visitors and other professionals such as general practitioners (GPs) have expressed concerns about the reduction in health visiting hours and the impact this is having on service delivery.

Immunisation concerns

Controversies surround immunisations and clearly affect the uptake which has fluctuated over many years particularly in the coverage of measles, mumps and rubella (MMR). Part of this can be attributed to the publication of Wakefield *et al.*'s research in 1998 suggesting a link between MMR, autism and bowel disorder. However, Polterak

Ethical and Philosophical Aspects of Nursing Children, First Edition. Edited by Gosia M. Brykczyńska and Joan Simons.
© 2011 Blackwell Publishing Ltd. Published 2011 by Blackwell Publishing Ltd.

et al. (2004) pointed out that other factors may influence parental decisions not to immunise including birth experience, feelings of control, family history, engagement with health services and friends. They go further in suggesting that professionals provide information to parents with the expectation that they will immunise, but parents have many ways of accessing information including the internet, parent groups and movements such as *Jabs* and the *Informed Parents*. These all help to influence parents' confidence in the MMR programme despite the fact that numerous studies such as Taylor *et al.* (1999), Madsen *et al.* (2002) and Polterak *et al.* (2004) have found no causal link between MMR and autism. Whatever the reason, evidence suggests that the media (Peltola *et al.* 1998) plays a pivotal role in shaping parents' decision.

We know that some parents refuse to have their children immunised possibly for reasons mentioned earlier but this should not deter health visitors, school nurses and practice nurses from promoting the vaccination programme. Equally, in applying ethical principles to immunisation which health visitors promote through their health promotion work, consequence-based theory or consequentialism can be applied. These are terms given to theorists who believe actions are either right or wrong based on their good and bad consequences (Beauchamp & Childress 2001). They drew attention to utilitarianism, the most well-known consequence-based theory and according to Jones & Cribb (1997), the most favoured ethical principle in health promotion is the utilitarian approach with the notion that benefits should outweigh the disadvantages for the majority of people. This approach therefore argues that we should act in such a way as to promote the greatest happiness for the greatest number of people (Rumbold 2002).

In exploring the ethical principle of non-maleficence according to Rumbold (2002), nurses have a duty not to harm their patients or clients, and can be extended to not imposing risks of harm (Beauchamp & Childress 2001). Referring to the immunisation programme, Rumbold states that we vaccinate in order to do good, benefiting not just the individual but the community as a whole. The benefit is that the individual will not contract the disease, and if enough people are immunised it will provide herd immunity thus protecting those who are not immunised from the disease

(Rumbold 2002; NHSII 2009). Rumbold, however, advises caution stating that risks include the fact that a minority of people may suffer harmful side effects to the vaccination, some of which can be serious or fatal. This notion of course becomes a dilemma for many parents and may influence their decision not to immunise. But, despite Rumbold's concerns, he counteracts this statement by suggesting that there would be greater harm caused if we did not immunise and the effects of this could be just as serious as potential vaccination side effects. He states that to apply the principle 'above all do no harm' to vaccinations is clearly illogical, and sees a correlation between beneficence and non-maleficence because not doing harm is sometimes an inevitable consequence of doing good.

As a health visitor, it feels that at times we are battling with so many viewpoints and whilst we know that having sound theoretical knowledge and information should enhance the clinical process, invariably some commentators reveal the types of ethical dilemma involved in immunising children. For example, Jones & Cribb (1997) referred to the fact that we cannot be sure that those who are immunised would have contracted the disease and in contrast that those who are harmed by being immunised may not have been harmed by the disease if they had not been immunised. Austin *et al.* (2008) in their study found that some participants felt pressurised into having vaccinations. This of course is unacceptable and health visitors must ensure that the advice they provide to parents does not remove their parental autonomy.

The Nursing and Midwifery Council (NMC 2008) bases part of its role in safeguarding the well-being of the public on ethical principles. It considers the principle of autonomy as central to nursing, and to remove clients' autonomy could be deemed as being in breech of the nurses' code of conduct particularly because it undermines clients' freedom to make their own choices. McHale & Gallagher (2003) see autonomy as *self-rule* or self-determination concerning our ability to control our lives. It also concerns individual choice, freedom and privacy. This includes acknowledging that a person has the right to hold their own opinion, make their own choices and that actions may be based on personal values and beliefs (Beauchamp & Childress 2001).

However, although health visitors must do good for their clients and ensure no harm, the

NMC (2008) states that nurses must also respect people's right to accept or decline treatment, to ensure that the best available information is given, and that it is evidence based. Equally, Bedford (2008) stipulates that health-care professionals, who are knowledgeable about immunisations and related issues, can be highly effective in gaining informed consent. This, however, is not as easy as it seems; Burnard & Chapman (2003) warn that sometimes there is the temptation to *water down* the information in our effort to explain medical and clinical matters without frightening the patients and clients.

Burnard & Chapman's (2003) suggestion could be applied to immunisations where health visitors may readily provide information on the programme, notify clients when the vaccinations are due and tell them why they should immunise but not necessarily give the full facts about side effects or efficacy. Health visitors are also very much aware of the *Green Book* (DoH 2006) which contradicts this, highlighting the importance of health professionals being able to adequately communicate the benefits, side effects, efficacy and safety of vaccinations to parents. The aim is to minimise fears whilst ensuring the facts are provided in a way that the clients will understand and in an environment where they feel able to ask questions and express concerns.

Health visitors and other nurses should move away from the notion that telling the truth may be too frightening for clients because it is probably more upsetting to the clients not to reveal all the facts, which may later become apparent. In contrast, the NMC (2008) tells us that we must be open and honest which ties in with Edwards' (1996) notion of veracity suggesting that professionals should be truthful in their interactions with clients. Beauchamp & Childress (2001) propose that when we communicate with our clients, we implicitly promise to be truthful including diagnosis, prognosis and procedures. This of course should be the case with immunisations. It is not, however, straightforward and some decisions made by parents will require the health visitors having discussions with members of the multidisciplinary team, in line with the NMC (2008). Equally, Austin *et al.* (2008) concluded that professionals must also listen to parents' concerns, respond to their fears and ensure that trust is a key interpersonal feature,

the rationale being, that trust can enhance the view that the information being provided is reliable and unbiased. However, despite all the information, the debate and controversies surrounding immunisation looks like it will continue. Health visitors can play their part by keeping themselves updated not just with the vaccination programme but with the research evidence so they can better support families with whatever decision they undertake.

Domestic abuse

Health visitors deal with various forms of abuse on a daily basis during the course of their work including domestic abuse. Definitions of domestic abuse include physical, psychological, sexual, and financial abuse between intimate adults and/or family members. The abuser has both power and control over the person who is being abused (DoH 2000; RCN 2000; Women's Aid 2009), and Buka (2008) points out that a causal link in all types of abuse is a breech of trust. Linked to abuse is the notion of vulnerability which creates a great challenge for health visitors who are constantly prioritising their workload in order to meet the needs of these clients. Whilst it is acknowledged that men may also experience domestic abuse, the main focus of health visitors' work is with women, and the Department of Health (DoH 2000) report that it is mainly women who experience this type of abuse, and it is largely men who are the perpetrators.

The impact of domestic abuse is well documented, not just on women but also on children who may experience the abuse or are passive observers. It is difficult to highlight how many women and children are affected as there is possibly underreporting of the violence (DoH 2000). Nevertheless, the Metropolitan Police (2004) reports that by the time it is brought to their attention, women would have experienced repeated patterns of abuse. It is estimated that on average, women experience 35 episodes of domestic abuse before seeking help (DoH 2000). Equally, domestic abuse starts to intensify during pregnancy and neonatal period (Mezey & Bewley 1997), and continues in the postpartum period (Stewart 1994). These findings are clearly important to health visitors who have a role in providing support to these women and children. However, such support may be less forthcoming during the antenatal period due to the pressures of health visitors' caseload and could mean an over-reliance on the midwifery services which may also be over-stretched.

Worms (2004) pointed out that raising public awareness of domestic abuse is often left to health visitors who provide varying degrees of information. This does not detract from the good work that is being done by voluntary organisations such as *Women's Aid* which has a great role to play, but health visitors may come into contact with the clients before referrals are made to other agencies. Like the Department of Health (DoH 2000), many health visitors believe that domestic abuse requires a multi-agency approach including working with social services, police, *Women's Aid* organisations and *Domestic Violence Forums*, whilst the Department of Health recognises the important role health visitors play in supporting those experiencing domestic abuse. Worms (2004) concurs but sees training as an important issue along with the importance of designated staff sitting on Domestic Violence Forums. Although training is usually available, getting time off work is often difficult, yet it could enhance effectiveness and may also help to provide the confidence needed to be able to ask clients about domestic abuse.

The Department of Health (DoH 2000) goes further in stating that health-care professionals must be aware of the risks in order to enhance their alertness as this may prevent or minimise further abuse. Health visitors and indeed other professionals involved in domestic abuse services must also combine the risks with the difficulties women have in reporting such abuse. According to the DoH (2000, 2005), factors deterring women from seeking help include fear of reprisals (perpetrator may threaten the woman), embarrassment, may not recognise they are being abused, cultural or religious barriers, fear the children will be taken into care and not knowing where to go for help. Some women and children may not reveal their experience but health visitors are well placed to identify non-verbal queues which will *sound alarm bells* and they must then find ways of approaching the subject, give appropriate advice and support and make suitable referrals.

Domestic abuse is an emotive topic and health visitors have a moral duty to act when abuse is taking place and, like other health professionals, are aware that the care provided must be in the best interest of parents and children. This is reinforced by Buka (2008) who wrote that health-care professionals owe their clients a duty of care not to harm them and to avoid omissions in care delivery which could lead to harm, and correlates this with the advice of the NMC (NMC 2008). There are, however, difficulties associated with domestic abuse; on the one hand, health visitors want to ensure the safety of women and children, but they also want to make certain that it is done in a way that the clients' wishes are respected. However, health visitors are very much aware that regardless of the woman's decision the needs of the children must be paramount as stated in the Children's Act (OPSI 1989).

Health visitors' dilemma is worsened with the revelation that some health-care professionals are reluctant to identify domestic abuse for reasons such as 'opening a can of worms', fear of not knowing what to do next and fear of offending the clients (DoH 2000). On the other hand, what seems to be missing from this list is the issue of inadequate resources to meet the clients' identified needs. From my own experience and conversations with colleagues, there is sometimes a sense of helplessness as referrals are made by health visitors to appropriate services who are themselves over-stretched. In spite of this, the Department of Health's recommendation is understandable, and health visitors would be failing in their duty of care if they choose to ignore abuse when they see it. Equally, the ethical principles highlighted earlier will come into play as failure to act could lead to harm not just to the women involved but also their children. Here we can also look at the ethical principle of beneficence which Beauchamp & Childress (2001) see as action done to benefit others. This notion is important in helping the survivors of domestic abuse in increasing their awareness of what constitute abuse, recognising abuse and where to turn to for help. Again this principle also applies to the children including the unborn child as some of these women will be pregnant.

Ethical dilemmas for health visitors often occur when they are faced with suspicions that domestic violence might be occurring but their gut feelings alone are not acceptable evidence to intervene and have something done about it. The NMC's (2007) guidance on record keeping states that records should be factual and accurate; gut feeling may not be either of these, yet documenting this feeling in some format could draw attention to problems within a family. Equally, the NMC (2008) states that the nurse must act if he/she feels that someone is at risk of harm but again it can be argued that the health visitor must have factual information in order to instigate proceedings such as social service involvement. This reinforces the need for even more multi-agency working as discussions should occur between various agencies, who may also have information that could support any ongoing concerns. Women and children's needs can then be explored and help given as needed.

Safeguarding children

In looking at child protection, UNICEF (2008) refers to it as preventing and responding to violence, exploitation and abuse against children whilst HM Government (2006) sees it as part of safeguarding and promoting the welfare of children. It is about the activity undertaken to protect specific children who are suffering, or are at risk of suffering, significant harm. The government identified significant harm as the threshold that justifies compulsory intervention in family life, in the best interests of children. It also gives local authorities a duty to investigate and decide whether action is needed to safeguard or promote the welfare of a child; the term safeguarding children is therefore increasingly being used. Whilst the focus here is not on the types of abuse, it should be noted that abuse is a form of maltreatment of a child and this may include physical, emotional and sexual abuse or aspects of neglect (HM Government 2006). NICE (2009) reinforces the importance of taking child maltreatment seriously and encourages health professionals to take this into account when making clinical judgement.

The Department of Health (DoH 2001) stated that health visitors' knowledge enables them to identify children in need of protection and that they are well placed to work with vulnerable families. They are also very much aware of child protection procedures and are used to making referrals to various agencies. One of the biggest concerns for health visitors is safeguarding children and this continues to prove challenging for them primarily because of increasing workloads/caseloads, cost cutting (efficiency savings) exercises, including the cutting of health visiting posts which are being frozen, reduction in their numbers due to retirement and vacant posts not being filled.

Although some of the issues in health visiting are national ones, the way services are managed locally will vary from locality to locality and tie-in with the Department for Children, Schools and Families' (DCSF) notion that decisions about resourcing are best done locally (Community Practitioner 2009a). This was in response to the suggestion that the money to be used for safeguarding children should be ring-fenced. On the other hand, bodies such as the *Care Quality Commission* in reviewing the National Health Service's (NHS) involvement in Baby Peter's care recommended not just basic requirements such as communication and training but also a sufficient number of staff (Community Practitioner 2009b). However, it often takes the death of innocent children for agencies such as NHS Trusts and local authorities to employ more staff, and sometimes increase their pay rates. Equally, it is incomprehensible that some of the issues which arose in Victoria Climbie's case were repeated in other child death cases including that of Baby Peter.

In looking at Baby Peter's untimely death, it is frightening that he was seen numerous times prior to his death in August 2007 (Community Care 2009) and is a cause for concern. Laming (2009) proposed that the death of children who are known to be in danger of harm is a reproach on society. The media provided much insight into Baby Peter's mother's life highlighting obvious generational abuse within her family. Baby Peter's maternal grandmother had alcohol and drug problems. His mother was known to social services as a child and was placed in a boarding school; she only found out the true identify of her father 4 years ago; when 16 years old, she moved in with Peter's father, 17 years her senior, and the relationship soon broke up; and when Peter was about 3 months old, his mother formed a relationship with her partner who was involved in the abuse of Peter. Peter's stepfather had previously attacked his grandmother in an attempt to have her change her will and is a convicted rapist (raping a 2-year-old girl). The lodger, who is the partner's brother, was also involved in the assault on their grandmother and was living in Peter's mother's house with a 15-year-old girl (BBC News Channel 2009).

There were numerous indications that Baby Peter's mother herself was vulnerable from childhood into adulthood and when Baby Peter became a child protection concern, his mother's past social history should have shown up a catalogue of complex needs but there seems to have been a lack of background/historical information which would have alerted professionals much earlier of Baby Peter's vulnerability and likelihood of suffering significant harm. Perhaps initiatives such as ContactPoint (DCSF 2009), an online directory (to be rolled out shortly) for people working with children and young people, would have helped. It allows practitioners to see just who is working with the child so they can communicate as needed and hopefully safeguard the children.

HM Government (2006) believes that to understand significant harm one must consider the nature of harm, the impact on the child's health and development including within the context of their family and wider environment, aspects that may affect his/her development and parenting capacity. If we return to Baby Peter, some of these patterns are clearly visible but their recognition still did little to protect him. The fact that Baby Peter was seen frequently and still experienced significant harm is frightening and it is easy to see why many health visitors are concerned about their own caseload. One tool which I strongly believe is important and helpful in getting our points across is the *Framework for the Assessment of Children in Need* (HM Government 2006) which takes a holistic approach to identifying the child and family's needs. Hopefully this approach would ensure that all aspects of a child's care are covered during our assessment of families.

Health visitors have many vulnerable clients on their caseloads but thankfully despite the reporting of fatalities in child-abuse cases, to be abused to the extent of Victoria Climbie and Baby Peter is still quite rare. The government's way of ensuring the safety of children is by stating that they should have the opportunity to achieve their full potential and sets out five key outcomes. These are to stay safe, be healthy, enjoy and achieve, make a positive contribution and achieve economic well-being (DfES 2004; HM Government 2006). Failure to provide these needs could deny children some of their basic human rights and possibly lead to abuse and neglect, which was evident in Baby Peter's case. It

is, however, easy to reflect on this whole catalogue of warning signs, but what is more difficult is how health visitors and others are to move forward to prevent such reoccurrences.

Standard five of the National Service Framework for Children, Young People and Maternity Services (DoH 2004) is about safeguarding and promoting the welfare of children and young people thus preventing harm. It goes further in stating that the services provided should address the children's needs. However, whilst some improvements such as children's centres and the child health promotion programme can be seen, the issues regarding safeguarding children remain a challenge not just for health visitors but for anyone working with children.

Domestic abuse and safeguarding children may require health visitors to act as advocates for clients who sometimes experience difficulties in articulating themselves. Mind (2009) sees an advocate as someone who has the ability to listen and speak out during a person's times of need, and therefore as someone who supports and enables people to articulate their wishes. Whilst Mind is referring to people with mental health problems, the notion of advocacy remains important throughout nursing and should be embraced by all nurses. Maud & Hawley (2007) stated that advocacy is the active support of clients or causes, and when adopted it can greatly enhance the standard and quality of care. This takes us back to the principle of beneficence or non-maleficence which includes our duty to do good and avoid harm, our duty of care to our clients and the duty of advocacy, thus defending the rights of those who are unable to do so themselves – the weak and vulnerable (Thompson *et al.* 2000).

Health visitors act as advocates for their clients all the time and it is an important part of our safeguarding role. Equally, health visitors are increasingly having to work with clients who have mental health problems or learning disabilities, and Rumbold (2002) highlights just how important it is to ensure that they are supported and empowered despite possible lack of comprehension or capacity issues. However, Rumbold believes that such clients are often denied the opportunity to make essential choices about very basic care needs. Health visitors must therefore not forget the notion of autonomy as prescribed by the NMC (2008). Because ethics is concerned among other things with what is considered acceptable moral conduct in society (Rumbold 2002; Tschudin 2003), our nursing code of professional conduct (NMC 2008) informs us as to what is ethically acceptable to the NMC in order to maintain public safety. Nurses must ensure that they are always safeguarding vulnerable children and adults.

Workload issues

Resource allocation is a major issue in health visiting and has been widely acknowledged as such. McHale & Gallagher (2003) argued that nurses are in a position to review resources and raise concerns when necessary, whilst the NMC (2008) states that nurses should inform managers whenever patients are being put at risk. However, fear of reprisal may deter many health visitors from reporting concerns (Community Practitioner 2009c). Professional Officer Dave Mundy in the journal *Community Practitioner* (2009c) reports that managers are telling employees that they should not raise awareness of poor services as this could adversely influence commissioning of future services. It could however be seen as breech of the NMC's (2008) ethical code if they do not report factors that impact negatively on care.

It is easy to empathise with Alston (2009), a health visitor from London, who wrote that she has never felt so demoralised or inadequate in her work as she did at the time of writing her article. She highlighted many health visitors' views regarding the bureaucracy which governs how they work and the fact that it was getting in the way of client care. It was disheartening to read that RIO – the electronic record system which has been introduced in a number of NHS trusts to enhance communication, encourage information sharing and standardising practice – has apparently served to remove health visitors from their clinical work with clients. Indeed, at this stage it would appear as one of the more time-consuming devises introduced to the NHS in recent years. Equally, our quest to meet targets and show evidence of just how much work we are doing could ultimately affect the very quality of our work, as clinicians' time is constantly being taken up by such administrative work.

Rumbold (2002) however states that demands for resources are limitless and that it is unrealistic to expect all demands to be met, suggesting that injustice in health care is inevitable where there are insufficient resources to go around. Ultimately, there will be some winners and some losers. However, from a safeguarding perspective, losing may have serious consequences for a child. In contrast, Chadwick & Tadd (1992) argue that traditionally nurses tended to cope regardless of the situation which sometimes put them under extreme pressure affecting their health and even ultimately patient-care delivery. Their call for nurses to become political activists is in line with the principles of health visiting, proposing they influence policies affecting health. Informing management of the detrimental effects on clients if services are inappropriately designed is just one aspect (Amicus-CPHVA 2007). Adams & Craig (2009), in a study conducted by CPHVA and Durdle Davis, highlighted the stresses that health visitors are working under and showed that there are serious consequences if the early years in children are ignored, particularly at a time when the government itself is concerned about negative parenting outcomes.

In looking at beneficence, Rumbold (2002) suggested that there are two main strands in health care: the first is to always do what is best for the patients and the second is that patients should be put before one's own needs, thus placing patients' needs above organisational needs. For example, giving care to patients is of a higher priority than carrying out administrative tasks which have no direct effect on patient care. Equally, Rumbold's argument can be linked to Alston (2009) writing about the stress of administrative work within health visiting, and its impact on client care. However, with the current lack of resources the ethical dilemma for health is spelt out by Rumbold's proposing that at times the question might be not how to do good for the patients but how to do the least harm to them. Whether this would receive support from the general population is open to debate.

Donaldson *et al.* (2007) drew attention of the fact that despite the NHS' quest for quality improvements, the vision has still not been fully realised. They go even further in stating that the Laming Report (2003) following the death of Victoria Climbie pointed to gross failure in the organisation, management and leadership of key public services which were specifically designed to protect her from deliberate harm. Consequently, changes have occurred following Lord Laming's investigation, but it is interesting to note that in 2009 in response to the death of Baby Peter, Laming again pointed out that health visitors need to take immediate action to increase their numbers, professional competence and work confidence.

The Getting the Right Start: National Service Framework for Children Standard for Hospital Services (DoH 2003) mentions quality and its link to clinical governance and places safeguarding children under the clinical governance umbrella, giving responsibility not just to *Safeguarding Boards* but also NHS Trusts. Therefore, information should be reported to Trust Boards on a regular basis and designated persons are to be held accountable, including for any failings. Nevertheless, it is difficult to know just what information is being fed to Trust Boards as this is usually done by senior managers, not front-line staff. It is even more worrying that Laming's (2003) investigation found discrepancies between the perceptions of front-line staff, and that of managers.

Conclusion

One needs therefore to ask the question, 'is it ethical for those in a position of authority to knowingly let a service deteriorate in a way that negatively impacts on client care?' The answer is *no*. Organisations have a duty of care not just to the clients but also the staff. It is interesting that Laming (2003) highlighted management failures in the Victoria Climbie's case, claiming that they failed to understand or accept their responsibility for the quality, efficiency and effectiveness of services. It is clearly time for managers to appreciate that health visitors must act within the NMC's (2008) code of conduct and safeguarding guidelines. Managers should, on the other hand, facilitate this through support in dealing with issues such as domestic abuse and vulnerable families; it is not only their duty to do this but it is also ours, and, most importantly, it is our clients who deserve it.

Reflective scenario I

You visited the home of a family who has a toddler with a medical condition who was asked to attend GP practice for immunisation of the Swine flu vaccine because she has a chronic medical condition which puts her in the *at-risk group*. The parents are unsure of the information provided in the media and has asked your opinion. They want to know if you would vaccinate your own child with this vaccine.

1. Would you openly admit whether you would consent to the vaccine being given to your child?
2. Would you provide her with all the information in order to facilitate her making her own choices?
3. How else could you have responded to the situation?

Reflective scenario II

A female client has attended your child health promotion clinic and informed you (in confidence) that her partner assaulted her the previous night and her toddler was pushed during the altercation, but neither had any obvious injuries and your client said that it was her fault and it was the first time this had happened. You saw the child who was her *normal self* happy, playful and talkative.

1. Would you inform your client that you would speak to the doctor and ask him/her to look at the child?
2. Would you inform your client that you would need to report the incident to social services?
3. Would you ignore the situation but note that you would need to monitor the family?
4. Are there any other ways in which you would manage the above situations?

Give reasons for arriving at your decisions to follow a course of action within the context of your own individual principles and those of *respect*, autonomy, non-maleficence and beneficence.

References

Adams, C. & Craig, I. (2009) Health visitor cuts affecting vulnerable families. *Community Practitioner*, **80** (5), 14–17.

Alston, M. (2009) Save the safeguarders. *Community Practitioners*, **82** (8), 15.

Amicus-CPHVA (2007) *The Distinctive Contribution of Health Visiting to Public Health and Well Being* [Online]. Amicus-Community Practitioner and Health Visitors Association, London. Available at: http://www.amicustheunion.org/cphva/docs/Complete%20HV%20Statement%20docFinal1.doc. Accessed 13 August 2009.

Austin, H., Campion-Smith, C., Thomas, S. & Ward, W. (2008) Parents difficulties with decisions about childhood immunizations. *Community Practitioners*, **81** (10), 32–35.

BBC News Channel (2009) *Baby Peter: Trio Who Caused His Death* [Online]. BBC, England. Available at: http://news.bbc.co.uk/1/hi/england/7727641.stm. Accessed 15 October 2009.

Beauchamp, T.L. & Childress, J.F. (2001) *Principles of Biomedical Ethics*, 5th edn. Oxford, London.

Bedford, H. (2008) Immunisation: Ethics, effectiveness, organisation. In: *Community Public Health in Policy and Practice a Sourcebook* (ed. Cowley) 2nd edn. Bailliere Tindall and Elsevier, Edinburgh.

Buka, P. (2008) The older person and abuse. In: *Patients' Rights, Law and Ethics for Nurses a Practical Guide* (ed. P. Buka). Hodder Arnold, London.

Burnard, P. & Chapman, C. (2003) *Professional and Ethical Issues in Nursing*, 3rd edn. Bailliere Tindall, Edinburgh.

Chadwick, R. & Tadd, W. (1992) *Ethics and Nursing Practice a Case Study Approach*. MacMillan, Houndsmills.

Community Care (2009) *Baby Peter Case in Haringey* [online]. Community Care, London. Available at: http://www.communitycare.co.uk/Articles/2009/08/11/109961/baby-peter-case-in-haringey.html. Accessed 16 August 2009.

Community Practitioner (2009a) No ring-fenced money for safeguarding. *Community Practitioner*, **82** (6), 4.

Community Practitioner (2009b) CQC outlines baby P trust failings. *Community Practitioner*, **82** (6), 5.

Community Practitioner (2009c) 'Too scared' to blow the whistle. *Community Practitioner*, **82** (6), 5.

DCSF (2009) *The Protection of Children in England: Action Plan the Government's Response to Lord Laming*. Crown, Department for Children, Schools and Families, London.

DfES (2004) *Every Child Matters: Change for Children*. Crown, Department for Education and Skills, London.

DoH (2000) *Domestic Violence: A Resource Pack for Healthcare Professionals*. Department of Health, London.

DoH (2001) *The Health Visitor and School Nurse Development Programme: Health Visitor Practice Development Resource Pack*. Department of Health, London.

DoH (2003) *Getting the Right Start: National Service Framework for Children Standard for Hospital Services*. Crown, Department of Health, London.

DoH (2004) *National Service Framework for Children, Young People and Maternity Services*. Crown, Department of Health, London.

DoH (2005) *Responding to Domestic Abuse: A Handbook for Professionals*. Crown, Department of Health, London.

DoH (2006) *Immunisation against Infectious Diseases*. Crown, Department of Health, London.

Donaldson, L., Halligan, A. & Wall, D. (2007) Clinical governance: Improving the child's experience of healthcare. In: *Ethical, Legal and Social Aspects of Child Healthcare*. Elsevier, Edinburgh.

Edwards, S.D. (1996) *Nursing Ethics a Principle-Based Approach*. Macmillan, Houndsmils.

Hawley, G. (2007) Start at 'go'. In: *Ethics in Clinical Practice: An Interprofessional Approach* (ed. G. Hawley). Pearson, Essex.

HM Government (2006) *Working Together to Safeguard Children: A Guide to Interagency Working to Safeguard and Promote the Welfare of Children*. Crown, London.

Jones, L. & Cribb, A. (1997) Ethical issues in health promotion. In: *Promoting Health: Knowledge and Practice* (eds J. Katz & A. Peberdy). Macmillan and Open University, London.

Laming, L. (2003) *The Victoria Climbie Enquiry Summary and Recommendations*. Crown, London.

Laming, L. (2009) *The Protection of Children in England: A Progress Report*. Her Majesty's Stationary Office, London.

Madsen, K.M., Anders, H., Vestergaard, M., Schendel, D., Wohlfahrt, J., Thorsen, P., Olsen, J. & Melbye, M. (2002) A population-based study of measles, mumps, and rubella vaccination and autism. *The New England Journal of Medicine*, **347** (19), 1477–1482.

Maud, P. & Hawley, G. (2007) Clients' and patients' rights and protecting the vulnerable. In: *Ethics in Clinical Practice: An Interprofessional Approach* (ed. G. Hawley). Pearson, Essex.

McHale, J. & Gallagher, A. (2003) *Nursing and Human Rights*. Butterworth Heinemann, London.

Metropolitan Police (2004) *'Getting away with it': A Strategic Overview of Domestic Violence Sexual Assault and 'Serious' Incident Analysis*. Metropolitan Police, London.

Mezey, G.C. & Bewley, S. (1997) Domestic violence and pregnancy. *British Medical Journal*, **314** (7090), 1295.

Mind (2009) *Mind Guide to Advocacy* [online]. Mind, England. Available at: http://www.mind.org.uk/ help/rights_and_legislation/mind_guide_to_advo cacy. Accessed 6 August 2009.

NHSII (2009) *What Is Herd Immunity?* [online]. National Health Service Immunisation Information, Scotland. Available at: http://www.immunisation.nhs.uk/ About_Immunisation/Science/What_is_herd_immu nity. Accessed 19 August 2009.

NICE (2009) *Quick Reference Guide: When to Suspect Child Maltreatment*. National Institute for Health and Clinical Excellence, London.

NMC (2007) *Record Keeping Advice Sheet*. Nursing and Midwifery Council, London.

NMC (2008) *The Code Standards of Conduct, Performance and Ethics for Nurses and Midwives*. Nursing and Midwifery Council, London.

OPSI (1989) *Children Act 1989*. Crown, Office of Public Sector Information, London.

Peltola, H., Patja, A., Leinikki, P., Valle, M., Davidkin, I., & Paunio, M. (1998) 'No evidence for MMR vaccine-associated inflammatory bowel disease or autism in a 14-year prospective study'. *Lancet*, **351**, 1327–1328.

Polterak, M., Leach, M. & Fairhead, J. (2004) MMR "Choices." In: *Understanding Public Engagement with Vaccination Science and Delivery*. Institute of Development Study, Brighton.

RCN (2000) *Domestic Violence Guidance for Nurses*. Royal College of Nursing, London.

Rumbold, G. (2002) *Ethics in Nursing Practice*, 3rd edn. Bailliere Tindall, London.

Stewart, D.E. (1994) Incidence of postpartum abuse in women with a history of abuse during pregnancy. *Canadian Medical Association Journal*, **151** (11), 1601–1604.

Taylor, B., Miller, E., Farrington, C.P., Petropoulos, M., Favot-Mayaud, I., Li, J. & Waight, P.A. (1999) Autism and measles, mumps and rubella vaccine: no epidemiological evidence for causal association. *The Lancet*, 353, 2026–2029 [online]. Available at: http://www. freenetpages.co.uk/hp/gingernut/lancet/Brent%20 Taylor%20June%201999.pdf

Thompson, I.E., Melia, K.M. & Boyd, K.M. (2000) Ethics in our everyday life and decision making. In: *Nursing Ethics* (eds. I.E. Thompson, K.M. Melia, & K.M. Boyd), 4th edn. Churchill Livingstone, Edinburgh.

Tschudin, V. (2003) *Ethics in Nursing: The Caring Relationship*. Butterworth-Heinemann, Edinburgh.

UNICEF (2008) *Child Protection Information Sheet: What Is Child Protection* [online]. United Nations Children's Fund, New York. Available at: http://www.unicef. org/protection/files/What_is_Child_Protection.pdf. Accessed 15 August 2009.

Wakefield, A.J., Murch, S.H., Anthony, A., Linnell, A., Casson, D.M., Malik, M., Berelowitz, M., Dhillon, A.P.,

Thomson, M.A., Harvey, A., Valentine, A., Davies, S.E., Walker-Smith, J.A. (1998) Ileal-lymphoid-nodular hyperplasia, non-specific colitis, and pervasive developmental disorder in children. *Lancet*, **351** (9103), 637–641.

Women's Aid (2009) *Domestic Violence Frequently Asked Questions Factsheet* [online]. Women's Aid, Bristol. Available at: www.womensaid.org.uk. Accessed 20 July 2009.

Worms, J. (2004) *Domestic violence and health: an audit of PCT practice in the Thames Valley* [online] Available at: http://www.thamesvalleypartnership. org/down loads/dvhaudit.pdf. Accessed 2 February 2009.

Suggested further readings

Powell, C. (2007) *Safeguarding Children and Young People: A Guide for Nurses and Midwives*. Open University Press, Berkshire.

This book although predominantly for nurses and midwives can be used by other professionals working with children and young people and focuses on education, practice and research. It is easy to read and each chapter provides learning outcomes for the reader to achieve as well as points for reflection.

Willson, K. & James, A. (2007) *The Child Protection Handbook*, 3rd edn. Bailliere Tindall/Elsevier, Edinburgh.

This book provides a multi-agency approach which is essential in child protection and is divided into three sections comprising understanding child protection, managing the process and intervention.

Sharpen, J. (2009) *Improving Safety, Reducing Harm: Children, Young People and Domestic Violence. A Practical Toolkit for Front-Line Practitioners*. DH, London.

This toolkit covers a range of issues relating to children and young people in particular domestic violence, but also other areas such as child protection, sexual abuse, bullying and risk assessment and is for front-line professionals.

Web sites

Home Office – Domestic violence. Available at: http:// www.homeoffice.gov.uk/crime-victims/reducing-crime/domestic-violence/

Provides information on other web sites/organisations relating to domestic violence including England, Scotland, Northern Ireland and Wales.

http://www.hpa.org.uk/

Provides information on immunisation including statistical evidence.

Local Safeguarding Children Board Haringey (2009) *Serious case review: baby Peter executive summary.*

Available at: http://www.haringeylscb.org/executive_summary_peter_final.pdf

This serious case review followed the death of Baby Peter and investigated the involvement of organisations and professionals with Peter and his family. It focused on lessons learnt and how agencies worked together. It is suitable reading for all professionals working with children.

6 Promoting the Health of School-Aged Children: An Ethical Perspective

Gill Coverdale

Introduction

There is an accepted presumption that the state has a responsibility towards reducing ill health and inequalities by reducing the causes of ill health, protecting and promoting the health of children and vulnerable people, helping people avoid unhealthy behaviours and ensuring healthy choices are the easiest choices. However, within this governmental challenge it is also important that professionals who work within government guidelines should not attempt to use coercion as a means to help people lead healthy lives and should work effectively with minimal intrusion on personal lifestyle choices. Therein lies a direct dichotomy, and this is made even more complex and challenging for health-promotion professionals working with children and young people of school age. Children start school at the beginning of the academic year in which they will be 5 years old – for some children this may be a day after their 4th birthday! This in itself poses challenges. Young people at present can leave school at 16 years of age but this is changing to 18 (Department for Education and Skills (DfES 2006)), though many young people do choose to stay on beyond the age of 16 in 6th form or further education college for a further 2 years. It is important to note that the majority of young people on leaving school are healthy, well informed about what a healthy lifestyle is and most do not or have not required any *clinical nursing* input. What they have had exposure to is health-promotion input to help them achieve this state of health and emotional well-being. This in itself contributes to the challenge faced by, among others, school nurses as one of the unique health professionals working in this arena.

The government's *Change for Children Programme: Every Child Matters* (Department of Health (DoH/DfES 2006)) stresses the magnitude of every child having the opportunity to fulfil their potential through being healthy, staying safe, enjoying and achieving, making a positive contribution and achieving economic well-being. School nurses working within this health-promotion role are faced with the dichotomy of ensuring that information is given at the appropriate time and in the correct manner and encourages action without it being perceived as coercion. This chapter will present some detailed debate and discussion on the challenges posed and how they are managed on a daily basis by those school nurses working with this predominantly *well* population group.

Ethical and Philosophical Aspects of Nursing Children, First Edition. Edited by Gosia M. Brykczyńska and Joan Simons.
© 2011 Blackwell Publishing Ltd. Published 2011 by Blackwell Publishing Ltd.

What is school nursing?

Many school nurses are specialist graduate nurses who are registered as Specialist Community Public Health Nurses (SCPHN) with the Nursing and Midwifery Council (NMC) on Part 1 and Part 3 of the register which

> ... recognises those nurses who work with populations and whose role is primarily public health focused – including the responsibility to work with both individuals and a population, which may mean taking decisions on behalf of a community or population without having direct contact with every individual in that community.
>
> (NMC 2004:4)

This provides a different emphasis to the role of the general nurse in that the SCPHN school nurse not only works with individuals but also a community or population group who are clients rather than patients. SCPHN provide care along the continuum of public health practice (DoH 2006a) working from the individual level to the population group level, with children and young people, laying down the foundations of good health, changing unhealthy lifestyles, improving knowledge or attitudes, empowering or influencing policy and developing community capacity (Elliott *et al.* 2004). The government document *Looking for a School Nurse* (DoH 2006a) advised that school nurses are in the ideal position to meet the health needs of the school age population, both within school and in the wider community, being the only health professional to uniquely straddle the health, social and educational arenas. This is supported by past and present government policy and contemporary literature (DoH 1999a, b, 2004a, b, c, 2006a, b, 2009; Lightfoot & Bines 2000; Wainwright *et al.* 2000; Madge & Franklin 2003; DfES/DoH 2004; Coverdale 2006; DoH, Department for Children, Schools and Families (DoH/DCSF 2007, 2008, 2009a, b).

The Children's National Service Framework (DoH 2004a) encourages the development of healthy lifestyles and the promotion of physical, emotional and mental well-being in tackling health inequalities. How school nurses do this is open to scrutiny and diversity. Other *well* population groups (adults, new Mum's, the elderly) can *choose* to engage in professional help and advice if they are not a captive audience in hospital or do not require care after illness or medical intervention. Yet, children and young people in school are arguably a captive audience, and the relationship they have with the health professional – school nurse, practice nurse, health visitor or GP – often shapes how they will access health services and value health and well-being as adults and often as parents themselves. There are also many children and young people who are not in school for various reasons and school nurses also have a joint responsibility for this vulnerable group. School nurses therefore have a responsibility to be fit for professional standing through adherence to the NMC code of professional conduct, performance and ethics (NMC 2008) and work to the NMC standards set for SCPHN (NMC 2004) which are explicitly to:

- Promote and protect health and well-being
- Reduce risky behaviours and health inequalities
- Prevent disease
- Assess and monitor the health of communities and populations to identify those at risk and those with health problems
- Assess priorities for action

The principles for practice are centred on equity, collaboration and participation with others to strengthen community action (Turton *et al.* 2000; Costello & Haggart 2003). As more and more concerns come to light about young people (Chief Medical Officer (CMO 2007)), the need for preventative action within this population group is increased, and the need for young people to engage in healthy lifestyles becomes apparent. An Essence of Care Benchmark on Promoting Health has been developed (DoH 2006b) to ensure quality is driven into service provision and provides school nurses with a framework for delivering effective and high quality health-promoting services. However, it is important to note that the face of services is changing, with young people acting as consumers and thus the power relationship between the consumers and the health professionals is also changing (Costello & Haggart 2003; Richman 2003). The advent of the internet and other information sources mean the health professional is no longer solely responsible for providing expert advice and support, and that children and young people are adept at seeking information in other places such as the internet.

The work of school nurses is population based and prevention focused and is underpinned by the ten key principles of public health practice (NMC 2004) which are grouped into four domains:

- Search for health needs
- Stimulation of awareness of health needs
- Influence on policies affecting health
- Facilitation of health-enhancing activities

The aim is to make services more responsive to what young people and their parents want; balancing greater opportunities and support while promoting young people's responsibilities; making services for young people more integrated, efficient and effective; and improving outcomes for all young people, while narrowing the gap between those who do well and those who do not. This requires involving a wide range of organisations from the voluntary, community and private sectors in order to increase choice, whilst securing the best outcomes and building on the best of what is currently provided. What is accepted is that holistic health and well-being must be achieved by the majority in the pursuit and promotion of a healthy future population. The most common aspects of the school nurse role that require careful exploration of the ethical challenges faced are in the provision of health promotion, vaccines, contraception and sexual health services and *drop in* services. These challenges will be explored within the chapter.

Health promotion and ethics

There are many threats to the development of happy, healthy children and young people. This may come from their own behavioural choices but also in the choices their parents/carers make. The CMO Annual report (CMO 2007) discussed the following key concerns:

- Alcohol use is increasing: consumption by increasingly younger children and young people, consumption of large amounts of alcohol in single sessions and increasing levels of consumption amongst girls.

- Illegal drugs are widely available and children and young people are increasingly exposed to them. Young people such as those who are truants, young offenders, children in care and homeless young people are at particular risk for problem drug use. Drug misuse is linked with other social problems such as unemployment and homelessness and cannot be seen in isolation.

Emotional health and psychological well-being have also been identified as priority areas in the Government's *Change for Children Programme: Every Child Matters* (DoH/DCSF 2006) and *National Service Framework for Children, Young People and Maternity Services* (DoH 2004a). *Choosing Health*, the Public Health White Paper (DoH 2004b), sets out priorities for action which have close links to low self-esteem and mental ill health. These include reducing obesity, drug and alcohol misuse and teenage pregnancy. The Public Service Agreement target for Child and Adolescent Mental Health Services (CAMHS) has been set to improve life outcomes for children with mental health problems, by ensuring that all those who need them have access to comprehensive CAMHS and comprehensive mental health and emotional well-being promotion (Department of Children's Schools and Families (DCSF 2008)).

School nurses do help children develop self-confidence, manage stress and solve problems to cope with vulnerable periods during transitions between primary and secondary schools and exams through various means on an individual and community basis. This may include not only providing information, educating, and empowering and enabling good health choices, but also advocating politically to help children and young people fulfil their health potential. However, it is argued that telling people how they should live is a moral and political process and this is a highly ethical issue; do we have a right to tell people especially young people how to live their lives? Buchanan (2006) believes that educating people about their health should be done through public forums (such as Personal, Social and Health Education [PSHE]), which provide everyone with the same knowledge and information, which he argues addresses the inequity in power distribution. The health professional is often seen as the powerful body that delivers the message yet it is accepted that health professionals need to give power to the public if they are to lead a healthy life. Laverack & Labonte (2000) also discusses the role power plays in health promotion and public health and argues that clients who have more power will gain more control over their lives.

Tones & Green (2004:3) promote the ideal that that empowerment is a reciprocal arrangement between individuals and the health professional, but emphasise that the environment must be 'conducive to their making empowered choices'. They suggest that empowerment requires voluntarism to succeed rather than coercion – the client acquiring control over their involvement in the activity through information, consultation and joint planning which leads to a high degree of empowerment. Rollnick *et al.* (1992), however, urge caution with the understanding of empowerment and argue that it is a jargon word well used in practice but question whether it is fully understood. He suggests that it needs to be seen as a liberating equalising of power and basic rights. Professionals need to be reminded that one cannot empower someone but one can enable clients to take control over their lives, the health professional acting as a catalyst for action (Rollnick *et al.* 1992). How much option for consultation and joint planning is there for children and young people is very much down to school nurses and their multi-disciplinary colleagues. The key aim is to empower children and young people with the possession of skills or competencies which enable them to exert control over their own lives, address environmental enhancing or inhibiting factors and in turn increase self-belief and self-worth (Tones 1993).

The ideologies of the empowerment model of health promotion according to Tones & Green (2004) are beneficence (i.e. helping people benefit) and non-maleficence (i.e. doing no harm). According the World Health Organisation (WHO), equity and empowerment are the twin pillars of health promotion along with voluntarism and social justice (WHO 1991). Giddens (1989, cited in Tones & Green (2004)) argues that 'the ideology of power' serves to legitimise the different power which groups hold. It is difficult to see how this can be done effectively with children and young people without first empowering parents and carers who may and often do require health-promoting advice. The challenge is to provide this without eroding confidence,

capability and capacity, which in turn de-powers and can 'destroy the potential of people' (Illich 1976:42, cited in Tones & Green 2004).

Advocacy is also a key concept within health promotion, and Campbell (2004:43) offers an all encompassing definition: any effort to influence policy and decision making, fight for social change, transform public perception and attitudes, mobilise human resources and modify behaviour and mobility. Yet, this may lead to ethical problems when the school nurse may advocate a particular action in a client (such as accepting a vaccine or utilising contraception) at the same time as empowering them to make their own decisions. Campbell (2004) suggests that the key is in developing the capacity in the client to undertake advocating activities. The Health Action Model (Tones & Green 2004) is a useful structured framework which guides health-promotion practitioners to address the concept of advocacy and empowerment through two strategies: one is to raise client's critical consciousness of issues and the second to create healthy public policy. The model also reminds us of the wide-ranging influences on health-related behaviours, such as the environment, lifestyle, beliefs, values, motivation and the normative pressure on individuals to conform. Knowledge of the beliefs, values and attitudes of those receiving the health promotion is vital, along with awareness of the concepts of self-belief, self-esteem, perception of perceived vulnerability, health locus of control, motivation and the capacity to change (Downie *et al.* 1996). The most commonly utilised health-promotion models which are used by school nurses are the Health Belief Model (Becker 1974), the Health Action Model (Tones & Green 2004); the Self-Efficacy Model (Bandura 1977); the Stages of Change Model (Prochaska & Diclemente 1984) and the Theory of Reasoned Action (Ajzen & Fishbein 1980), and all provide a framework for effective health promotion.

Professional versus personal values

The terms *values* and *ethics* are often used interchangeably along with *morals* and *judgements*. Beauchamp & Childress (2009:5) argue that ethics is a general term referring to both morality and ethical theory. Burnard & Kendrick (1998) argue that the term *ethics* is ambiguous. Professionals are influenced by their personal values and these have the potential to impact upon the decisions and judgements they make on a daily basis (Peate 2007). There are several key influencers on our ability to make a professional decision: religion, culture, the law, personal experience and values, social convention and the professional code of conduct to name a few. Often the health professional is faced with an ethical issue that brings into conflict their personal and professional values. A good example of this is when school nurses may be challenged in the provision of sexual health and contraceptive services to young people and none more challenging than being faced with a 13-year-old requesting contraceptive advice. Personally, one may believe that providing contraceptives to a 13-year-old is morally wrong yet it is vital that other aspects are taken into account when deciding on the outcome. This example will be utilised to explore the four principles of healthcare ethics in helping professionals achieve the correct balance in relation to client/patient rights and professional responsibilities. Conflict only occurs when the actions go against the discussion below or indeed when there is harm done.

Respect for autonomy

Autonomy is defined as the 'capacity to think, decide and act on the basis of such thought and decision … freely and independently without let or hindrance' (Gillon 1985:6). The key question here then is whether or not the young person is capable of making his/her own decision and is not being coerced into a sexual relationship. The best way to protect young people who are sexually active is to reaffirm their rights to access confidential sexual health services while empowering and supporting professionals to make an effective assessment as to whether they are at risk of harm or exploitation (Collyer & Whitehead 2008). Being able to offer confidentiality except in exceptional circumstances is crucial in encouraging the development of a relationship of trust, where young people are able to talk freely and honestly about their situation; it allows appropriate steps to be taken to safeguard their well-

being. However, if the nurse did believe the young person to be at risk of abuse it would require referral to social services (Collyer & Whitehead 2008).

Key words that are used with reference to autonomy are: independence, individuality, self-choice and freedom of will (Cuthbert & Quallington 2008). Harris (1985) argues that defects in the young person's control, reasoning, information and stability will limit the individual's ability to remain autonomous. The school nurse will need to sensitively explore whether the young person is making an autonomous request and has made an informed and correct decision. It is important that they are not attempting to please someone else or are adversely influenced by peer group norm. The NMC (2008) states that nurses will make the care of patients their first concern, treating them as individuals and respecting their dignity. Arguably, a 13-year-old should be treated with respect as an individual, but it is also important that the school nurse is confident that the young person understands the information they are being given and the disadvantages and advantages of that course of action. It is always good practice to encourage the young person to discuss the actions with a parent to ensure support is there if necessary, but it is not required according to the Fraser law (House of Lords 1986), which will be discussed later in the chapter.

Beneficence

Beneficence is the duty to *do good* and avoid doing harm to others, either physically or psychologically (Benbow & Jordan 2009), and requires the school nurse to act in the best interests of the client/patient. Young people are provided with sex education in school to ensure they do have information and know where to access sexual health and relationship advice and support. It is carried out within a comprehensive framework of legislation and professional guidance and school nurses are also guided by legislation and the professional infrastructure; however, it is a role which remains fraught with professional and ethical dilemmas (Collyer & Whitehead 2008). A recent report by the National Children's Bureau showed that school nurses frequently give advice, condoms, pregnancy tests and morning-after pills to children without their parents being informed (Emmerson 2008). The argument from this perspective then is whether providing the contraception to the young person is *doing good*. Beauchamp & Childress (2009) purport that beneficence is an obligation to ensure that the other person receives help to achieve their legitimate interest or to act in a way that will positively benefit someone else. It can also be seen as an act of kindness. In this case, the beneficence is about preventing unintended pregnancy and it may be about reducing the risk of Sexually Transmitted Diseases which has arguably got to be a good thing, whether or not we feel it is a good thing for a 13-year-old to be engaged in the risky activity in the first place. However, what is important is ensuring that *truthful* information, presented in a way it can be understood (NMC 2008), is vital if the young person is to acknowledge the risks associated with certain contraceptives.

Non-maleficence

The NMC *Code* (2008) says the nurse may *do no harm*, which is difficult in some nursing situations. The key question in this example is whether by refusing to provide contraception the nurse would be doing more harm, and that could include psychological harm. If there is doubt that the young person understands the information being given about the contraception then it may be necessary to refuse the request and encourage parent attendance. This in itself causes problems as the young person may refuse and will be at risk of becoming pregnant or if the young person received such advice or treatment their physical or mental health was likely to suffer. Can this action be justified? It may be argued that it is not justified but the legal position according to Gillick (House of Lords 1986) is that any young person under 16 must be able to understand the information and its impact, and if they have sufficient maturity and judgement to enable them to fully understand what is proposed. The NMC *Code* (2008) states that nurses must provide a safe standard of care that avoids or minimises risk. In this case, risk of pregnancy, or worse, risk of complications? This puts the school nurse often in a challenging situation and often in moral conflict.

Justice

This relates to whether the action can be seen as fair, equitable and appropriate. An important element of this principle is *Respect for the Law*. School nurses must act within legal boundaries at all times and the provision of sexual health services is one which is more complex and less clear cut. Home Office guidance published in 2004 on the Sexual Offences Act 2003 stated that 'although the age of consent remains at 16, the law is not intended to prosecute mutually agreed sexual activity between two young people of a similar age, unless it involves abuse or exploitation' (Home Office 2004).

However, misinterpretation of the Sexual Offences Act and of the context of recommendations made by the Bichard Inquiry (The Stationery Office 2004) have resulted in a situation where the confidentiality of younger people is being undermined (Collyer & Whitehead 2008). The Bichard Inquiry made two recommendations concerning how social services handled allegations of underage sexual activity. It called on the government to reaffirm the guidance in *Working Together to Safeguard Children* (HM Government 2006) on handling allegations of criminal activity and, in particular, recommended that national guidance be produced to inform the decision as to whether or not to notify the police (The Stationery Office 2004).

School nurses must be very clear about their understanding of legal issues as well as compliance with the professional code of conduct when providing contraceptive and sexual health services. It is also important to ensure safety and evidence-based practice, as well as ensuring that such confidential advice and treatment is only given to children with decision-making capacity. School nurses must also ensure that their actions cannot be seen as encouraging sexual activity with a child under 16 which is unlawful (Griffith 2008).

The Sexual Offences Act 2003, Section 14(3) does provide a school nurse with a defence against aiding, abetting or counselling such an offence if the purpose is to

- Protect the child from sexually transmitted infection;
- Protect the physical safety of the child;
- Protect the child from becoming pregnant'

- Promote the child's emotional well-being by the giving of advice unless the purpose is to obtain sexual gratification or to cause or encourage the relevant sexual act.

This defence allows school nurses to be free from prosecution (Griffith 2008).

Confidentiality

The fundamental part of the relationship between the nurse and the patient/client is trust and the *duty of confidence* that any information given by a patient should not be passed on without consent (Caulfield 2005). Young people are entitled to the same rights for confidentiality as adults. Health professionals such as school nurses will be aware of their own professional codes of conduct not to disclose information about individual patients without their consent except in exceptional circumstances. Even if the young person is not considered sufficiently mature to consent to contraceptive treatment, the consultation itself can remain confidential unless there are child-protection concerns (Collyer & Whitehead 2008). The Teenage Pregnancy Unit's guidance on the provision of effective sexual health services reaffirms that the duty of confidentiality to young people is the same as for older patients (Teenage Pregnancy Unit 2000).

The Sexual Offences Act 2003 stated that 'Young people, including those under 13, will continue to have the right to confidential advice on contraception, condoms, pregnancy and abortion' (Home Office 2004). A school nurse who considers a child to be Gillick competent owes that child a duty of care. However, within school nursing services the NMC *Code* (NMC 2008), which has endorsed Caulfield's statement of respecting people's right to confidentiality, is often in conflict as it is necessary always to inform young people that their right to confidentiality can be breached if the nurse believes that they are at risk of harm or that they are at risk of harming someone else. There is no right to notify the parents against the wishes of the child unless it can be justified by one of the exceptions to the duty of confidence (R (on the application of Axon) v Secretary of State for Health [2006]). The need for a duty of confidence is seen as crucial to a child's treatment. If a duty of confidentiality was not

imposed, this 'would probably or might well deter young people from seeking advice and treatment' (R (on the application of Axon) v Secretary of State for Health [2006] per Justice Silber at 46 cited in Griffith 2008). The duty of confidence also extends to access to health records. Disclosure of a Gillick competent child's health record cannot occur without the consent of the child (*Data Protection Act* (HM Government 1998)).

School nurses offer confidential *drop in* services to school children which may or may not be in the school environment. These are open for children and young people and often parents/carers and teachers to access health and social care advice on an ad hoc basis. Much of the advice is physical, sexual or mental health related and a listening ear is important. Confidentiality is made explicit through poster or other types of information advertising the service. Sometimes leaflets may be given or children and young people are signposted to other services. It is explained that the school nurse will maintain confidentiality at all times *unless* they are at risk of harm or that they are at risk of harming someone else. This is made very clear so that if a child or young person discloses abuse or behaviour that the school nurse deems significantly harmful, the child knows the school nurse cannot keep it confidential and it will require sharing. It is always important to ensure that children and young people are informed about why and how information may be shared by those providing the care (NMC 2008).

Sharing information

The NMC guidance on disclosing information (NMC 2007) states that disclosure of information can only happen in exceptional circumstances and should only be done to protect individuals, groups or society as a whole from significant harm, such as child abuse, drug trafficking or serious crime. In school nursing work, this is more likely to be child abuse but could be drug trafficking or even crime.

Informed consent

In his article on Consent and Children, Richard Griffith (2008) states that Kennedy & Grubb (1998) argue that children pass through three developmental stages on their journey to becoming an autonomous adult:

1. The child of tender years – children of tender years will not have the decision-making capacity to give or withhold consent to treatment and the school nurse will rely on a person with parental responsibility to give consent on behalf of the child.
2. The Gillick competent child – discussed above and below.
3. Young people 16 and 17 years of age who are able to consent to treatment as if they 'were of full age' (Family Law Reform Act (HM Government 1969), Section 8; Mental Capacity Act (HM Government 2005), Section 1).

The NMC *Code* (2008) states that a nurse must ensure the patient/client has given consent before treatment or care. It is also the nurse's professional duty to provide sufficient information to allow the patient/client to make an informed decision. Consent can be verbal, written or implied within competent adult services, but children's services are much more complex. When a young person is being provided with health care, the law on consent is different to that of an adult. It is clear that a 16- and 17-year-old are able to give consent to treatment under the Family Law Reform Act (HM Government 1979). However, under 16 years of age there are considerations to be made. If the young person has sufficient understanding and intelligence to enable them to understand the proposed treatment or investigation, they are felt to have the capacity and deemed competent to consent (DoH 2001) and are said to be *Gillick competent*. Mrs Gillick was a mother who raised stringent objections at her teenage daughter receiving sexual health advice without her knowledge and the case became a landmark for assessing young people's ability to consent to treatment independently of their parents/carers. This is sometimes called Fraser competent after the judge who heard the case between Mrs Gillick and West Norfolk and Wisbech Area Health Authority (House of Lords 1986). Lord Fraser set out guidance to protect health professionals from prosecution when giving contraceptive advice and treatment. The Fraser guidelines state that such advice and treatment are

clinically indicated and therefore lawful where the school nurse is satisfied that:

- The child understood the advice.
- They could not persuade the child to tell or allow them to tell the parents.
- The child was likely to have sexual intercourse with or without contraceptive treatment.
- Unless the child received such advice or treatment, their physical or mental health was likely to suffer.
- The child's best interests required such advice or treatment without the knowledge or consent of the parents.

It is recommended that school nurses continue to follow Lord Fraser's guidance and record as evidence that the purpose of the advice and treatment was clinical and not to obtain sexual gratification or to cause or encourage the relevant sexual activity (Griffith 2008).

Most vaccine programmes given in the school setting by school nurses seek consent from parents via consent forms that are sent to parents beforehand with a range of questions that seek information about past medical history, allergies and previous vaccinations. Parents are given the option to opt their children in or out of the vaccination programme. In the secondary school setting, if the form is not returned the young person can consent at school on the day if the nurse is satisfied that they have sufficient understanding and intelligence to enable them to understand the proposed treatment. However, the Human Papillomavirus infection (HPV) vaccine was a school-based vaccine that had required full parental consent and was not allowing young people to consent independently due to the prolonged duration of the vaccination programme (three doses over 6 months). The HPV vaccination programme was introduced at the beginning of the 2008/2009 school year in order to reduce a female's risk of cervical cancer in the future (Green & Catlow 2009). It has been successful at immunising 12–13-year-old girls in the UK and many of these vaccines have been given by school nurses in the school setting. As the most common viral infection in sexually active men and women, persistent infection with a high-risk type of HPV can cause abnormalities of the cervix, which, if left undetected and untreated, can lead to cervical cancer. The vaccine (Cervarix) used for the national immunisation programme protects against HPV types 16 and 18. Three doses of HPV vaccine are given over a period of 6 months. The vaccine has been found to be well tolerated in extensive clinical studies (Paavonen *et al.* 2007; MHRA 2009).

Interestingly recent research (Racktoo & Coverdale 2009) found that participants who had received the vaccine reported that they had not had enough information about the vaccination programme and therefore had experienced fear and anxiety especially about painful injections and about the safety record of the vaccine and possible long-term side effects. Written information had been given and has an important role to play, but the authors felt that more is needed in the context of easily accessible and user-friendly information. In this research, the participants also reported an overall positive response from their parents and that the majority of parents had encouraged uptake of the vaccine. Parents had influenced many of the

participants in their decision to be vaccinated. Therefore, accessible and user-friendly information is important for parents as well as for young people (Sturm *et al.* 2005).

Conclusion

This chapter has explored some of the current ethical and moral complexities faced by health professionals when dealing with predominantly well children and young people. It has shown that delivering health-promotion services to this age group is not without its challenges. Being clear about professional role boundaries and legal constraints is vital in the delivery of school nursing services which need to ensure that the *Every Child Matters* outcomes for children and young people are reflected in all of their work, making services more responsive to what young people and their parents want and ensuring that children and young people's health and well-being is safeguarded and promoted.

Reflective scenario

Ginny is 14 and has been persuaded into your *drop in* service at school by her friends. She is hostile and non-communicative. Her best friend informs you that she has heard that Ginny was at a party at the weekend where she got drunk and woke up in bed with a bloke. She thinks she may have had unprotected intercourse.

- What concerns would you have for Ginny?
- How might you approach Ginny given her hostility?
- What challenges lie ahead in terms of your ethical responsibility towards Ginny?

References

Ajzen, I. & Fishbein, E. (1980) *Understanding Attitudes and Predicting Social Behaviour*. Prentice Hall, Englewood Cliffs.

Bandura, A. (1977) *Self Efficacy Towards a Unifying Theory of Behaviour Change. Psychological Review*, **64** (2), 191–225.

Becker, M.H. (1974) *The Health Belief Model and Personal Health Behaviour*. Charles B Slack, Thorofare, New Jersey.

Benbow, W. & Jordan, G. (2009) *A Handbook for Student Nurses*. Reflect Press, Devon.

Beauchamp, T.L. & Childress, J.F. (2009) *Principles of Biomedical Ethics*, 6th edn. Oxford University Press, Oxford.

Buchanan, D.R. (2006) A new ethic for health promotion: Reflections on a philosophy of health education for

the 21st century. *Health Education and Behaviour*, **33** (3), 290–304.

Burnard, P. & Kendrick, K. (1998) *Ethical Counselling: A Workbook for Nurses*. Edward Arnold, London.

Campbell, S. (2004) Advocating Immunisations. *Primary Health Care*, **14** (7), 43–49.

Caulfield, H. (2005) *Vital Notes for Nurses: Accountability*. Blackwell, Oxford.

Cuthbert, S. & Quallington, J. (2008) *Values for Care Practice*. Reflect Press, Exeter.

Chief Medical Officer (2007) *Annual report: UNDER THEIR SKINS tackling the health of the teenage nation*. Department of Health, London.

Collyer, N. & Whitehead, S. (2008) Safeguarding and confidentiality: Protecting children and young people. *British Journal of School Nursing*, **3** (6), 301–303.

Costello, J. & Haggart, M. (eds) (2003) *Public Health and Society*. Palgrave Macmillan, Hampshire.

Coverdale, G.E. (2006) School nursing for the future: Principles and strategy. *British Journal of School Nursing*, **1** (1), 29–31.

DfES (2006) *Raising Expectations: Supporting All Young People to Participate Until 18*. Department for Education and Skills, London.

DoH (1999a) *Saving Lives – Our Healthier Nation*. The Stationary Office, London.

DoH (1999b) *Making a Difference: Strengthening the Nursing, Midwifery and Health Visiting Contributions to Health and Healthcare*. The Stationary Office, London.

DoH (2001) *Reference Guide to Consent for Examination or Treatment*. Department of Health, London.

DoH (2004a) *National Service Framework for Children, Young People and Maternity Services*. Department of Health, London.

DoH (2004b) *Choosing Health-Making Healthier Choices Easier*. HMSO, London.

DoH (2004c) *The Chief Nursing Officer's Review of the Nursing, Midwifery and Health Visiting Contribution to Vulnerable Children and Young People*. Department of Health, London.

DoH (2006a) *School Nurse Practice Development Resource Pack revised edition*. The Stationary Office, HMSO, London.

DoH (2006b) *Essence of Care for Health Promotion*. The Stationary Office, HMSO, London.

DoH (2009) *Getting It Right for Children and Families*. Department of Health, London.

DoH/DCSF (2007) *The Children's Plan*. Department of Health, Department for Children, Schools and Families, London.

DoH/DCSF (2008) *The Children's Plan One Year on: A Progress Report*. Department of Health, Department for Children, Schools and Families, London.

DoH/DCSF (2009a) *Healthy Lives, Brighter Futures: The Strategy for Children's and Young People's Health*. Department of Health, London.

DoH/DCSF (2009b) *Securing Better Health for Children and Young People through World Class Commissioning. A Guide to Support the Delivery of Healthy Lives, Brighter Futures: The Strategy for Children and Young People's Health*. Department of Health, Department of Children, Schools and Families, London.

DoH/DfES (2006) *Every Child Matters: Change for Children in Health Services*. Department of Health, Department for Education and Skills, London.

DCSF (2008) *Children's Workforce Strategy*. Department for Children, Schools and Families, London. www.everychildmatters.gov.uk/deliveringservices/workforcereform/childrensworkforcestrategy/. Accessed 11 November 2009.

Downie, R.S., Tannahill, C. & Tannahill, A. (1996) *Health Promotion: Models and Values*, 2nd edn. Oxford Medical Publications, Oxford.

Elliott, L., Crombie, I.K., Irvine, L., Cantrell, J. & Taylor, J. (2004) The effectiveness of public health nursing: The problems and solutions in carrying out a review of systematic reviews. *Journal of Advanced Nursing*, **45** (2), 117–125.

Emmerson, L. (2008) *National Mapping of Onsite Sexual Health Services in Education Settings*. National Children's Bureau, London.

Giddens, A. (1989) *Sociology*. Polity Press, Cambridge.

Gillon, R. (1985) *Philosophical Medical Ethics*. Wiley, Chichester.

Green, D. & Catlow, D. (2009) Immunisation against human papillomavirus in a primary care trust: A report on the first three months of the national campaign. *British Journal of Infection Control*, **10** (3), 112.

Griffith, R. (2008) Consent and children. *British Journal of School Nursing*, **3** (6), 281–283.

Harris, J. (1985) *The Value of Life*. Routledge & Keegan Paul, London.

Home Office (2004) *Working within the Sexual Offences Act 2003*. Home Office, London. www.voiceuk.org.uk/docs/careworkers.pdf. Accessed 24 September 2009.

HM Government (2006) *Working Together to Safeguard Children*. HM Government, London. www.everychildmatters.gov.uk/resources-and-practice/IG00060/. Accessed 24 September 2009.

HM Government (1969) *Family Law Reform Act, 1969*. Stationary Office, London.

HM Government (1998) *Data Protection Act 1998*. Stationary Office, London.

HM Government (2005) *Mental Capacity Act 2005*. Stationary Office, London.

House of Lords (1986) Gillick v West Norfolk and Wisbech Area Health Authority. House of Lords, England. Accessed at http://www.hrcr.org/safrica/childrens_rights/Gillick_WestNorfolk.htm on 7/11/09 at 20.03.

Illich, I. (1976) *The Limits to Medicine Medical Nemesis: The Expropriation of Health*. Penguin, Harmondsworth.

Kennedy, I. & Grubb, A. (1998) *Principles of Medical Law*. OUP, Oxford.

Laverack, G. and Labonte, R. (2000) A planning framework for community empowerment goals within health promotion. *Health Policy and Planning*, **15** (3), 255–262.

Lightfoot, W. & Bines, J. (2000) Working to keep children healthy: The complimentary roles of school staff and school nurses. *Journal of Public Health*, **22** (1), 74–80.

Madge, N. & Franklin, A. (2003) *Change, Challenge and School Nursing*. National Children's Bureau, London.

MHRA (2009) *Human Papillomavirus (HPV) Vaccine.* Medicines and Healthcare Products Regulatory Agency, UK. http://tinyurl. com/klv883.

NMC (2004a) *Standards of Proficiency for Specialist Community Public Health Nurses.* Nursing and Midwifery Council, London.

NMC (2007) *NMC Record Keeping Guidance.* Nursing and Midwifery Council, London.

NMC (2008) *The Code: Standards for Conduct, Performance and Ethics for Nurses and Midwives.* Nursing and Midwifery Council, London.

Paavonen, J., Jenkins, D., Bosch, F.X., *et al.* (2007) Efficacy of a prophylactic adjuvanted bivalent L1 virus-like-particle vaccine against infection with human papillomavirus types 16 and 18 in young women: An interim analysis of a phase III double-blind, randomised controlled trial. *Lancet,* **369** (9580), 2161–2170.

Peate, I. (2007) *Becoming a Nurse in the 21st Century.* Wiley, Chichester.

Prochaska, J.O. & Diclemente, A. (1984) *The Transtheoretical Approach: Crossing Traditional Boundaries of Theories.* Dow Jones Irwin, Homewood.

Racktoo, S. & Coverdale, G.E. (2009) 'HPV? Never heard of it' Students and the HPV vaccine. *British Journal of School Nursing,* **4** (7), 328–334.

Richman, J. (2003) Holding public health up for inspection. In: *Public Health and Society* (eds J. Costello & M. Haggart), Chapter 1. Palgrave Macmillan, Hampshire.

Rollnick, S., Heather, N. & Bell, A. (1992) A Quality v taking clients through the system – Payments or targets? *Journal of Mental Health,* **1**, 25–37.

Sturm, L., Mays, R. & Zimet, G.D. (2005) Parental beliefs and decision making about child and adolescent immunization: From polio to sexually transmitted infections. *Journal of Developmental and Behavioral Pediatrics,* **26** (6), 441.

The Stationery Office (2004) *The Bichard Inquiry Report.* The Stationery Office, London.

Teenage Pregnancy Unit (2000) *Best Practice Advice on the Provision of Effective Ontraception and Advice Services for Young People.* Department of Health, London.

Tones, K. (1993) *The Theory of Health Promotion: Implications for Nursing.* In: *Research in Health Promotion and Nursing* (eds J.M. Wilson-Barnett & J. Clark). Macmillan, Basingstoke.

Tones, K. & Green, J. (2004) *Health Promotion: Planning and Strategies.* Sage. London.

Turton, P., Peckham, S. & Taylor, P. (2000) Public health in primary care. In: *Nursing for Public Health. Population Based Care* (eds P.M. Craig & G.M. Lindsay). Churchill Livingstone, Edinburgh.

Wainwright, P., Thomas, J. & Jones, M. (2000) Health promotion and the role of the school nurse: A systematic review. *Journal of Advanced Nursing,* **32** (5), 1083–1091.

WHO (1991) *Sundsvall Statement on Supportive Environments for Health.* World Health Organisation, Geneva.

Suggested further readings

Griffith, R. (2008) Consent and children. *British Journal of School Nursing,* **3** (6), 281–283.

Collyer, N. & Whitehead, S. (2008) Safeguarding and confidentiality: Protecting children and young people. *British Journal of School Nursing,* **3** (6), 301–303.

Thurtle, V. & Wright, J. (eds) (2008) *Promoting the Health of School Aged Children.* Quay Publishers, London.

Web sites

Young Minds http://www.youngminds.org.uk
Sainsbury Centre for Mental Health www.scmh.org.uk
Every Child Matters: www.everychildmatters.gov.uk

7 'To Be Like the Others': Children's Views of Nursing in Community Settings

Duncan Randall

Introduction

Advances in medical and nursing understanding and technology have led to more and more children living today with complex health-care needs than was previously the case (Glendinning *et al.* 2001; DES/HM Treasury 2007; DoH/DCSF 2009). Children are surviving the neonatal period, or serious illness and trauma, when previous generations would not have done so. These children present a challenge to traditional hospital-based care, because hospital-based medically orientated care assumes that children will be returned, by the administration of clinical care, to a state of health where they return to their parents' care and lead *normal* children's lives. However, children with complex health needs have ongoing medical and nursing needs which their parents or other carers may not be able to provide for, without professional support.

Gradually, there has been an acknowledgement that children with such ongoing nursing and medical needs will require accommodation and support to live in their communities instead of in hospitals, or other institutions. Perhaps, in part because of the shift in health policy rhetoric towards community settings (DoH 1997, 2000,

2008), and in part because of a recognition of children's rights to a family life and to social and educational opportunities arising from children's rights agenda and human rights legislation (Noyes 2000; DES/HM Treasury 2007). This relocation of care from hospital or institutions to community settings produces a number of complexities surrounding the provision of care, equipment, workforce development and physical environment. One of these complexities is how to listen to children's experience of receiving nursing care in community settings. Community settings are defined here as settings other than health-care institutions in which children interact socially with others (e.g. the child's own home, school, street, etc.).

This chapter considers the findings of a study which sought to elicit the views of children about how they experienced receiving nursing care in community settings (Randall 2008). The chapter does not detail the methods or methodology of the study, but considers instead the moral and ethical implications for children's nursing of listening to children. In essence, it considers how we can understand what is *good* children's nursing in community settings from the perspective of children who receive nursing care in the community.

Ethical and Philosophical Aspects of Nursing Children, First Edition. Edited by Gosia M. Brykczyńska and Joan Simons.
© 2011 Blackwell Publishing Ltd. Published 2011 by Blackwell Publishing Ltd.

The chapter begins by arguing that listening to children involves understanding the social contexts of children's lives, which in turn is helped by understanding children as social actors who interact in a social world shared with adults. The concepts of ethical symmetry (Christensen & Prout 2002) and cultures of communication (Christensen 2004) are proposed as useful approaches to interacting with children. The chapter then considers the findings of an exploratory study (Randall 2008) which suggested that children's main concern when receiving nursing care in community settings is to portray themselves as being like other children, with access to the same opportunities as their peers. Whether these attempts to be like the others can be conceptualised as *passing strategies* as described by Carnevale (2007) is discussed. Finally, it is argued that for children their attempts to be like other children is central to their experience of living with illness, and has wide-ranging implications for children's nursing practice, education, research and policy.

Listening to children and hearing their voice in community settings

The past decade has seen an increasing willingness on the part of adults involved in delivering services to children to listen to children's own views about the services they receive (DoH 2002; Coad & Shaw 2008). Although arguably this movement has been led by social and education services (Mayall 1993, 2002), health has now embraced the fact that children are willing and able to evaluate the services they receive and can offer critical and insightful analysis of services which can lead to service improvements (DoH 2002; Coad & Houston 2006; DoH/DCSF 2009). The move to respect the views of children has, perhaps, been enhanced by commentaries in the sphere of research *with* children such as the work by Scott (2000), who argued that adult voices are not a proxy for children's experience and the 5–15 program supported by the European Social Research Council (ESRC), which demonstrated that children can comment very effectively on their social worlds (Prout 2001).

Listening to children in community settings may have some particular difficulties. Children receiv-

ing care in hospital settings are in a sense a captive audience. Children are often grouped by medical label in ward areas. Parents and children attend outpatients, or are on wards often for long periods with little to do and there is opportunity to speak to them, or involve them in activities. In community settings, care is often delivered to children in isolation. The nurse will interact with a child on a one to one basis. This interaction may be short. Children in the study gave the impression that nurses came, delivered the intervention and left. This was also evident from the observation of nurses in this study (Randall 2008, 2009). Having another visit to gather children's views may not therefore have been appropriate. Kirk (2001) has written about the burden on children and carers of professionals who visit the home, yet another professional visiting may not always be welcomed. While hospital visits are made with the purpose of attending to health matters, a home visit may well interrupt a child's normal routine and social interactions.

Studies which have sought a user view have normally asked adults as well as children about the services they receive, but have not always focused on the children's voice. For instance, Sartain *et al.'s* (2001) account of an evaluation of a community children's nursing services gives only half a page to the children's views while adult views warrant two pages. Similarly, Lewis's (1999) study gives more weight to adult views than to children's. There has also been a lack of focus on the effect of the relationships between adults as members of one generation and children as members of another generation. Very few studies state how the researcher takes account of the influence that adults may have had on the data children give. Gardner & Randall (2009) have argued that interviewing children in the presence of an adult can affect the data given by the child. By comparing interviews from two separate projects, they showed that children's interview conversations gave richer data when children were interviewed alone, and that some adults acted to limit what children said if they were present during the interview – although they also found that in some contexts the presence of a familiar adult may help children to express themselves. Negotiating a conversation with children in community settings seems to pose particular difficulties. Research with children in the home setting and in schools would seem to suggest that the power relationships between adults and children are important in determining the extent to which children are allowed a voice (Connolly 2008; Mayall 2008). A factor in these power relationships is the perception of adults of the abilities of children. In their consideration of ethical symmetry, Christensen & Prout (2002) suggest that adult researchers need to be reflexive about their attitudes towards children's abilities. (For a more detailed overview of the ethics of research with children, see Chapter 17.)

Ethical symmetry

The concept of ethical symmetry is described by Christensen & Prout (2002) in relation to the approach of researchers to research that involves children. However, this approach may prove useful for health-care workers who work with children (see Chapter 20). Christensen & Prout (2002) argue that the development of the sociology of childhood and the view that children are social actors should lead to a re-evaluation of the ethics for those working with children. Further, they use the ideas of Bauman to argue that in the postmodern era, individuals need to reflect on their role in taking responsibility for others whose voices have been neglected. This would suggest that nurses need to take account of the context of their work with children, and children's social/cultural and political position. Also, using Bauman's conceptions, Christensen and Prout argue that those working with children need to take responsibility *for* children, but not take responsibility *away* from them. They suggest avoiding paternalistic behaviour and treating children and adults symmetrically, while not treating all children as though they are the same. Rather, Christensen and Prout argue that adults need to enter into a dialogue with children which recognises both commonalities and differences. This requires that adults explore their assumptions about children and attempt to employ the same ethical processes when working with children as they would with adults, but also take account of the context of the children's lives, their social networks and their social/cultural/political positions within their families and communities.

Christensen & Prout (2002) explicitly reject categorising children's abilities by age or developmental progression. Instead, they advocate those working with children attempt to understand the *cultures of communication* that children employ. Christensen (2004) has described cultures of communication thus:

... my work emphasised the importance of seeing fieldwork as a practical engagement with local cultural practices of communication. Thus, by observing children's language use, their conceptual meanings and their actions, I pieced together a picture of the social interactions and the connections between people.

(Christensen 2004:170)

The concept of *cultures of communication* would suggest that listening to children is more than attending to the words spoken by children, but rather that those working with children need to attend to the behaviour of children and adults, looking for patterns of communication set in a social context (see Chapter 20 for an elaboration of this theme). The cultures of communication of children and adults and the ethical symmetry between healthcare professionals and children may be different in community settings when compared with hospital settings. The behaviour of children acting as hosts and of visiting professionals as guests has been described in the research context (Coad *et al.* 2008; Mayall 2008). These behaviours can also be seen in clinical practice where community children's nurses and other community nurses are often permitted access to the *public* areas of the home, and offered food and drink. Community settings are perhaps perceived of as belonging to the child, their family or their community as *their* home or *their* school. This is perhaps in contrast to hospital settings which Bluebond-Langner's (1978) study would suggest children recognise as being under professional control. The act of being a host to professionals in your own space alters the dynamic between children and health-care workers. It not only alters the way children communicate with health-care workers, but also with other adults and peers within the home, or community setting. The findings of the study reported here may also suggest that to some extent it alters the relationship between children, nursing and nurses.

'To be like the others'

A qualitative exploratory study, which followed seven children for over a year using Clark's (2004) mosaic approach, found that children focused on portraying themselves as being like other children (Randall 2008, 2009). The children were all receiving nursing care at home and had been doing so for at least 6 months. Early on in the study, it was decided to try to minimise the influence adults had on children's involvement with the research. Ethical approval was granted for the research team to interview children away from their main carers; group work with children was also conducted without their main carer present. Parents were asked that they allow their children to keep their own diary of when the nurse visited, only helping their child if asked. While this strategy of separation was not wholly successful, with adult carers influencing the children's participation in various ways, it did arguably allow the children the space to express views which perhaps would not be *sanctioned* by their parents. For instance, some children expressed negative views of nurses which their parents tried to prevent.

The children had a range of medical labels and received different interventions from community children's nurses. In total, the children had almost 11 years experience of receiving care. The project used a mosaic of qualitative methods and methodology, but across the whole project children consistently seemed to portray themselves as being like other children. They took pictures of their family and friends, of their schools and the places where they played, of their pets, but made few images of nurses. Some of the children seemed reluctant to talk about nursing and some refused to talk about nurses at all:

[after repeated attempts to talk
about *carers*]

RESEARCHER   *About the carers, when the carers come what happens?*
MOHAMMED[1]   *Umm [pause].*
RESEARCHER   *Can you tell me what happens when the carers come?*

MOHAMMED   Na na na na na naahh [singing]…
RESEARCHER   *Do you not want to talk about that? [pause] Shall we talk about some thing else?*
MOHAMMED   *Yeah.*

Mohammed: interview after observation.

When asked if they talked to their friends about having a nurse visit them at home, the children evidently did not tell their friends much about the nurse's visit:

RESEARCHER   *… Do you talk to them about why you have a nurse come and see you at home?*
NANNY   *No.*
RESEARCHER   *No, ok, you just say 'I've got to go home now because the nurse is coming'.*
NANNY   *Yeah.*

Nanny: Photo Talk Diary interview.

The message from the children seemed to be that they wanted to present themselves as being like other children. Even the children like Nanny who spoke enthusiastically about her nurse would rather be playing with friends:

NANNY   *When you're sitting in the house whatever you are doing with the nurse. The nurse is fun with you, but you would rather be playing outside with some friends.*

2nd Children's group.

The children in the study were presented with summary statements which were simplified statements that attempted to capture the sense of the early analysis of the data from the study (known as member checking, Colaizzi 1978; Beck 1994). The children felt the following two statements reflected what it was like to have a nurse visit them at home:

- I don't like to think about being ill. I prefer to think about playing with my friends and being with my family.
- I would rather have my mum or dad do all the things I need to keep me well, than have nurses visit me at home.

It would seem reasonable that these statements could come from any child. They focus on doing

---

[1]   *The names used here are names chosen by the children and used with their agreement; they are not the children's real names.*

the things that children do, playing with friends, being with their families and seem to resist the intervention of nurses, instead looking to parents to provide care.

In the study, nurses were interviewed and their practice in the community observed. What emerged from the work with children and with the community children's nurses was that nurses seemed to have an almost task-orientated approach, they arrived at the home, they performed a task and left:

RESEARCHER *What happens when the nurses come?*

JOANNE *First they come and they get all the stuff out, and then they get the stuff ready, and then I go in the other room cause I feel sick, and then they get the injection, and when they are ready they call me, and I have the injection, and then I go to the room, and then they put their things away, and then they wash their hands, and then they write in their book, and then they go.*

Joanne: Photo Talk Diary interview.

Both children and the nurses agreed that a purely technical performance of tasks would be unacceptable:

KELLY *Because some nurses might just Umm, might just go in and they are not as good, they might just go in wash their hands. Don't ask if they are allowed to use the bathroom, or anything. Which would make them a bit angry and then they just give the needle without asking if they were alright, or not giving them time to do the Mr Bump.*

Kelly: Interview after observation.

However, some of the nurses recognised that a more task-orientated approach could help to support children in their efforts to be like other children:

CCN *Sometimes they don't want that relationship. They just actually want what needs doing at home as quickly as possible and just go out. While you are there you are stopping them going shopping, stopping them meeting their friends, stopping them doing what ever. Actually, what you are*

there to do is to prevent them having a hospital admission, travelling 2 hours to [names city regional centre] or wherever that would be. Actually you are just there to do a job to get it done, so they can go back to a normal life, thank you very much.

CCN Group interview area 2.

The nurses were observed and spoke about supporting children to be like other children, in a number of ways. Some of which were more visible than others, although often for the children, these interventions were less visible. Often, nurses taught other family members to enable them to deliver care, for example, nurses taught mothers how to perform complex wound care and overnight enteral feeding regimes. The children, however, did not recognise this teaching role of nurses. The community children's nurses arranged for children to be treated at local hospitals when on holiday, arguably making family holidays a possibility. For one young man, the nurses helped his mother to do complex daily dressings so that he could arrive at school with his peers. In another example, the nursing team worked with teachers and carers to teach them how to care for an oxygen-dependent young woman, who required overnight ventilation, so that she could join her peers on a school outward-bound trip. Proudly displayed on her school walls were photographs of the young women abseiling with her oxygen cylinder!

Although this facilitation, or boundary work, which perhaps bridges health, social care and education is less visible to children and some professionals than work which supports the practice of medicine, it seems vital for the children's attempts to be like their peers. The work of nurses, often carried out behind the scenes, allowed these children to attend school, go on family holidays and maintain their social friendships.

Other studies have also reported on children's focus on family, friends and school both in community settings and in hospital. In hospital studies by both Coyne (2006) and Carney et al. (2003), children focused on their families and their home life including their friends and pets. For instance in Carney et al. (2003), 52.1% of the children referred to how they attempted to manipulate the hospital environment to be more like their own home. In Coyne's study, a girl of 13 commented:

> Miss my mum, my dog, my sister, the atmosphere, my own bed, the living room, the telly and the garden. I miss school? miss friends at school? Like, I'm worried about my schoolwork if I stay too long in hospital. What will happen next?
>
> (Coyne 2006:329)

In community settings, Carter found that children measured the performance of the nurse by the standard of their parents (Carter 2005); this too could be seen as children attempting to suggest that just like other children they should be cared for by their parents rather than by nurses.

Passing strategies?

What is meant by *being like other children* perhaps needs to be explored further. The children in these studies were all living with illness, sometimes these were long-term conditions or chronic illnesses, for some these health problems were life-limiting and/or life-threatening. The children did not attempt to be like other children living with illness, rather they tried to portray themselves as being like their perception of what healthy, or perhaps ordinary children are like. Arguably, the children attempted to portray themselves as being like a hegemonic child, an idealised image of what contemporary children should be like.

Are these children attempting to *pass*? Carnevale (2007) has suggested that children living with illness do use passing strategies as outlined by Goffman (1968). Although Goffman was writing about adults with mental health problems, Carnevale has suggested that Goffman's concept of passing, by the use of passing strategies, can be applied to children living with illness. Passing strategies involve someone living with illness, who is stigmatised by society as ill, attempting to portray themselves as being a *normal*, just like everyone else, in order to access the same social interactions as those not stigmatised by illness. For

adults, it could be argued that this is a social trick. Those living with illness who are stigmatised trick those not stigmatised into thinking that they are in the non-stigmatised category.

While being seen as *normal* or un-stigmatised may carry certain advantages for adults, it can be argued that for children being categorised as a child, like other children, is integral to the child's childhood and to gaining social and educational skills. For children, such behaviours may be more than a social trick, as without access to the social interaction that play and education afford to children, the child's developmental progress may be jeopardised. Children who are unable to play or attend school can fail to develop social skills which would help them to build relationships. Interrupted schooling not only affects educational progress but disrupts children's social networks making it difficult for them to maintain or establish friendship networks (Sandeberg *et al.* 2008).

Being perceived as a child like other children who attend school and have a peer friendship network carries, for children living with illness, immense advantages as opposed to isolation and a lack of access to social interactions which facilitate the learning of educational and social skills. It is perhaps no wonder then that children are keen to portray themselves as being like other children.

This analysis of children's attempts to portray themselves as being like other children – being a form of *passing strategy* – relies on children considering illness as a stigma to be avoided. However, Admi (1995) has argued that this may be overstating the negative aspects of illness for children. Her retrospective study of growing up with cystic fibrosis showed that children and young people's attitudes to disclosing information about their illness changed over time. Until around age 10–13, children tended to rely on adults for their strategies in disclosing information. A particularly important landmark was telling their first boy/girl friend. Within this progression, young people described a process of selecting their audience such that if they felt that the other person had similar experiences then they would disclose more details, dependant on the context in which they found themselves. Thus, if time and the social situation allowed, and they felt the audience would be sympathetic, they might disclose their diagnosis, but if the inter-action was brief and the audience judged not par-ticularly sympathetic they would offer a partial explanation or claim to have a cold rather than cystic fibrosis. Admi suggests that rather than denying their illness as is implied by Goffman's analysis, children seek an *ordinary* life where their illness is 'nothing to hide and nothing to adver-tise'. However, for the young people in Admi's (1995) study, behaviour around disclosing infor-mation does seem to support the idea that young people recognise the potential for stigma that being deemed ill can have. If they did not recog-nise the potential for social stigma, one would assume that they would reveal full details of their illness in most situations. The careful selection of an audience, the complex social negotiations around disclosing information, including mak-ing judgements on how sympathetic the audi-ence is likely to be, implies that the young people recognise the potential for them to be stigma-tised. It could be argued that they are attempting to select people to tell about their illness in situations where they think the other person is going to be sympathetic and therefore less likely to apply social sanctions or stigma of illness to them.

It may be more accurate to consider children's attempt to be like other children as attempts to access the same social interactions as their peers rather than conceptualising their behaviour as *passing* in the sense that Goffman sets out. Children's attempts 'to be like the others' are then a social justice issue, where children living with illness are attempting to assert their rights to a family life (articles 8.1, 9.1, 16 of the *UN Convention on the Rights of the Child* (United Nations 1989)), to an education (articles 28 and 29) and to social association (article 15), as well as other aspects covered by the United Nations Convention, such as religious and cultural identity (see Appendix II). These children who may also be considered as disabled are attempting to access the same social interactions and life opportunities as their peers. This would seem to be more complex than simply *passing* as described by Goffman or Carnevale. While for adults passing is about a social trick, whereby a person who may be in danger of being stigmatised manages to portray themselves as being like normal or un-stigmatised people, for

children attempting 'to be like the others' is about social justice in society, such that children living with illness are able to access the same opportunities as their peers to a childhood and to acquiring social skills and education.

Supporting children 'to be like the others'

For children then it seems important, both person-ally and socially, that they succeed in their attempts to portray themselves as being like other children. Nurses would appear to agree and act to support children to be like other children, albeit in a somewhat covert way. This last section of the chapter will explore the implications for children's nursing of this finding. Firstly, it will be argued that supporting children to be like other children holds a dilemma for nurses in clinical practice, in that these attempts by children may jeopardise their health. Then, the implications for education will be explored and it will be argued that sup-porting children in this way requires an inter- or multidisciplinary approach which needs to be supported by educational programmes, taught across disciplines. The research agenda should seek to understand what effect nurses' support for children's attempts to be like other children would have on health outcomes. Finally, policy needs to address how children's nursing is measured to support children's access to social and educational opportunities.

Implications for practice

Although nurses in the study reported here acted in some instances to support children's attempts to be like other children, there are potential diffi-culties in facilitating children accessing the same social interactions as their peers. Firstly, this work is less visible than work which overtly supports the practice of medicine. Liaschenko (1997) sug-gests that when nurse's work is less visible, it makes the work vulnerable, such that when resources are reduced the work may be lost. As discussed above, in supporting children to be like other children the nurse almost needs to disap-pear, as children not living with illness do not have nurses. The more time spent with the nurse, the more visible the care and the less likely it is that the child will succeed in being like children not living with illness. Thus, supporting children to be like the others requires the nurse to be less visible and this may threaten the very work which enables these children to access the same opportunities as their peers.

Secondly, there is perhaps a tension between children attempting to be like other children and health outcomes. Children who live with illness may need to take medication or submit themselves to interventions which children not living with illness do not. In attempting to be like other children, encouraged by children's nurses, children may not take their medication or avoid interventions which may place their health at risk. Perhaps the most obvious example would be a child who is diabetic not injecting insulin in order not to appear different, resulting in poor blood glucose control. Another example might be children staying on to play with their friends rather than making their excuses to go home for the nurses' visit and thereby missing their injection or wound dressing. Thus, while nurses may want to support children's attempts at being like other children this cannot be done without some limits and critical thought. How nurses determine the balance between supporting the practice of medicine and supporting children in accessing social and educational opportunities has yet to be explored and detailed.

Re-balancing children's nursing, to make more visible the boundary work of supporting children to be like other children, will challenge the current high visibility of nurse's work which supports the practice of medicine. Focusing more on how nurses facilitate children access to social care and education will also have implications for the education of future nurses.

Implication for nursing education

Helping children living with illness to access social care and education seems to logically suggest an interdisciplinary approach. Health, social work and education disciplines would need to work together to facilitate children living with illness being able to access the same opportunities as their peers. Although there are isolated examples of good practice, the curriculum for children's nursing set out by statutory bodies and suggested by current textbooks often focuses on the practice of medicine, with the occasional mention of child psychology. Children's nursing courses are by and large taught in nursing faculties of universities rather than as joint ventures across health, social and educational faculties. If nurses are to help children to access social and educational opportunities, they need to learn with and from other disciplines how to do so. Such learning will need to be theorised in academia, but practiced in health, social and educational settings.

A first step would be to understand the thinking and skill-set used by health, social and educational workers who already successfully facilitate the social integration of children who live with illness. Then learning experience packages need to be designed to help students to acquire these skills and understanding, along with appropriate student assessments. This will require much pedagogic research and a thorough rethink of the present curricula.

Implications for research

A number of programmes of research would seem to arise from this agenda to support children living with illness. Perhaps the most important would be to investigate whether supporting children 'to be like the others' is of any benefit to children. Currently there is little evidence to indicate whether children's health, social or educational outcomes are affected by how successfully they are able to access social and educational opportunities. Sandeberg *et al.* (2008) have shown that self-assessed quality of life measures are improved by school attendance. However, this may only demonstrate that children with less symptoms and side effects from their illness and treatment were able to attend school more often. Such children are perhaps likely to report a better quality of life in comparison to those with more debilitating symptoms who were unable to attend school.

A second important question would be whether nurses can support children's attempts to be like other children. Although nurses may facilitate children accessing social and educational opportunities in line with those of their peers such as the cases reported here, where nurses facilitated school attendance and family holidays, this may still not be enough for those children living with illness to be accepted by their peers, or by society – as being like other children. It seems likely that nurses alone will not be effective, but that acting together with social workers and educationalists they could be more effective, although such a collaborative model has yet to be tested (Sloper 2004).

Once an evidence base is established that for children living with illness:

1. Children's successful attempts at being like other children improves their health, social or educational outcomes.
2. Professional health workers, social carers and educationalist can help children in their attempts to be like other children.

Then policy makers may be influenced to design policies to support children being like other children.

Implications for policy

As well as policies which would support the implications detailed above for practice, education and research, policy which acknowledged the importance of being like other children would address how to take account of this issue in the metrics of children's nursing and reflect its importance in the contracting of services for children and young people.

A performance measure for nursing services could be introduced which measured how well children living with illness were facilitated to access social and educational opportunities. This would form part of the monitoring of standards for services alongside established health indicators of quality. Without being prescriptive, quality measures could be designed to monitor school attendance, or attendance at pre-school facilities. Work already being done such as facilitating family holidays or attendance at social clubs would be valued as a success measure for nursing services rather than an extra and unappreciated nursing intervention.

Perhaps beyond the boundaries of nursing and health, policy makers need to acknowledge that more and more children are living with illness, often with complex and long-term health problems. If these children are to live in communities and not be effectively housebound, but to be able to achieve their rights under the *United Nations Convention on the Rights of the Child* to a family life, to free association, to education and to cultural and religious identity, then policy makers across health, social care and education will need to adopt an interdisciplinary approach that considers children as children. While progress has been made towards such an approach (DES/DoH 2004; Young *et al.* 2008), it has been perhaps slow, disjointed and divided by professional and disciplinary divisions.

Conclusion

Hearing children's voices in community settings presents challenges which may have many features in common with listening to children in other settings, but which also has features unique to community settings. A sociological understanding of children and childhoods in line with Christensen & Prout's (2002) ethical symmetry and which incorporates Christensen's ideas on cultures of communication may be useful frameworks to aiding nurses in listening to children.

When we do listen to children, we find that they are focused on portraying themselves as being like other children. Arguably, the other children they wish to be are idealised conceptions of children from within their own cultures. However, nurses seem to support the view of children, that they should have access to the same social and educational opportunities as their peers. Taking on board this message from children has far-reaching implications for children's nursing practice, education and policy, and requires further research to provide an evidence base which could be used to advocate for children's nursing to respond to children's desire 'to be like the others'.

Reflective scenario

As a community children's nurse you are delivering care to Eleanor (aged 5); she has a painful abscess which you are dressing. When you arrive at Eleanor's house, she is standing in the hallway obviously scared. As you enter the house she dashes past her mother and runs upstairs, crying. Eleanor's mother apologises for her daughter's behaviour and having shown you into the living room goes upstairs to her crying daughter. After 10 min Eleanor is brought downstairs still visibly upset.

- Is Eleanor refusing treatment?
- Using the concept of ethical symmetry, explain how and why the care offered to Eleanor would be different from that offered to an adult.
- How could you support Eleanor to be a child in this situation?

References

Admi, H. (1995) "Nothing to hide and nothing to advertise" managing disease related information. *Western Journal of Nursing Research*, **17** (5), 484–501.

Beck, C.T. (1994) Phenomenology: Its use in nursing research. *International Journal of Nursing Studies*, **31** (6), 499–510.

Bluebond-Langner, M. (1978) *The Private Worlds of Dying Children*. Princeton University Press, Princeton.

Carnevale, F.A. (2007) Revisiting Goffman's stigma: The social experience of families with children requiring mechanical ventilation at home. *Journal of Child Health Care*, **11** (1), 7–18.

Carney, T., Murphy, S., McClure, J., *et al.* (2003) Children's views of hospitalization: an exploratory study of data collection. *Journal of Child Health Care*, **7** (1), 27–40.

Carter, B. (2005) "They've got to be as good as mum and dad": Children with complex health care needs and their siblings' perceptions of a Diana Community Nursing service. *Clinical Effectiveness in Nursing*, **9**, 49–61.

Christensen, P.H. (2004) Children's participation in ethnographic research: Issues of power and representation. *Children and Society*, **18** (2), 165–176.

Christensen, P. & Prout, A. (2002) Working with ethical symmetry in social research with children. *Childhood*, **9** (4), 477–497.

Clark, A. (2004) The Mosaic approach and research with young children. In: *The Reality of Research with Children and Young People* (eds V. Lewis *et al.*), pp. 142–161. Sage/ The Open University Press, London.

Coad, J. & Houston, R. (2006) *Voices of Children and Young People*. Action for Sick Children, London.

Coad, J. & Shaw, K. (2008) Is children's choice in health care rhetoric or reality? A scoping review. *Journal Advanced Nursing*, **64** (4), 318–327.

Coad, J., Twycross, A., Milnes, L., Randall, D., Gibson, F., Horstman, M. & Carter, B. (2008) "Be my guest!"

Challenges and practical solutions of undertaking interviews in the home with children and young people. In: *Royal College of Nursing Research Society Conference*, pp. 113–114. Royal College of Nursing Events, London.

Colaizzi, P. (1978) Psychological research as the phenomenologist views it. In: *Existential Phenomenological Alternatives for Psychology* (eds R.S. Valle & M. King), pp. 48–71. Oxford University Press, New York.

Connolly, P. (2008) Race, gender and critical reflexivity in research with young children. In: *Researching with Children: Perspectives and Practices* (eds P. Christensen & A. James), 2nd edn., pp. 173–189. Routledge, Abingdon.

Coyne, I. (2006) Children's experiences of hospitalization. *Journal of Child Health Care*, **10** (4), 326–336.

DES/DoH (2004) *Every Child Matters: Change for Children in Health Services*. Department of Education and Skills and Department of Health, London.

DES/HM Treasury (2007) *Aiming High for Disabled Children: Better Support for Families*. Department of Education and Skills & HM Treasury, Office of Public Sector Information, Norwich.

DoH (1997) *The New NHS Modern, Dependable*. The Stationery Office, Department of Health, London.

DoH (2000) *The NHS Plan: A Plan for Investment, a Plan for Reform*. The Stationery Office, Department of Health, London.

DoH (2002) *Listening, Hearing and Responding*. The Stationery Office, Department of Health, London.

DoH (2008) *High Quality Care for All: NHS Next Stage Review Final Report*. Department of Health, London.

DoH/DCSF (2009) *Healthy Lives, Brighter Futures: The Strategy for Children and Young People's Health*. Department of Health, Department for Children, Schools and Families, London.

Gardner, H. & Randall, D. (2009) Interviews with children: Notes from the field. Paper presented at *Royal College of Nursing International Research Conference*,

Royal College of Nursing, Cardiff. Wednesday 25th March 2009.

Glendinning, C., Kirk, S., Guliffrida, A. & Lawton, D. (2001) Technology dependent children in the community definition, numbers and costs. *Child Care Health and Development*, **27** (4), 321–334.

Goffman, E. (1968) *Stigma: Notes on the Management of Spoiled Identity*. Harmondsworth, Penguin.

Kirk, S. (2001) Negotiating lay and professional roles in the care of children with complex health care needs. *Journal of Advanced Nursing*, **34** (5), 593–602.

Lewis, M. (1999) The lifetime service: A model for children with life threatening illness and their families. *Paediatric Nursing*, **11** (7), 21–23.

Liaschenko, J. (1997) Ethics and the geography of the nurse-patient relationship: Spatial vulnerabilities and gendered space. *Scholarly Inquiry for Nursing Practice*, **11** (1), 45–59.

Mayall, B. (1993) Keeping healthy at home and school: "It's my body so it's my job". *Sociology of Health and Illness*, **15**, 464–487.

Mayall, B. (2002) *Towards a Sociology for Childhood: Thinking from Children's Lives*. Open University Press, Birmingham.

Mayall, B. (2008) Conversations with children: Working with generational issues. In: *Research with Children: Perspectives and Practices* (eds P. Christensen & A. James), 2nd edn., pp. 109–125. Abingdon, Routledge.

Noyes, J. (2000) Are nurses respecting and upholding the human rights of children and young people in their care? *Paediatric Nursing*, **12** (2), 23–27.

Prout, A. (2001) Representing children: Reflections on the children 5–16 programme. *Children and Society*, **15**, 193–201.

Randall, D. (2008) Children's views of being nursed at home. In: *Community Children's Nursing Forum Conference 2008*. Royal College of Nursing, Birmingham 13/03/08. Children's version available online from http://www.abpn.org.uk/Portals/_Rainbow/Documents/87299ChildViewsbook.pdf. Accessed 17/4/09.

Randall, D. (2009) *"They just do my dressings": Children's perspectives on community children's nursing*. Unpublished thesis, The University of Warwick Conventry.

Sandeberg, M., Johansson, E., Bjork, O. & Wettergren, L. (2008) Health-related quality of life relates to school attendance in children on treatment for cancer. *Journal of Pediatric Oncology Nursing*, **25** (5), 265–274.

Sartain, S.A., Maxwell, M.J., Todd, P.J., Haycox, A.R. & Bundred, P.E. (2001) Users' views on hospital and home care for acute illness in childhood. *Health and Social Care in the Community*, **9** (2), 108–117.

Scott, J. (2000) Children as Respondents: The challenge for quantitative methods. In: *Research with Children: Perspectives and Practices* (eds P. Christensen & A. James), pp. 98–120. Falmer Press, London.

Sloper, P. (2004) Facilitators and barriers for coordinated multiagency services. *Child Care Health and Development*, **30** (6), 571–580.

United Nations (1989) *Convention on the Rights of the Child*. United Nations, Geneva.

Young, A., Temple, B., Davies, L., Parkinson, G. & Bolton, J. (2008) Disabled children (0–3 years) and integrated services – The impact of early support. *Health and Social Care in the Community*, **16** (3), 222–233.

Suggested further readings

Carter, B. (2005) "They've got to be as good as mum and dad": Children with complex health care needs and their siblings' perceptions of a Diana Community Nursing service. *Clinical Effectiveness in Nursing* **9**, 49–61.

James, A., Jenks, C. & Prout, A. (1998) *Theorizing Childhood*. Polity Press, Cambridge.

Mayall, B. (2002) *Towards a Sociology for Childhood: Thinking from Children's Lives*. Open University Press, Birmingham.

Web sites

Youth health talk http://www.youthhealthtalk.org/

Children first for health by Great Ormond Street Hospital http://www.childrenfirst.nhs.uk/

Every child matters http://www.dcsf.gov.uk/everychildmatters/

8 Care of the Severely Disabled Child: A Moral Imperative

Vicki Rowse

Introduction

If I knew then what I know now I would have made very different decisions. (Mother of a child with severe neonatal encephalopathy who died aged 5 years.)

Over the past two decades, the nature of disabled children and their needs has changed significantly. Advances in technology and medical science, such as the human genome, IVF, neonatal care and antenatal screening techniques have given parents a choice around pregnancy and care of their baby. However, they have also given rise to a different kind of disabled child, one who is increasingly complex and dependent on a high level of technology for their daily life. This coupled with the modern way of life where both parents work, the extended family no longer lives nearby and society has a *throwaway* mentality, means that raising children is very different today from the past; and raising a disabled child presents significant challenges. Supporting parents in this endeavour also raises practical and ethical challenges – for organisations to work together, for professionals to be multiskilled and for the government to ensure that money is spent effectively.

A definition of disability is given in the Disability Discrimination Act (OPCS 1995) as follows:

… a physical or mental impairment which has a substantial and long-term adverse effect on his or her ability to carry out normal day to day activities.

There are around 770,000 disabled children in the UK, with 570,000 of those children in England (DCSF 2007b). Amongst the population of disabled people, children aged 0–16 are the fastest growing group and over the past 10 years there has been a significant increase in the number of children with autism and complex health needs. This is due to the survival of preterm and low birth weight babies, and advances in medicine, leading to both earlier diagnosis of congenital and genetic conditions and a greater range of treatment options and technological developments for children, resulting in better outcomes and longer life expectancy following severe illness or injury. It is estimated that there are around 100,000 children in England with complex care needs, who need support from a wide range of services (EDCM 2009). Modern disabled children fall into two very clear groups: those

Ethical and Philosophical Aspects of Nursing Children, First Edition. Edited by Gosia M. Brykczyńska and Joan Simons.
© 2011 Blackwell Publishing Ltd. Published 2011 by Blackwell Publishing Ltd.

who are learning disabled, particularly with the increase in autistic spectrum disorders, and those who are physically disabled – a large number of whom are also learning disabled and have multiple facets to their health needs. The needs of these two groups are quite disparate, and it is becoming apparent that different approaches are needed to deliver their care. John Rawl's *Theory of Justice* (Rawls 1972) and his mind experiment concerning social justice comes closest to offering an intellectual exercise which could help the reader to start appreciating the moral and practical problems encountered when trying to provide adequate services for this group of children. When reflecting on services for this group of children and young people, we are predominantly entering the debate about justice, resource allocation and aspects of basic human rights. In addition, several of the articles in the United Nations Convention on the Rights of the Child (UNCRC) speak directly to the concerns of these children, most significantly, the right to the best possible care and the right to be heard.

Nature of their care needs

Historically disabled children would have had poor life expectancy and many died as babies. As health care improved and survival rates increased, disabled children required education and care so homes and long-stay hospital units developed, often as rural branches of children's hospitals such as Tadworth Court and Great Ormond Street Children's Hospital. These were commonly referred to as institutions and children lived there receiving education and care, probably not seeing their parents much, if at all. When children were in hospital, they were cared for by nurses and visitors as parents were actively deterred from visiting their children due to concerns about infection control, a situation which prevailed until the 1950s. Children who were at home were often isolated from their peers and those with high nursing care needs would not have survived infanthood; life expectancy was short for many, and disabilities tended to be grouped as mental, physical, deafness, blindness or epilepsy.

In the 1980s there was a greater recognition of the needs of disabled children, and in particular the need for inclusion, following the Warnock (HMSO 1978) report into special education. This had the knock-on effect of changing the delivery of care as well as education, as it was recognised that disabled children learned in every aspect of their daily life. As a result, many care homes were closed in favour of small homes from home units with house parents and a greater focus on a normal life rather than a rigid care routine. Further to this, the Children Act of 1989 directed that all children should be within a family unit if at all possible, and all efforts were put into achieving this. This is a laudable and correct aim, which is good for children, but it has coincided with the increase in dependency of disabled children and there is now a care gap. It could be argued that it is not in the best interests of parents and siblings as it appears that no one really considered that the families may need significant help to manage these children. In recent years, the use of technology to support children's heath needs has grown enormously, and it was estimated in 2001 (Glendinning *et al.* 2001) that there were 6000 children dependent upon technological equipment to maintain their lives. It is now common for children to be at home with equipment such as enteral feed pumps, nebulisers, suction machines and oxygen concentrators, and it is very likely that there are significantly more than 6000 such children today as evidenced by the rise in the number of children cared for at home with ventilators. In 1999, Jardine (Jardine 1999) identified 136 children under the age of 16, by 2000 this had risen to 241 (House of Commons 2004) and in 2009 Breathe On UK, a charity set up to support families of ventilated children, reported that there were 1000 ventilated youngsters up to the age of 25 in the UK (www.breatheon.org.uk). Initially, teams of qualified nurses were put together to help manage these children, but this has gradually changed due to the relative lack of available nursing staff, and also a re-evaluation of the care of the children, which has determined that although they are technology dependent, they are essentially stable, and with proper treatment protocols, training and supervision, they could be cared for by trained, but unqualified staff. The effect of this has been that it is now expected that parents will learn a wide range of skills including managing their child's dialysis, total parental nutrition (TPN), suction, subcutaneous infusions and invasive ventilation via tracheostomy, as well as routine nursing tasks and supervision of health-care assistants to enable their children to live at home rather than in hospital!

Nature of respite and palliative care

Families are clear that they need help and a break from the caring role, they are also clear that they need a range of options to meet the needs of their child and family. Respite care is gradually being seen as more than a break for parents, it is now recognised as an opportunity for the disabled child to have time away from their parents, to develop their own friendships and social network and to experience a range of activities not necessarily possible in a family group. It is also becoming recognised that siblings are marginalised in families where there is a disabled child – their needs usually taking second place to those of their disabled sibling – and many of them becoming young carers to help the family function. Respite should recognise the needs of all members of a family and be available in a flexible format to the best advantage of all. However, there are in effect three different types of respite (1) that provided by Social Services to help the family manage basic care needs, such as washing and dressing, (2) that provided for the child to access out of home activities and (3) that provided by the health-care system to help manage the nursing care of their child. This latter nursing care help is what sometimes is viewed as respite, but in fact may not be, as it is often no more than an extra pair of hands needed to deliver a therapy programme or to ensure that a ventilated child is safe, and as a result is not a break for the parents.

The range of respite care has varied over the years. Traditionally, disabled children left home to receive care, often in boarding schools or units attached to hospitals, or they were supported at home by the extended family. Gradually, institutional care was replaced by small units for 3–4 children, closer to their parents' homes and children were encouraged to go to day schools. As health care improved and survival rates for disabled children increased, parents wanted their children at home within the family unit, and started to request home-based respite and this has been the focus of the past 10–20 years. While there are some special-

ist residential units, it is increasingly difficult to get places at them as they are full, and are extremely expensive, with few families able to afford them and local authorities/primary care trusts (PCTs) reluctant to fund places unless it can be proven beyond doubt that the child's needs cannot be met locally. However, it seems as if the pendulum has swung too far towards home care and the availability of residential or short break care is very limited, particularly if a child is of pre-school age. The impact of long-term stress on parents' mental health is poorly acknowledged and it is not at present considered to be a valid reason for a child to be placed in a residential unit, even though it is known that disabled children at are greater risks of abuse. The likelihood of abuse is increased with social isolation, mental health issues and poverty, all of which occur in these families as will be discussed later (Powell 2007).

The Children Act (DoH 1989) stated that children should be cared for within a family environment as far as possible. If this imperative were applied to families requiring respite care or short breaks, there would need to be a pool of willing family link or foster parents and the reality is that there are very limited numbers of people able or willing to take on such a role in our modern society. In addition, this work is poorly paid which does not attract people to take on the responsibility for a child with complex health-care needs or with behavioural difficulties. Due to the lack of such carers, families wait many months for a placement and then even more time for equipment to be available – if in fact it can even be funded. This type of home-based care can also be problematic for older children with physical disabilities as significant building adaptations are generally required to make a house fit for their specific care needs – and these adaptations are usually only funded for the child's main residence. However, access to the family link person can be very rewarding for both the disabled child and the adults involved, and it can be therapeutic for the parents to have a bond with someone who understands their child and the daily difficulties they have to face. In addition, the child has time with a family other than their own and as a result has new experiences and a broader social network (DoH/DfES 2004).

It is, however, poorly recognised that some families feel they have failed if they see another family *managing* the child successfully when they have struggled. Often, residential respite is more acceptable to families who view it as a choice they have made for their child, much the same as boarding school or holiday clubs for non-disabled children, with professionals caring for their child. In the current climate of *choice* and participation, where all agencies have to consult with users over the development and evaluation of services, the wishes of parents of disabled children are likely to become more overt and less easy to ignore (DCSF 2007a; DoH/DCSF 2009).

New models of respite or short breaks, as it is now fashionable to call respite, are being developed in response to local needs. These include:

- Short-term care in the children's own homes, including overnight and daytime sitting services.
- Contract carers: a network of contract carers who are paid a retainer fee throughout the year and offer placements on a more or less full time basis to a number of children. This has the advantage of providing a suitably equipped, resourced and skilled carer, with knowledge of the individual children and ability to comprehensively meet their care needs.
- Family-based care, such as family link schemes.
- Hospice and hospice at home schemes.
- Short-term residential care.
- Day care, including specialist child minders and holiday play schemes.
- Befriending: schemes include adult befriending to help young people experience new social activities, belong to clubs or learn new skills; and peer befriending in which young able bodied people take part in group activities with disabled youngsters of similar age.

The government, in Aiming High for Disabled Children (AHDC) (DoH/DfES 2008), recommends that all of these options are considered for development by commissioners in order to meet the needs of disabled children in their area. However, something that is poorly recognised is that holiday periods and in particular the 6-week summer holidays are extreme pressure points for many families and there is little extra provision at this time for disabled children. There is a paradox of parents being expected to take on complex care of their children, but those same children are then deemed too dependent or unstable for family link schemes, or play schemes when risk assessments are undertaken.

For many years, there has been a health versus social care debate over who is responsible for which aspects of care and this seriously inhibits the effective planning of care for this group of children. In particular, the rise in the number of children with autism is introducing a new problem, as it is unclear whether they have a social-care need or a health-care need. Is autism a health problem or a learning problem? As Social Services referral criteria become more stringent in the light of increased workload, those children with nursing needs that can be met at home are falling through a provision of service gap (EDCM 2009). There is also pressure from social-care agencies for health-care workers to exclusively support these children, particularly since the new *Continuing Healthcare* criteria for adults was introduced (DoH 2007), and children began to be assessed against these in the absence of a child-specific assessment process. This has proved disastrous for children assessed to have fully funded health-care needs, as they were then excluded legally from Social Services support. The launch of the *Children's Continuing Healthcare Framework* is currently running at least a year behind schedule, but must be comprehensive in order to overcome the issues faced by professionals and families in developing and delivering appropriate packages of care.

In the past, the types of nursing tasks these children required were considered to be very specialised and to be undertaken only by qualified children's nurses, but now it is becoming the norm for these children to be cared for away from hospital and there is a considerable body of knowledge and skill around their care. Some of these tasks, such as gastrostomy feeding, are increasingly considered to be social care because they are relatively uncomplicated procedures and meet basic human needs. In the current and worsening economic situation of the public sector budget, the debate about who should pay for what will escalate rather than diminish. While there are moves towards shared budgets and joint commissioning, the results of this are not yet available to children and families. For example, many families who received social care did so in the form of direct payments; but provision of health care under this scheme is currently illegal. This gives rise to the situation of a child having at least two sets of carers, one set chosen by the family under direct payments, a second set provided by the health sector with limited options for choice of carer and often a third set at school! It is also possible that the assessed risks around safeguarding children will have an impact on the provision of care in multiple settings, with professionals trying to minimise risk, possibly at the expense of the child's social and personal development needs. (Example: a pre-school child with severe cerebral palsy and failure to thrive, whose parents are struggling to cope, is not allocated residential respite on the grounds of age, as social workers feel that the parents will not bond with their child and multiple carers put the child at risk. If the child were given out of house respite, the parents would have a break, the child would be removed from a stressful situation and their relationship may well improve as a result.)

In reality, respite care needs to be made up of a combination of options and children should have a variety of choices to meet their needs as well as those of their parents. Pooled budgets and integrated teams are the way forward for good communication, cost-effective and efficient service delivery and child-centred care planning (EDCM 2009; DoH 2008a).

Issues surrounding paediatric hospices

The Children's Hospice movement, started in the UK by Sister Frances Dominica in 1982 with the opening of Helen House in Oxford, has steadily grown and spread worldwide (Children's hospices (CHUK) UK 2009a). Today there are 42 hospices in the UK (CHUK 2009a). The Association for Children's Palliative Care (ACT) has been influential in developing definitions and care pathways for this group of children, and it is clear that the focus of care needs to be on *living* with a palliative diagnosis, rather than on end of life concerns. However, children's hospice care has historically been exclusively charitably funded and currently receives only 12% of their costs from the government (CHUK 2009a). Fund-raising is

becoming more and more difficult with the increasing demand for care and the number of children eligible for hospice care rising steadily due to improvements in health care and life expectancy. This has resulted in an urgent need to provide similar facilities for young people over the age of 16. To help meet this need, Douglas House was opened in Oxford in 2004 and similar facilities are being built at other UK children's hospices to meet the needs of people aged 16–35 (CHUK 2009a). The reason for the unique development of these respices, as they are beginning to be known, is that the needs of these young people cannot be met in traditional adult hospices where the services are focused almost exclusively on adults with a life expectancy of 6 months or less. The 2008 financial recession hit charitable organisations as much as private individuals and businesses. One example is a children's hospice that lost £5 million in The Icelandic Bank scandal (CHUK 2009b), and as a result they have had to reduce service to children and families in order to make ends meet. While this is understandable, the people who lose out are the children and their families. For several years, ACT has been lobbying the government for contributions to hospice running costs and there was some progress with the announcement in February 2008 of £20 million over 3 years specifically for children's hospices, and £30 million in February 2009 for children's palliative care. However, this latter sum is allocated via PCT funding streams and is not ring fenced, so it remains to be seen how much will actually be invested in children's palliative care services (EDCM 2009; DoH/DCSF 2009).

Hospices are also increasingly faced with the assumption on the part of statutory agencies, that they will automatically contribute to care packages for children with palliative care diagnoses, with no contribution from the agencies themselves towards the costs of the care. This is becoming more noticeable with the financial constraints on both Health and Social Service budgets, while hospices are under pressure from families to help them even more – particularly in emergency situations such as illness of a parent (DoH 2008a). Another difficulty for hospices is the recruitment and retention of nursing staff as it is a specialist role and not suitable for everyone as it can be emotionally draining and challenging. The nurses can also end up isolated from other health providers and colleagues. There is also the problem of maintaining and developing clinical skills, as much of the hands-on-care is provided by health-care assistants and volunteers, with the trained nurses working in a supervisory and management capacity (DoH 2008a).

Appropriate education of paediatric nurses

The education of nurses is currently under review, and it seems as though children's nursing will remain a discrete entity. However, the increased number of student nurses needing placements over the past few years has resulted in much creative thinking on the part of the universities, but also some bizarre placements for students who qualify to care for sick children. Placements have included pre-school nurseries, special schools and even NHS Direct (Richardson *et al.* 2006). While a good grounding in child development is essential and an understanding of the more generic needs of children in primary care is important, there needs to be a balance of the type of placement the student is allocated to. Child health students have qualified with as few as two acute paediatric ward placements during their training and consequently have had little exposure to or experience of critically ill children, or children with severe disabilities or complex care needs. Nursing students are in theory qualified to work in the community when they graduate, but in practice they do not have the skills or experience to underpin the level of autonomous practice required in these community roles. It must be also questioned whether the overemphasis on public health is in the best interests of those children with disabilities and/or complex health-care needs. Since the introduction of the Third part of the NMC register and a greater focus on public health, there been a steady increase in children's nurses working in primary care, as part of health-visiting teams. As a result, there are some recruitment problems for secondary care, which is caught in the middle between the apparent glamour of tertiary referral units and the family-friendly working hours of primary care. The main drawback in this scenario is that the secondary units, namely, the district general hospitals, tend to

be the places where disabled children are regularly admitted to and often for significant periods of time, and are then discharged back into the community. It appears that some nurses working in the acute sector do not understand disabled children and the increasing drive for community care and ever shorter stays in the hospital, meaning that the necessary skills to care for these children are not developed in the acute sector. In addition, these children tend to be much sicker when they are admitted and require more high-dependency care, resulting in a focus on their health and physical needs rather than their overall person-centred needs.

Children's Community Nurses (CCNs) have become pivotal in the care of children with complex health care or palliative care needs, resulting in a range of nursing procedures and interventions taking place in the community and often by health-care assistants. This has had the effect of de-skilling nurses in the acute sector in procedures such as changing gastrostomy buttons and accessing implanted ports. As a result, a ventilated child, or one requiring TPN, could be admitted to a District General Hospital children's ward because the child happened to live in the catchment area and find that the staff do not have the skills to be able to manage their care safely. The current change in focus of care can be clearly seen in CCN teams who have evolved from Generic to Specialist teams to meet the needs of the caseload. CCN training has evolved into an advanced practitioner model and it could be argued that elements of this model should be included in pre-registration training so that nurses are prepared to manage both palliative and complex care needs.

Role of government in sustaining respite and palliative care

Since the early 1990s, thanks to ACT, children with palliative care needs have crept up the political agenda. Initiated by the Diana Princess of Wales Memorial Fund through to funding for Diana Nursing Teams in 1998, children's palliative care received dedicated funding via the Big Lottery in 2003 which led to the development of local services (Craft & Killen 2007). These were all favourably evaluated (Big Lottery 2007) resulting in a higher profile and government interest in palliative care, to the extent that an independent review was commissioned and undertaken by Professor Sir Alan Craft and Sue Killen (2007). Their report detailed what should be available and has been backed up by *Better Care: Better Lives* (2008) detailing the Department of Health's vision for these children and families.

Key messages from this review are that (DoH 2007):

- Children and young people's palliative care is not well understood and often confused with end of life care;
- There is considerable overlap between children and young people with palliative care needs and those with disabilities and complex needs;
- There is little evidence of effective joint planning, commissioning and delivery of services between health, education and social care;
- There is a lack of information on the number of children with palliative care needs, their location and future trends;
- There is a lack of transition services to manage the transfer to adult services;
- Short-term funding, for example, Big Lottery, whilst prompting innovation, did not lead to long-term sustainability.

Worryingly, there is an end-of-life strategy focusing on adults (DoH 2008b), which is receiving a great deal of attention nationally and locally, but is not including children's palliative care, which is being subsumed into the AHDC agenda (DoH/DfCSF 2009).

A plethora of policy documents and initiatives with the core focus on redesigning services for children have appeared since 2002. These include The National Service Framework for Children and Young People (DoH/DfES 2004), The Children's Plan (DCSF 2008), Every Child Matters (DoH 2003) and AHDC (DCSF 2007b) and a variety of other documents. Since 2008, children have become one of the four national priority areas and there has been specific investment. Particularly relevant is the investment of £340 million for the period 2008–2011 (DoH/DfCSF 2009), in addition to the £340 million already allocated to Local Authorities under the AHDC programme. Hospices have received a little of this money, but still rely on charitable donations for 88% of their funding.

But how much of this is being translated into reality? With lack of ring-fenced budgets, continual reorganisation of PCTs and constant pressure on financial balance, this small group of children are unlikely to be high priority, and this has serious ethical implications for the care of the children concerned. In addition, the AHDC (DFCS 2007b) agenda is looking at all disabled children with an increasing emphasis on those with Autistic spectrum disorders. This is partly driven by the increase in the number of children diagnosed with autistic spectrum disorders, and also by the needs of society and parents in particular, to work and enable their children to experience a range of opportunities to enhance their potential development to adulthood. Palliative care has been included under this large umbrella and the concern is that these children and families will be lost in the wider agenda. It is possible that those with severe and multiple disabilities will become marginalised, due to their relatively small numbers and that service development will meet the greatest number of children rather than those with the greatest need, a seemingly utilitarian approach to the situation. A fundamental ethical issue is that the needs of this group of children and their families are poorly recognised and understood, although at government level there has been a shift lately in understanding and a definite policy move towards the improvement of service delivery for children with palliative care needs. A key message, delivered in *Better Care: Better Lives* (DoH 2008a) is that 'Palliative care services need to be designed around the needs of children and families' (DoH 2008a:8).

The very nature of childhood means that children are growing, developing and changing at a fast pace and require services and activities to keep pace with them. Children's lives are multifaceted and involve a wide range of people, making the provision of respite a challenging and complex issue, not least because there is no clear definition of what *respite* actually means. To parents and carers it means having a break from caring for their child, and allowing someone else to undertake this role for a short time, and for the children it is the chance to be independent of their parents and to broaden their range of experiences.

It has become unfashionable in Children's Services to recognise *respite* as a need; the preference seems to be in favour of the term *short break*, which moves the focus from the needs of the parents and family to the needs of the child. There is a danger that the need of the parents to have a break or *respite* from caring for their child may be ignored or dismissed, leading to even greater isolation and stress amongst families. A ministerial foreword in *AHDC: Short Breaks Implementation Guidance* highlights the current situation with the statement as follows:

> … children who have the greatest need for breaks often seem unable to access provision because of the challenges posed by their disability.
>
> P1 (DCFS 2008)

A key factor in the provision of care for disabled children and young people is individual knowledge of their care and needs. Many of the aspects of their care are easy to teach to carers, but it is less easy to provide a flexible range of respite options as the knowledge of the individual is vital in providing safe effective care. This means that considerable time has to be spent setting up and preparing respite provision, and emergency care is therefore only available to those children and young people already known to respite facilities. Further compounding the issue of access to respite is the lack of common eligibility criteria and, as noted already, no clear definition of disability or complex healthcare needs. This results in a lack of cohesive strategy in the development of services, variable thresholds and as a result inequitable provision of services across the country and even within one county (DCSF 2007b).

Children's and parents' concerns

Parents continually report having to contact multiple agencies and professionals and having to fight to get services and equipment (e.g. a child with severe cerebral palsy). There is, however, growing research into the views of children, young people and their families and a recurring theme is that they want to be heard or at least listened to (EDCM 2009; Grant & Hamlyn 2009). This is also a fundamental right of the children concerned – enshrined in the UNCRC and confirmed in the Children Act. Organisations such as Contact a Family, Mencap and the Council for Disabled Children are very active in campaigning for the rights of these disabled children and in providing support and advice for their families, while the Joseph Rowntree Foundation actively supports social research. What the studies are showing, not surprisingly, is that families with disabled children face a number of challenges compared to families without disabled children. The Every Disabled Child Matters campaign, led by an alliance of charities has reviewed the evidence of the families' lives and the findings give a stark picture of their plight (EDCM 2007, 2008, 2009). A key message is that there is a strong association between low income, social exclusion and disability in families who have a disabled child. Examples of this include employment, income and expenses and housing.

- Employment: They are 50% more likely to be in debt and 50% less likely to be able to afford holidays, extras at school, new clothes and treats, than other families. Only 16% of mothers of disabled children work compared with 61% of non-disabled children; while 85% of parents with disabled children say they want to work. Reasons for this lack of employment are many and varied, but key difficulties are the availability of suitable, affordable childcare; lack of understanding by employers and the difficulties of single parenthood – since 29% of lone parents have a sick or disabled child.
- Income and Expenses: 55% of families are living in or almost in poverty as it costs three times as much to bring up a disabled child compared to a non-disabled child and state benefits do not meet their costs. For example, childcare costs are higher due to higher staff ratios, in the region of £8 compared to £4 per hour for non-disabled children, and working tax credit does not make up the difference. Other contributory factors are the additional expenses of travelling, equipment, adaptations in the home and childcare, coupled with the actual difficulties in securing and maintaining employment. Many parents give up employment as there are no viable options for childcare and work is not flexible enough to allow

time off for the vast number of appointments with therapists, hospital consultants, social workers, schools, etc.

- Housing is reported to be inadequate in three quarters of families with disabled children according to the government's own report (Cabinet Office 2005). Features identified include poor conditions, lack of space for undertaking therapies and storage of equipment, lack of mobility access both within and without the home and lack of space for other family members. Poor housing also impacts on the physical and mental health of other family members, with carers reporting injuries as a result of trying to move their children in inadequate space, and mental health problems due to lack of time away from the pressures of managing the whole family needs. Siblings are also disadvantaged, often having to share a room with their disabled brother or sister, and having no space to themselves. One positive step has been the abolition of the means test for disabled facilities grants, the main grant to fund housing adaptations, which frequently disadvantaged those in employment with their own homes.

In August 2009, a national survey was published of research undertaken with families to assess progress against the five elements of Core Offer described in AHDC (Grant & Hamlyn 2009).

The elements of the core offer are as follows:

- Good provision of information;
- Transparency in how the available levels of support are determined;
- Integrated assessment;
- Participation of disabled children and their families in local services;
- Feedback and complaint procedures that are accessible.

The research asked for feedback in each of the elements of the core offer around the three agencies providing services to these children: health, education, and care and family support services. It is interesting that only 30% of the 12,226 respondents received disability living allowance (DLA) for their child, and the majority of the children had cognitive impairment. Depression, seizures and palliative care needs were the least reported diagnoses and only 18% had mobility difficulties. This supports the view that children with learning and other cognitive impairments are now a significantly large group within the population and highlights that their needs are being poorly met. Significant findings are dissatisfaction at lack of resources and difficulty accessing services and poor communication, while transparency was the highest rated and feedback rated the lowest across the three agencies.

These findings echo an earlier study by Beresford *et al.* (2007) against the Every Child Matters (DoH 2003) five outcomes, which are to be healthy, stay safe, enjoy and achieve, make a positive contribution and achieve economic well-being. Children and parents stated that they wanted the same outcomes as non-disabled children, although they interpreted the outcomes differently to non-disabled children and families. It appeared that the ECM outcomes could only be met if underpinning principles were in place. These included the ability to communicate and be understood, comfort and physical health, and emotional well-being – all these were considered necessary to any further achievement. Communication in particular was highlighted as a fundamental principle, without which progress in meeting the outcomes for disabled children would be slow. Parents wanted an identity other than that of a parent of a disabled child, which included having employment and social activities; they wanted more time to be a parent to their disabled child and less time as a nurse or carer; access to information and advice on a variety of subjects including managing behaviour, supporting communication and developing independence; access to financial and practical resources; and access to a quality-consistent service for their child's ongoing needs.

Transition to adult care

Craft and Killen (DoH 2008a) highlighted the lack of transition services to manage the move of children and young people with palliative care needs to adult services. Increasing but small numbers of young people with complex needs are surviving into adulthood and families are experiencing difficulty in making the transition.

The reasons for this include:

- The different ages at which transition takes place within agencies. Health services move young people on from 16 years of age, although Payment by Results includes 19-year-olds and Continuing Healthcare criteria states 18 as the upper age limit for accessing paediatric care; Children's Services transfer young people on their 18th birthday; and education at the end of the academic year in which they are 16, or if profoundly disabled 19 years of age. However, if properly managed this staged transfer of services may be of benefit to the young people and their families, as it enables a gradual transition by agency rather than a complete change overnight.
- The change in model of health care from the general specialist (paediatrician) to general practitioner (GP). In health, a fundamental problem is the change in focus from a paternalistic model of care to one led by young people themselves.
- The move from education to employment, with often poor opportunities for those with complex health-care needs.

While health practitioners are willing to manage transition, there is no clear pathway and often no clear destination. The current message is that transition includes those aged 14–25 years, and there appears to be a move, particularly within health, that services currently designed for children should develop to care for young people up to the age of 25. While this has some value, it also has serious drawbacks. One of the problems of transition is the different style of service delivery in adult care, and keeping young people in a service whose roots are within paediatric practice will only compound the problem, with the risk that they will be kept as children due to the nature of their disabilities impeding communication and understanding of their individual wishes and needs. Children's nurses, paediatricians and social workers cannot meaningfully manage a caseload aged 0–25 and be effective in delivering services appropriate for all ages, stages of development and encompassing emotional, mental and physical health. There is also the difficulty of having sound knowledge of the services available in adult care to enable good

transitional plans to be developed (e.g. a young person requiring 24-h care and nursing).

A fundamental problem of transition, particularly with severely or multiply disabled young people, is that paediatricians have a long term, unique relationship with each child and family, and have a large body of knowledge about them. Where transition pathways are not obvious, there may be pressure to keep the young person within the paediatric system as it is easier for the professionals and parents. However, this is unlikely to be in the best interests of the young person as it only delays the time when transition has to be made, and it is then unlikely to be smooth, coordinated or planned well, so the experience becomes traumatic for the family. This age group have significant and encapsulated needs and issues that, coupled with long-term disabilities or health problems, require understanding expertise and a certain amount of innovative thinking to better meet their needs in our present society.

It is suggested that an effective model would be a designated young people's service, perhaps based on the CCN model, with integrated interagency working with Connexions, and adult services but delivered by a community matron (DoH/DCFS 2008). This would enable a service with comprehensive knowledge of adult care in all agencies, alongside a developed knowledge of the specific needs of young people and individuals in particular.

Conclusion

The government has made the welfare of children a key policy area, and has started to recognise disabled children and young people within these plans. This is an ethical response to the plight of very many of our children in the community. It is also acknowledged that they have increasingly unique needs and require collaborative working and innovative thinking by professionals and politicians in order to have their needs met. However, much still needs to be done to bring care and opportunities in line with the rhetoric, and it is unclear as to how progress will be measured when there are no distinct targets and a very poor financial climate ahead over the next few years. As demonstrated, the ethical imperative to care for these children is fraught with difficulties.

Reflective scenario

Simon is a 4-year-old and requires skilled 24-hour care as a result of severe learning difficulties and complex health-care needs including complex epilepsy, global developmental delay, tracheomalacia and failure to thrive. He has gastrostomy and tracheostomy, requires emergency seizure medication 3–4 times per week and has 100+ small seizures per day. He lives in local authority housing, with his mother and two older siblings, financially supported by benefits. Simon's father no longer lives with the family and provides little practical support.

1. How can his social, emotional, educational, housing and care needs be effectively met?
2. What ethical issues might you have to reflect upon?

Consider his changing needs, cooperation with multiple agencies, the need for respite, care and support of siblings, working with parents and their needs, family finances and the social economics of looking after a child in the community, the skills required to adequately care for Simon and safeguarding issues.

References

Beresford, B., Rabiee, P. & Sloper, P. (2007) *Priorities and Perceptions of Disabled Children and Young People and Their Parents Regarding Outcomes from Support Services.* DH 2147. Social Policy Research Unit, University of York, York. www.york.ac.uk/spru

Big Lottery (2007) *Evaluation of the Big Lottery Fund Palliative Care Initiative.* Final Report.

Cabinet Office (2005) *Improving the Life Chances of Disabled People.* Prime Minister's Strategy Unit, HMSO, Norwich.

CHUK (2009a) *Facts and Figures about Children's Hospices.* Accessed 28/8/09: www.childhospice.org.uk

CHUK (2009b) link to http://www.naomihouse.org.uk/news/index.aspx

Craft, A. & Killen, S. (2007) *Palliative Care Services for Children and Young People in England: An Independent Review for the Secretary of State for Health.* Department of Health, London.

DCSF (2007a) *The Children's Plan, Building Brighter Futures.* HMSO, Norwich.

DCSF (2007b) *Aiming High for Disabled Children: Better Support for Families.* HMSO, Norwich.

DCSF (2008) *Aiming High for Disabled Children: Short Breaks: Implementation Guidance,* HMSO, Norwich.

DfES (2003) *Every Child Matters.* Department for Education and Skills Publications, Nottingham.

DoH/DfCSF (2008) *Transition: Moving on Well. A Good Practice Guide for Health Professionals and Their Partners on Transition Planning for Young People with Complex Health Needs or a Disability.* HMSO, London.

DoH/DfCSF (2009) *Healthy Lives, Brighter Futures: The Strategy for Children and Young People's Health.* HMSO Norwich.

DoH/DfES (2004) *National Service Framework for Children, Young People and Maternity Services: Disabled Children and Young People and Those with Complex Health Needs.* Department of Health, London.

DoH (1989) *The Children Act.* The Stationery Office, London.

DoH (2007) *The National Framework for NHS Continuing Healthcare and NHS-funded Nursing Care.* HMSO, London.

DoH (2008a) *Palliative Care Strategy Better Care: Better Lives.* DoH Publications Orderline PO box 777, London SE1 6XH.

DoH (2008b) *End of Life Care Strategy: Promoting High Quality Care for all Adults at the End of Life.* HMSO, London.

EDCM Campaign (2007) *Disabled Children and Child Poverty.* Briefing paper. London. http://www.edcm.org.uk/pdfs/disabled_children_and_child_poverty.pdf 28/8/09

EDCM Campaign (2008) *Disabled Children and Housing* http://www.edcm.org.uk/pdfs/disabled_children_and_housing.pdf 28/8/09

EDCM Campaign (2009) *Disabled Children and Health.* Campaign Briefing. www.edcm.org.uk/pdfs/edcm_disabled_children_and_health.pdf 2/8/09

Grant, C. & Hamlyn, B. (2009) *Parental Experience of Services for Disabled Children; National Survey.* BRMB Social Research. www.dcsf.gov.uk/research Research Report DCSF-RR146

Glendinning, C., Kirk, S., Guffrida, A. & Lawton, D. (2001) Technology-dependent children in the community: definitions, numbers and costs. *Child: Care, Health and Development,* **27,** 321–334.

HMSO (1978) *Special Educational Needs: Report of the Committee of Enquiry into the Education of Handicapped Children and Young People* (Warnock Report). Her Majesty's Stationery Office, London.

House of Commons (2004) *Select Committee on Health Written Evidence* Appendix 26 Letter from Jan Morrison to the Clerk of the Committee (PC 30) 26 July 2004.

Jardine, E., O'Toole, M., Paton, J. Y. & Wallis C. (1999) Current status of long term ventilation of children in the United Kingdom. *BMJ*, **318**, 295–299.

OPCS (1995) *Disability Discrimination Act.* The Stationery Office, London.

Powell, C. (2007) *Safeguarding Children and Young People. A Guide for Nurses and Midwives.* Open University Press, England.

Rawls, J. (1972) *A Theory of Justice,* Revised Edition. Harvard University Press, Cambridge, Massachusetts.

Richardson, J., McEwing, G.& Glasper, E.A. (2006) Pre-registration children's and young people's nurse preparation. A SWOT analysis. *Paediatric Nursing*, **18** (10), 34–37.

Suggested further readings

Clare Conners and Kirsten Stalker. (2003) *The Views and Experiences of Disabled Children and their Siblings.* Kingsley Publishers, London, ISBN:1-84310-127-0.

McLaughlin, J., Goodley, D., Clavering, E.K. & Fisher, P. (2008) *Families Raising Disabled Children: Enabling Care and Social Justice.* Palgrave Macmillan, Basingstoke. ISBN: 13 978-0-230-55145-9.

Teare, J. (ed.) (2008) *Caring for Children with Complex Needs in the Community.* Blackwell Publishing, Oxford. ISBN 978-14051-5-5177-1.

Web sites

Every Disabled Child Matters Campaign: www.edcm.org.uk

Joseph Rowntree Foundation: www.jrf.org.uk

The Social Policy Research Unit, York University: www.york.ac.uk/inst/spru

9 Ethical Aspects of Care of the Adolescent

Yvonne Dexter

Introduction

When we study, we learn what is ideal, what is optimal. In life we sometimes fall short of the ideal. This semester reminded me that it is part of my contract with society and my profession to always strive for ideal practice and, if my practice is not ideal, then to figure out to the best of my ability why not, and make an honest attempt to correct it.

(Student nurse cited by Noveletsky-Rosenthal & Solomon 2001:25)

It has gradually been accepted that the health-care needs of adolescents are significantly different from those of younger children and adults and that their unique care needs are related to their in-between status as neither child nor adult. Practitioners caring for this group face distinct ethical challenges and controversies. Despite the plethora of guidance that exists to clarify ethical issues, practitioners may still experience personal and professional conflict. This chapter aims to identify key issues in adolescent health, policy and practice and explore ethical issues and dilemmas that arise in working with this group; it will also suggest how education can provide opportunities to develop knowledge, skills and attitudes to enhance practice.

Adolescence

Briggs (2008) observes that adolescence is organised around two phases: 'The transition from childhood to early adolescence, through the impact of puberty, is a period of intense growth and far-reaching changes – physically, cognitively, emotionally. This is followed by a long transition into adulthood, which, though inclusive of diverse "pathways", is usually extended, lasting approximately for a decade from mid/late teens until the mid-twenties. Primarily affected by social changes, this long transition to adulthood severely tests traditional thinking about the adolescent process' (p. 1). It is very different from the *age between* described in the middle of the twentieth century as 'a relatively short period of transition' (p. 2).

This extended transition creates challenges for adolescents, parents, practitioners, researchers and policy and law makers and highlights the unsuitability of age-related definitions. The question of how to legally define when a child is deemed to be responsible enough to make decisions is often debated. Brooks (2009:40) ponders the 'panoply of

Ethical and Philosophical Aspects of Nursing Children, First Edition. Edited by Gosia M. Brykczyńska and Joan Simons.
© 2011 Blackwell Publishing Ltd. Published 2011 by Blackwell Publishing Ltd.

mismatched legislation that governs ages of majority in this country'. Connexions Direct (2009) provides information and advice for young people on this puzzling state of affairs, for example, ages they can purchase alcohol or tobacco, vote and so on: 'You might not be seen as an adult in the eyes of the law until the age of 18, but as you get older you are legally allowed to do certain things. That can also mean you are legally responsible for your actions, so it's important to know what's what'.

Policy makers and practitioners face similarly taxing questions related to age. Webster *et al.* (2004:41) studied the long-term transitions of young adults in neighbourhoods beset by the problems of extreme social exclusion and concluded that 'problems associated with youth transitions do not conclude at neat, age-specific points and therefore age-related policies … do not "fit" harmoniously with the realities of the extended transitions that our sample members have undertaken'. The Social Exclusion Unit (2005:3) also recognised that 'services which are restricted to a particular age group often work against the principle that resources should follow need … 16- and 17-year-olds may receive inappropriate mental health services. They can find themselves falling between adolescent and adult services and losing continuity in treatment as a result'. In reality, policy and provision need to be flexible enough to respond to this extended transition and provide services which respond to need rather than age group.

Essential to engaging with adolescents is an understanding of key developmental issues affecting this transition, for example, risk taking, development of autonomy and decision-making ability (Steinberg 2008), and an awareness that development occurs 'against a backcloth of changing social and political circumstances' (Coleman & Hendry 1999:2). The patterns of transition to adult independence have changed dramatically in the past 50 years or so; they have 'become not only more extended, but also more complex, more "risky", and more polarised' with some young people 'catapulted into some forms of independence at a young age', for example, young carers; change has been caused by a drive for more young people to go to university, a decline in jobs and high house prices (Jones 2005:3). In practice, it is best to assess individual adaptation and adjustment to adolescence (Holmbeck 2002).

Attitudes to young people

'The British stand accused of not liking children. They seem to like teenagers even less' (Hall 2002:9). Indeed, Byron (2009) suggests that ephebiphobia (fear of youth) is a historically nurtured and culturally damaging phenomenon that is worse today than ever. The media play a significant role in demonising adolescents, making judgements and stereotyping them. Thompson *et al.* (2006:64) see the media as 'an example of a social structure that exerts powerful influences over the way in which human beings view themselves and others. The depiction by the media of healthcare is influential in forming the expectations of both healthcare providers and recipients'; in competing for customers they 'present eye-catching images and unusual or sensational storylines, accompanied by short and easily-assimilated explanatory accounts of the issues involved. The result is that … issues are often misleadingly oversimplified and alternatives presented in an adversarial manner, in order to make an impact'. Discussions about adolescent behaviour and risk taking often problematise them (boys are trouble and girls are in trouble) creating moral panic and affecting policy and practice, for example, headlines like 'Children's rights? What about the rights of those who live in fear of young thugs?' (Phillips 2008). A responsible media could inform and encourage discourse about adolescents and health issues but it is questionable whether this is achievable. The Child Poverty Action Group identified that stereotypes were a problem to which a responsible media was a solution (Dennehy *et al.* 1998) and The Children's Society (2009) urged the media to rethink the 'exaggerated picture they portray of young people threatening our social stability'. Batchelor & Raymond (2004:226) suggest that it is possible to work with and through the media to promote adolescent health. 'Press and public relations work can have an impact at both national and local level. Using the media to raise the awareness of sexual health matters can be effective but comes with risks since it is impossible to control the headlines. But by building positive relations, providing informative briefings and choosing media outlets carefully, you can begin to maximize the positives and minimise the negatives'.

Young people are aware that they are stereotyped and stigmatised. They say 'Treat us with respect – see beyond our labels' (Young Minds 2009) and 'Every child should be listened to, no matter how difficult they are to talk to' (Lord Laming 2009:78). Practitioners face the reality of working with this group and the ethical issues and dilemmas that they pose on a daily basis. They do not know what to say to an adolescent who has self-harmed; they are annoyed by a young binge drinker being nursed next to an acutely sick child; they are distressed by a teenage mother making her decision about whether to keep her baby; they are unsure about whether to breach confidence if a young person discloses risk-taking behaviour; they are caught between the needs of adolescents and their parents; they are frustrated by a lack of resources or expertise to care for vulnerable young people. As a result 'uncertainty over ethical and legal rights and responsibilities may lead professionals to refuse to see adolescents aged under 16 years on their own for fear of incurring parental wrath or even legal action. Disputes may arise in relation to an adolescent's competence to seek, consent to, or refuse medical treatment, and his or her right to confidentiality. In most cases these disputes can be resolved by discussion, compromise, and partnership, but in extreme circumstances the courts may be involved' (Larcher 2005:5). Donovan & Suckling (2004) explore how to address issues like these by exploring case histories of difficult consultations with troubled adolescents in primary care.

Health issues

'Adolescents are the only age-group in the population in which every priority health indicator (e.g. mental health, obesity and cardiovascular risk, smoking, alcohol use, drug use, sexual health) is either adverse or static. The health of adolescents has changed little in the past 40 years, in striking contrast to the dramatic strides made in the health of children and the elderly' (Viner 2007a:vii). This situation has stimulated significant interest in adolescent health (Jones and Bradley 2007; Coleman et al. 2007). In addition to adverse trends in key public health indicators, common long-term illnesses such as diabetes and asthma are increasing, 'advances in the treatment of congenital conditions have resulted in new cohorts with diseases largely unknown to adult physicians' and there is reason for concern about health inequalities and the coexistence of problems (Viner & Barker 2005:901). There is increasing awareness of the needs of disadvantaged, vulnerable and hard-to-reach groups (e.g. learning disabilities, looked after, young offenders, asylum seekers), bereaved adolescents (Dexter 2008) and issues of risk and resilience (Coleman & Hagell 2007; Pomerantz et al. 2007). Nurses are increasingly caring for adolescents with chronic illness and responding to the challenges of their care; compliance with treatment and transition to adult care have received much attention (Valentine & Lowes 2007). Providing for the health needs of adolescents is complex; Jones (2007:433) draws attention to the fact that 'adolescents are not a homogenous group, and it is therefore not surprising that interventions designed to influence their behaviours, which do not take into account variations in maturity and life experiences, are unlikely to be successful'. Viner & Barker (2005) make significant suggestions for investing in adolescent health, for example, a specific public health focus on adolescent health ending the focus on single issue approaches, direct engagement with adolescents through information technology and clinical services that engage young people.

Policy

Interest in adolescent health has increased since 1997 when it was identified that adolescent care was given insufficient priority, lacked focus and had poorly developed services (DoH 1997). New Labour's social investment strategy and drive to modernise and improve services has driven significant child welfare policy development and intervention in recent years; previous Conservative governments introduced some important measures, for example, the Children Act 1989, but they were much less interventionist (Fawcett et al. 2004). However, as Broadhurst et al. (2009:2) suggest, while it appears that recent UK governments have been 'genuinely concerned with the well-being of children' some findings 'clearly raise questions about a seeming incongruence between discursive commitments to children and young people and the realities of their lives, particularly those who are most vulnerable'.

The *Every Child Matters: Change for Children Programme* (DfES 2004) attempted to transform preventative and protective services for children and families, for example, through targeting socially excluded groups and early intervention. The Green Paper *Youth Matters* (DfES 2005a:3) laid out a vision for young people: 'to see services integrated around young people's needs helping all teenagers achieve the five *Every Child Matters* outcomes to the greatest extent possible'. Attempts to translate such ambitious policies into practice can be seen in the National Children's Bureau *Healthier Inside Programme* (NCB 2009) that aims to reduce the risks of repeat offending and social exclusion by ensuring that the *Every Child Matters* agenda is embraced within secure settings; a toolkit has been developed to help with reviewing and improving services (Lewis & Heer 2008) and guidelines have been produced for supporting bereaved young people who are over-represented in the criminal justice system and can consequently be vulnerable in secure settings (NCB 2008).

The *National Service Framework* (NSF) *for Children Young People and Maternity Services* (DoH 2004) is a 10-year programme to improve children's health in England and set standards for services; a Foreword by Sir Al Aynsley-Green reflects the discourse about children as investments and the 'moral dimension of child health policy' (Foley 2008:79): 'Children and young people are important. They are the living message we send to a time we will not see; nothing matters more to families than the health, welfare and future success of their children. They deserve the best care because they are the life-blood of the nation and are vital for our future economic survival and prosperity' (p. 4). The NSF targeted adolescents in *Standard 4: Growing Up into Adulthood*: 'All young people have access to age-appropriate services which are responsive to their specific needs as they grow into adulthood' (DoH 2004:6). *You're Welcome Quality Criteria, Making Health Services Young People Friendly* (DoH 2007) was developed to support the implementation of this standard; criteria included accessibility, confidentiality and consent; the environment, staff training, skills, attitudes and values; joined-up working; monitoring and evaluation; and involvement of young people. *Walk the Talk* (NHS Scotland 2009) is another initiative to help health professionals caring for adolescents to develop services that are more youth-friendly.

Pressure groups, champions and the voice of young people

Professional groups, charities, individual practitioners and adolescents themselves have important roles in influencing policy. The Royal College of Nursing Adolescent Health Forum has produced guidance on caring for adolescents (RCN 1994, 2002, 2008a), and the British Medical Association (BMA 2003, 2006) reviewed evidence surrounding nutrition, exercise and obesity; smoking, drinking and drug use; mental health; and sexual health. An intercollegiate consensus of views about adolescent health-care needs was achieved in *Bridging the Gaps: Health Care for Adolescents* (RCPCH 2003). Young People in Focus is a charity that helps individuals and organisations working with young people and families through research, training and publications; it regularly produces *Key Data on Adolescence* (Coleman & Brooks 2009) which is an invaluable source of information about young people and their lives. The recently formed charity and membership forum, the Association for Young People's Health, brings together professionals and organisations to share learning and best practice to promote better services to meet young people's health needs and campaigns to improve the coverage teenagers receive in the media. Individuals, too, can act as change agents and champions, campaigning and speaking out, researching and implementing evidence-based practice. Most importantly, the voice of young people is increasingly being heard; examples of adolescent *voice* include participation in research (Fraser *et al.* 2004) and 11 MILLION, the organisation led by the Children's Commissioner for England, a role created by the Children Act (2004) to promote the views of children. Through 11 MILLION, young people's views can be used to shape policies and decision-making. Sir Al Aynsley-Green, the first commissioner, has raised awareness of many issues including children with mental health problems being placed in adult wards and, most recently, bereavement; however, there is debate about the power and future of this office which is seen by some as an expensive *quango* (Wilby 2009).

Rights

The United Nations Convention on the Rights of the Child (United Nations 1989) has been a powerful driver for promoting the development of adolescent health-care policy and practice; its principles are reflected in UK policy and law, for example, the Children Act 1989, *Every Child Matters* and the appointment of a children's commissioner. It identifies a wide range of rights for children; these are often reduced to the *3Ps* providing a simplistic, but useful, framework for examining adolescent health issues: '(1) The right to *provision* of basic needs. (2) The right to *protection* from harmful acts and practices. (3) The right to *participation* in decisions affecting their lives' (Lurie 2003). Balancing these rights in practice often leads to tensions and contradictions. 'This is particularly the case with protection and participation rights, where the desire to protect children from too much responsibility, or from decisions that are too difficult may often result in limits on their right to participate in decision-making (Flekkoy & Kaufman 1997)' (Lurie 2003). This is apparent in the debate about providing sex education and presents barriers to practice leaving practitioners in a vulnerable position caught between opposing views (Brown & Simpson 2000; RCN 2005; Staines 2009); following research and consultation, the government has made personal social and health education compulsory from 2011 and lowered the age at which parents have the right to withdraw their children from sex education classes to 15 in an attempt to develop policy that balances the rights of adolescents and parents and has the potential to empower practitioners with clear guidance (DCSF 2009a).

Provision

Nurses have had an important role in the debate about providing care for adolescents in hospital since the Platt Report (DHSS 1959:8) identified that 'adolescents need their own accommodation, but if the numbers admitted do not permit this it is better for them to be nursed with children than with adults'. Viner & Keane (1998) identified that commissioning and provision of care for adolescents in hospital was poor and provided practical evidence-based guidance for establishing and operating adolescent inpatient units; they found the nursing literature on caring for adolescents in hospital was large and made up the largest proportion of the studies in their review. A national survey of use of hospital beds by adolescents in the UK found use of beds increased rather than decreased through adolescence, contradicting 'the assumption that adolescents use hospitals rarely and do not merit separate facilities' (Viner 2001:958). In response, Macfarlane & Blum (2001:942) acknowledged the case for separate units but recommended that even if numbers did not justify a separate ward 'a multidisciplinary approach from health professionals with interest and expertise in adolescent health is still feasible in every hospital … to truly realise a vision where all young people can receive the comprehensive services they need to become healthy adults we need to ensure that all health professionals in both primary and secondary care have the training they need to provide optimal care'; both recommendations are key elements of *Every Child Matters*, that is, integrated working and the Common Core of Skills and Knowledge for the Children's Workforce (DfES 2005b).

Research has demonstrated that adolescent inpatient wards improve quality of care for adolescents compared with children's or adult wards; however, 'few young people in the UK are currently managed on adolescent wards. These data support the further development of adult wards in larger general hospitals and children's hospitals' (Viner 2007b). Provision of such units has been boosted by funding from the Teenage Cancer Trust which also promotes awareness raising and education. The Scottish Government (2009) has reinforced the need for improved adolescent hospital services emphasising that 'service provision needs to be responsive to the emerging autonomy and independence of adolescent patients and to encourage them to take responsibility for their own health' (p. 2) but acknowledging that 'progress has been slow and incomplete' (p. 4). Nurses may not be able to control resources for optimum care but can attempt to implement evidence-based practice and participate in research to develop and evaluate practice.

Protection

In *The Protection of Children in England: A Progress Report* (2009) Laming acknowledged the 'vulnerability of adolescents, regardless of their bravado' (p. 2); he credited the Government for recent legislation and guidance: '*Every Child Matters* clearly has the support of professionals, across all of the services, who work with children and young people. The interagency guidance *Working Together to Safeguard Children* provides a sound framework for professionals to protect children and promote their welfare' and recognised that 'the need to protect children and young people from significant harm and neglect is ever more challenging' (pp. 3–4). Chally & Loric (1998:17) define an ethical dilemma as 'a moral problem involving two or more mutually exclusive, morally correct actions'. In safeguarding adolescents, the disclosure of risk-taking behaviour is a typical dilemma raising issues of confidentiality and information sharing.

Rogstad (2007) explores the ethical dilemma practitioners face when deciding whether to report sexually active adolescents to child protection services. The *Sexual Offences Act* (HMSO 2003) introduced measures to protect children, making sexual activity in under-16-year-olds illegal and classifying sexual activity with under-13-year-olds as rape; however, evidence demonstrates that adolescents are becoming sexually active at a younger age with associated health risks and that without confidentiality they are unlikely to attend health services. The situation is perplexing for adolescents, parents and practitioners. Confidentiality and information sharing are problematic in practice; Lord Laming (2009:40) found 'Despite the fact that the Government gave clear guidance on information sharing in 2006 and updated it in October 2008, there continues to be a real concern across all sectors, but particularly in the health services, about the risk of breaching confidentiality or data protection law by sharing concerns about a child's safety. The laws governing data protection and privacy are still not well understood by frontline staff or their managers. It is clear that different agencies (and their legal advisers) often take different approaches'. This highlights the challenge of integrated working and, for individual practitioners, the tension of the duty of care and the duty of confidentiality. There is a plethora of statutory, professional and lay guidance for those caught in this dilemma.

Government (DCSF 2009b) guidance is helpful and includes *seven golden rules*, case examples and a flowchart with key questions to guide practitioners in the decision whether to share information or not. Guidance is also available from Local Safeguarding Children Boards, Caldicott Guardians and professional bodies, for example, NMC and RCN. *Working within the Sexual Offences Act 2003* (Home Office 2004:6) offers useful clarification for practitioners in relation to sexual health work with adolescents: 'although the age of consent remains at 16, the law is not intended to prosecute mutually agreed teenage sexual activity between two young people of a similar age, unless it involves abuse or exploitation. Young people, including those under 13, will continue to have the right to confidential advice on contraception, condoms, pregnancy and abortion'. The third sector again has an important role to play in promoting good practice in adolescent healthcare; NSPCC and Brook offer clear interpretations of policy and law and guidance for practice. Despite this abundance of guidance, adolescents, parents and practitioners can be faced with difficult situations. Rogstad (2007) concludes that best practice involves providing individualised care, basing decisions on the best interests of the adolescent, asking advice within or outside the team, always being able to justify each decision to refer or not, and keeping appropriate records. Decision-making could be enhanced further by research into how to identify at-risk adolescents who should be referred to child protection services (McGough *et al.* 2006; Sykes & O'Sullivan 2006).

Participation

Participation rights are of more recent origin than provision and protection rights and are 'more controversial and more difficult to implement than protection rights because these rights are seen as threatening by many adults, who fear that they will undermine parental authority and family stability' (Lurie 2003). Viner & Barker (2005:901) emphasise that a 'prominent theme in recent government policy has been supporting self care for patients with long term conditions. Self management behaviours in long term illness are … laid down in adolescence. It makes sense to focus "expert patient" initiatives on young people, in whom the payback will be greater over longer periods'. This approach is crucial in the care of adolescents who are surviving into adulthood with chronic, complex conditions and can be achieved through their participation in consent, decision-making and planning transition from children's to adults' services. Despite clear guidance (DoH 2009) which outlines the legal position concerning consent and refusal of treatment by children and young people under the age of 18, the challenge of assessing competence still taxes practitioners (Hedley 2007; Vernon & Welbury 2007). Real difficulties arise, for example, when a young person wants to discontinue treatment; nurses may not be individually responsible for making a decision in this event, but will be part of the inter-professional team contributing to decision-making. Thompson *et al.* (2006) highlight the need for good communication and clarity about roles, rules, responsibilities and reporting in ethical decision-making in teams to avoid conflict and problematic power relationships; they conclude that understanding the ethics of complex situations 'may have more to do with analysing the power relations involved, than questions of disagreements of principle' (p. 97). Interprofessional education (IPE) could provide opportunities for practitioners to learn about each other's roles and explore power relationships.

Court (DHSS 1976:175) recognised that the 'transfer of health care and surveillance from the child-oriented to adult services is a cause of much concern. It would be neither possible nor desirable to set rigid demarcation lines ... we recognise the need for flexibility and for ascertaining the adolescent's own wishes'. Since then, the development of transition care has received much attention (McDonagh 2009). Guidance has been produced (DoH 2006, 2008; DCSF/DoH 2007) to show that the handover from children's services to adult services for adolescents with complex health needs or a disability should be planned and managed as a process based on individual needs rather than as an event at a particular age. Practical guidance (RCN 2004, 2008b) recognises that adolescents should be encouraged to participate at every stage. One young man (Warham 1998) who has experienced transition highlights the adolescent's role: 'Let people know what you think and feel, if you don't tell them, they can't help'. Despite wide recognition of the need for children to participate in health care there is limited evidence to suggest that

it is widely practiced (Franklin & Sloper 2005). However, there are many frameworks nurses can use to develop and evaluate participatory work and avoid tokenism, for example, Hart's Ladder of Participation (Smith & Coleman 2009) and *Involving Children and Young People in Health Care: A Planning Tool* (ASC 2009).

Education

'Fifty per cent of nurses admit to having difficulty meeting the needs and demands of teenage patients' (Norwich Union 2001). Literature and policy consistently highlight the need for specialist education, before and after qualification, for practitioners working in adolescent health care (De Sousa 2002; DoH 2007), but there is still limited provision (Coleman *et al.* 2007). Post-qualification nursing courses exist, for example, *Adolescent Health CPPD* provided by Thames Valley University, and the importance of IPE is recognised in the interactive e-learning *Adolescent Health Project* (RCPCH 2009) which is funded by the Department of Health and aimed at all health professionals involved with adolescents. Balint groups are a way of learning about and reflecting on the emotional content of working with adolescents. The Balint method involves regular case discussions in small groups under the guidance of a qualified leader; most commonly used by GPs for teaching, learning and research, a recent development has been the introduction of multidisciplinary groups. The Balints, who started these groups in the 1950s, aimed at 'a free give-and take atmosphere in which everyone could bring up his problems in the hope of getting some light on them from the experience of others' (Donovan & Suckling 2004:114).

Education needs to provide practitioners with opportunities to develop the knowledge, skills and attitudes that are needed for coping with ethical issues in adolescent care. Practitioners need to be able to define and analyse ethical issues in everyday practice and dilemmas, such as confidentiality and consent. They need to understand ethical approaches, for example, debating the advantages of principalism and narrative ethics (McCarthy 2003), and to develop the critical and reflective skills needed for ethical decision-making. Opportunities are also needed to develop communication skills, self-awareness and the ability to cope with the emotional labour and challenges of working with adolescents. Quallington (2000:6) found that nurses recognised ethical situations 'because of the feelings that they engendered; negative feelings of discomfort, anxiety and confusion'. Reflection is a useful device for exploring ethical issues and is recognised as an educational strategy to develop emotionally competent practitioners by encouraging them to 'challenge beliefs by applying deductive reasoning with the unique addition of considering feelings' (Horton-Deutch & Sherwood 2008:947).

Reflection

There has been remarkable worldwide acceptance of the potential of reflection to help nurses to develop and learn from practice individually or in groups (Bulman & Schutz 2008). It involves 'reviewing experience from practice so that it may be described, analysed, evaluated and consequently used to inform and change future practice. Importantly, reflection also involves opening up one's practice for others to examine, and consequently requires courage and open-mindedness as well as a willingness to take on board and act on criticism (Dewey 1933). In this context, reflection involves more than "intellectual thinking" since it is intermingled with practitioners' feelings and emotions and acknowledges an interrelationship with action' (Bulman 2008:2). Johns' model (Johns 2009) is useful in learning about adolescent care as it cues reflection on feelings and ethical issues through The Model for Structured Reflection (MSR) and use of ethical mapping. The model has been demonstrated to be helpful in developing students' self-awareness and caring potential (Noveletsky-Rosenthal & Solomon 2001).

The MSR offers reflective cues that can be used to trigger reflection on the feelings aroused by a situation including 'How do I interpret the way people were feeling and why they felt that way? How was I feeling and what made me feel that way? What was I trying to achieve and did I respond effectively? What were the consequences of my actions on the patient, others and myself? What factors influence the way I was/am feeling, thinking and responding to this situation?' (Johns 2009:51). The cue that triggers exploration of ethical issues is 'To

what extent did I act for the best and in tune with my values?' (Johns 2009:51); Johns developed ethical mapping and the ethical map trail to guide practitioners in exploring *acting for the best*, that is, 'Frame the dilemma; Consider the perspective of different actors, commencing with your own perspectives. Consider which ethical principles apply in terms of the best (ethically correct) decision. Consider what conflict exists between perspectives/values and how these might be resolved. Consider who had authority for making the decision/taking action. Consider the power relationships/factors that determined the way the decision/action was actually taken' (Johns 2009:65–66). Johns (1999:289) explains that ethical mapping 'guides the practitioner to view the various perspectives and contextual factors within any ethical decision' and illustrates its use through an account of a nurse reflecting on the care of a university student who had attempted to commit suicide and whether to inform the parents of the extent of his injuries. This model, used in practice in clinical supervision or in nurse education in reflective groups, can facilitate practitioners in reflecting on issues that concern them in adolescent care, whether it is the challenge of providing the best possible care in the less than ideal environment of a children's ward for an adolescent who has self-harmed, or the dilemma of whether to report a sexually active 13-year-old to child protection services.

Conclusion

Few client groups can provoke debate the way that adolescents can. They defy classification by age and are difficult to define leading to problems even in the terminology we use to describe them; but whatever label we apply to them it is clear that practitioners face unique ethical challenges in working with them. There has been significant interest in their health at policy and practice level in recent years with recognition that it is imperative to address deficits in their health care. Rights to provision, protection and participation have been used in this chapter to analyse key issues in adolescent care and it has been suggested that reflection using Johns' MSR provides a constructive means of facing the challenges of working with this thought-provoking group.

Reflective scenario

Stacey, a 13-year-old girl, tells you that she had unprotected sex for the first time with her boyfriend yesterday when they were at a party and they had been drinking. She wants to take the *morning after pill* but does not know how to get it and wants to know what she should do in future so that she does not get pregnant. Her boyfriend is 14 years old and they have been together since she started secondary school. She does not want her parents to know as she says they will be very angry and will try to end the relationship.

1. What are Stacey's rights in this situation?
2. What action would you take and why?
3. What would your feelings be about providing Stacey with contraceptive advice without informing her parents?

References

ASC (2009) *Involving Children and Young People in Health Care: A Planning Tool.* Action for Sick Children, London. Accessed at http://actionforsickchildren.org/assets/children%20guide.pdf on 24/10/2009.

Batchelor, S. & Raymond, M. (2004) 'I Slept with 40 Boys in Three Months.' Teenage sexuality in the media: Too much too young? In: *Young People and Sexual Health, Individuality, Social and Policy Contexts* (eds E. Burtney & M. Duffy), Chapter 14. Palgrave Macmillan, Basingstoke.

BMA (2003) *Adolescent Health.* British Medical Association, London. Accessed at http://www.bma.org.uk/images/Adhealth_tcm41-19549.pdf on 6/8/2009.

BMA (2006) *Child and Adolescent Mental Health.* British Medical Association, London. Accessed at http://www.bma.org.uk/health_promotion_ethics/child_health/Childadolescentmentalhealth.jsp on 6/8/2009.

Briggs, S. (2008) *Working with Adolescents and Young Adults, A Contemporary Psychodynamic Approach*, 2nd edn. Palgrave Macmillan, Basingstoke.

Broadhurst, K., Grover, C. & Jamieson, J. (eds) (2009) *Critical Perspectives on Safeguarding Children.* John Wiley & Sons Ltd., Chichester.

Brooks, L. (2009) You can't buy a hamster, but you can be tried as an adult. *The Guardian,* 2 October, p. 40.

Brown, E.J. & Simpson, E.M. (2000) Comprehensive STD/HIV prevention targeting US adolescents: Review of an ethical dilemma and proposed ethical framework. *Nursing Ethics,* 7 (4), 339–348.

Bulman, C. (2008) An introduction to reflection. In: *Reflective Practice in Nursing* (eds C. Bulman & S. Schutz), Chapter 1, 4th edn. Blackwell Publishing Ltd., Oxford.

Bulman, C. & Schutz, S. (eds) (2008) *Reflective Practice in Nursing*, 4th edn. Blackwell Publishing Ltd., Oxford.

Byron, T. (2009) *We See Children as Pestilent.* Accessed at http://www.guardian.co.uk/education/2009/mar/17/ephebiphobia-young-people-mosquito on 6/4/2009.

Chally, P.S. & Loric, L. (1998) Ethics in the trenches: Decision making in practice. *American Journal of Nursing,* **98** (6), 17–20.

Coleman, J. & Brooks, F. (2009) *Key Data on Adolescence, The Latest Information and Statistics about Young People Today.* AYPH Ltd and TSA Ltd., Brighton.

Coleman, J. & Hagell, A. (eds) (2007) *Adolescence Risk and Resilience, Against the Odds.* John Wiley & Sons, Chichester.

Coleman, J. & Hendry, L.B. (1999) *The Nature of Adolescence*, 3rd edn. Routledge, London.

Coleman, J., Hendry, L.B. & Kloep, M. (eds) (2007) *Adolescence and Health.* John Wiley & Sons, Chichester.

Connexions Direct (2009) *Your Rights, When Can I?* Connexions Direct, Cumbria. Accessed at http://www.connexions-direct.com/index.cfm?catalogueContentID=176&pid=161&render=detailedArticle on 29/10/2009.

Dennehy, A., Smith, L. & Harker, P. (1998) *Not to Be Ignored: Young People, Poverty and Health.* Child Poverty Action Group, London.

DCSF/DoH (2007) *A Transition Guide for All Services: Key Information for Professionals about the Transition Process for Disabled Young People.* Department for Children, Schools and Families/Department of Health, London.

DCSF (2009a) *Ed Balls: All Children to Learn about Personal Finance and Healthier Lifestyles.* Department for Children, Schools and Families, London. Accessed at http://www.dcsf.gov.uk/news/content.cfm?landing=ed_balls_all_children_to_learn_about_personal_finance_and_healthier_lifestyles&type=1 on 9/11/09.

DCSF (2009b) *HM Government Information Sharing Guidance.* Department for Children, Schools and Families, London. Accessed at http://www.dcsf.gov.uk/everychildmatters/resources-and-practice/IG00340/ on 9/11/09.

De Sousa, M. (2002) Generation gap. *Nursing Standard,* **16** (38), 96.

Dexter, Y. (2008) Responding to the needs of younger people: The bereaved adolescent. In *Contemporary Issues in Mental Health Nursing* (eds J.E. & S. Trenoweth), Chapter 14. John Wiley & Sons, Chichester.

DfES (2004) Every *Child Matters: Change for Children Programme*. Department for Education and Skills, The Stationary Office, London.

DfES (2005a) *Youth Matters: Summary*. Department for Education and Skills Publications, Nottingham.

DfES (2005b) *Common Core of Skills and Knowledge for the Children's Workforce*. Department for Education and Skills Publications, Nottingham.

DHSS (1959) *The Welfare of Children in Hospital*. Her Majesty's Stationary Office, London.

DHSS (1976) *Fit for the Future: Report of the Committee on Child Health Services*. HMSO, London.

DoH (1997) Health Committee Third Report, *Health Services for Children and Young People in the Community*. Department of Health, Home and School, Her Majesty's Stationary Office, London.

DoH (2004) *National Service Framework for Children, Young People and Maternity Services: Executive Summary*. Department of Health, London. Accessed at http://www. dh.gov.uk/dr_consum_dh/groups/dh_digitalassets/ @dh/@en/documents/digitalasset/dh_4090552.pdf on 7/11/09.

DoH (2006) *Transition: Getting It Right for Young People, Improving the Transition of Young People with Long Term Conditions from Children's to Adult Health Services*. Department of Health, London.

DoH (2007) *You're Welcome Quality Criteria, Making Health Services Young People Friendly*, 2nd edn. Department of Health, London. Accessed at http://www.dh.gov. uk/en/Publicationsandstatistics/Publications/ PublicationsPolicyAndGuidance/DH_073586   on 6/8/2009.

DoH (2008) *Transition: Moving on Well, A Good Practice Guide for Health Professionals and Their Partners on Transition Planning for Young People with Complex Health Needs or a Disability*. Department of Health, London. Accessed at http://www.dh.gov.uk/en/Healthcare/ Children/Transitionfromchildrenstoadultservices/ index.htm on 22/10/2009.

DoH (2009) *Reference Guide to Consent for Examination or Treatment*, 2nd edn. Department of Health, London. Accessed at http://www.dh.gov.uk/en/ Publicationsandstatistics/Publications/Publications PolicyAndGuidance/DH_103643 on 6/8/2009.

Donovan, C. & Suckling, H. (2004) *Difficult Consultations with Adolescents*. Radcliffe Publishing Ltd., Oxford.

Fawcett, B., Featherstone, B. & Goddard, J. (2004) *Contemporary Child Care Policy and Practice*. Palgrave Macmillan, Basingstoke.

Foley, P. (2008) Health matters. In: *Promoting Children's Wellbeing, Policy and Practice* (eds J. Collins & P. Foley), Chapter 3. The Policy Press and Milton Keynes, The Open University, Bristol.

Franklin, A. & Sloper, P. (2005) Listening and responding? Children's participation in health care within England. *International Journal of Children's Rights*, **13**, 11–29.

Fraser, S., Lewis, V., Ding, S., Kellett, M. & Robinson, C. (eds) (2004) *Doing Research with Children and Young People*. Sage Publications in association with The Open University, London.

Hall, D. (2002) Foreword in RCPCH (2003). *Bridging the Gaps: Health Care for Adolescents*. RCPCH, London. Accessed at http://www.rcpsych.ac.uk/files/pdfversion/cr114.pdf on 6/8/2009.

Hedley, M. (2007) Treating children: Whose consent counts. In: *Ethical, Legal and Social Aspects of Child Healthcare* (ed. P. Cartlidge), Chapter 39. Elsevier, Edinburgh.

HMSO (2003) *Sexual Offences Act (2003)*. Her Majesty's Stationary Office, London. Accessed at http://www. opsi.gov.uk/acts/acts2003/ukpga_20030042_en_1 on 8/11/09.

Holmbeck, G.N. (2002) A developmental perspective on adolescent health and illness: An introduction to the special issues. *Journal of Pediatric Psychology*, **27** (5), 409–416.

Home Office (2004) *Working within the Sexual Offences Act*. Home Office, England. Accessed at http://www. teachernet.gov.uk/_doc/6674/care-workers.pdf   on 9/11/09.

Horton-Deutch, S. & Sherwood, G. (2008) Reflection: An educational strategy to develop emotionally-competent nurse leaders. *Journal of Nursing Management*, **16**, 946–954.

Johns, C. (1999) Unravelling the dilemmas within everyday nursing practice. *Nursing Ethics*, **6** (4), 287–298.

Johns, C. (2009) *Becoming a Reflective Practitioner*, 3rd edn. Wiley-Blackwell, Chichester.

Jones, G. (2005) Young adults and the extension of economic dependence. National Family and Parenting Institute Policy Discussion Paper. Accessed at http://www.familyandparenting.org/Filestore/ Documents/publications/YouthDep.pdf on 20/09/2010.

Jones, R. & Bradley, E. (2007) Health issues for adolescents. *Paediatrics and Child Health*, **17** (11), 433–488.

Larcher, V. (2005) Consent, competence and confidentiality. In: *ABC of Adolescence* (ed. R. Viner), Chapter 2. Blackwell Publishing, Oxford.

Lewis, E. & Heer, B. (2008) *Delivering Every Child Matters in Secure Settings, A Practical Toolkit for Improving the Health and Well-Being of Young People*. National Children's Bureau, London. Accessed at http://www.

ncb.org.uk/dotpdf/open_access_2/hein_toolkit_final.pdf on 4/11/09.

Lord Laming (2009) *The Protection of Children in England, A Progress Report*. The Stationary Office, London.

Lurie, J. (2003) The tension between protection and participation, general theory and consequences as related to rights of children. *IUC Journal of Social Work*, **7**, 7.7. Accessed at http://www.bemidjistate.edu/academics/publications/social_work_journal/issue07/articles/Tension.htm on 23/10/2009.

Macfarlane, A. & Blum, R.W. (2001) Do we need specialist adolescent units in hospitals? Possibly. *British Medical Journal*, **322**, 941–942.

McCarthy, J. (2003) Principlism or narrative ethics: Must we choose between them? *Medical Humanities*, **29**, 65–71.

McDonagh, J. (2009) *Growing Up Ready for Emerging Adulthood, An Evidence Base for Professionals Involved in Transitional Care for Young People with Chronic Illness and/or Disabilities*. Department of Health, London. Accessed at http://www.dh.gov.uk/en/Healthcare/Children/Transitionfromchildrenstoadultservices/index.htm on 22/10/2009.

McGough, P., Thow, C., Butt, A., Lamont, M. & Bigrigg, A. (2006) Recording what happens in the under-16 consultation. *Journal of Family Planning and Reproductive Health Care*, **32** (2), 95–99.

NCB (2008) *Bereavement in the Secure Setting, Delivering Every Child Matters for Bereaved Young People in Custody*. National Children's Bureau, London. Accessed at http://www.ncb.org.uk/dotpdf/open_access_2/bereavement_secure_setting.pdf on 4/11/09.

NCB (2009) *Healthier Inside*. National Children's Bureau, London. Accessed at http://www.ncb.org.uk/resources/free_resources/healthier_inside.aspx on 7/11/09.

NHS Scotland (2009) *Walk the Talk*. NHS Scotland, Scotland. Project accessed at http://www.walk-the-talk.org.uk/index.aspx on 10/11/09.

Norwich Union (2001) *The Views of Adolescents and Nurses on the Provision of Healthcare in Hospital*. Norwich Union, Norwich.

Noveletsky-Rosenthal, H. & Solomon, K. (2001) Reflections on the use of Johns' model of structured reflection in nurse-practitioner education. *International Journal for Human Caring*, **5** (2), 21–26.

Phillips, M. (2008) *Children's Rights? What about the Rights of Those Who Live in Fear of Young Thugs?"*. The Daily Mail, London. Accessed at http://www.dailymail.co.uk/debate/columnists/article-515469/Childrens-rights-What-rights-live-fear-young-thugs.html on 6/11/09.

Pomerantz, K.A., Hughes, M. & Thompson, D. (eds) (2007) *How to Reach 'Hard to Reach' Children, Improving*

Access, Participation and Outcomes. John Wiley & Sons Ltd., Chichester.

Quallington, J. (2000) Ethical reflection: A role for ethics in nursing practice. In: *Empowerment through Reflection, The Narratives of Healthcare Professionals* (eds T. Ghaye, D. Gillespie & S. Lillyman), Chapter 1. Quay Books, Wiltshire.

RCN (1994) *Caring for Adolescents*. The Royal College of Nursing, London.

RCN (2002) *Caring for Young People, Guidance for Nursing Staff*. The Royal College of Nursing, London.

RCN (2004) *Adolescent Transition Care, Guidance for Nursing Staff*. The Royal College of Nursing, London.

RCN (2005) *Signpost Guide for Nurses Working with Young People, Sex and Relationships Education*. The Royal College of Nursing, London.

RCN (2008a) *Adolescence: Boundaries and Connections*. The Royal College of Nursing, London.

RCN (2008b) *Lost in Transition, Moving Young People between Child and Adult Health Services*. The Royal College of Nursing, London.

RCPCH (2003) *Bridging the Gaps: Health Care for Adolescents*. Royal College of Paediatrics and Child Health, London. Accessed at http://www.rcpsych.ac.uk/files/pdfversion/cr114.pdf on 6/8/2009.

RCPCH (2009) *Adolescent Health Project*. Royal College of Paediatrics and Child Health, London. Accessed at http://www.rcpch.ac.uk/Education/Adolescent-Health-Project on 9/11/09.

Rogstad, K.E. (2007) Confidentiality versus child protection for young people accessing sexual health services: "To report or not to report, that is the question." *Journal of Family Planning and Reproductive Health Care*, **33** (1), 7–9.

Smith, L. & Coleman, V. (eds) (2009) *Child and Family-Centred Healthcare, Concept, Theory and Practice*. Palgrave Macmillan, Basingstoke.

Social Exclusion Unit (2005) *Transitions, A Social Exclusion Unit Interim Report on Young Adults*. Office of the Deputy Prime Minister, London.

Staines, R. (2009) New government approach for tackling teenage pregnancies. *Paediatric Nursing*, **21** (8), 6–7.

Steinberg, L. (2008) *Adolescence*, 8th edn. McGraw Hill, Boston.

Sykes, S. & O'Sullivan, K. (2006) A 'mystery shopper' project to evaluate sexual health and contraceptive services for young people in Croydon. *Journal of Family Planning and Reproductive Health Care*, **32** (1), 25–26.

The Children's Society (2009) Recommendations from *The Good Childhood Inquiry*. The Children's Society, England. Accessed at http://www.childrenssociety.org.uk/all_about_us/how_we_do_it/the_good_childhood_inquiry/recommendations/14606.html on 16/2/2009.

The Scottish Government (2009) *Better Health, Better Care, Hospital Services for Young People in Scotland*. The Scottish Government, Edinburgh.

Thompson, I.E., Melia, K.M., Boyd, K.M. & Horsburgh, D. (eds) (2006) *Nursing Ethics*, 5th edn. Churchill Livingstone Elsevier, Edinburgh.

United Nations (1989) *United Nations Convention on the Rights of the Child*. United Nations, Geneva.

Valentine, F. & Lowes, L. (2007) *Nursing Care of Children and Young People with Chronic Illness*. Blackwell Publishing Ltd., Oxford.

Vernon, B. & Welbury, J. (2007) Consent for the examination or treatment of teenagers. In: *Ethical, Legal and Social Aspects of Child Healthcare* (ed. P. Cartlidge), Chapter 38. Elsevier, Edinburgh.

Viner, R. (2001) National survey of use of hospital beds by adolescents aged 12 to 19 in the United Kingdom. *British Medical Journal*, **322**, 957–958.

Viner, R. (2007a) Preface. In: *Adolescence and Health* (eds J. Coleman, L.B. Hendry & M. Kloep). John Wiley & Sons, Chichester.

Viner, R. (2007b) Do adolescent inpatient units make a difference? Findings from a national young patient survey. *Archives of Disease in Childhood*, **92** (Suppl. 1), A69.

Viner, R. & Barker, M. (2005) Young people's health: The need for action. *British Medical Journal*, **330** (16 April), 901–903.

Viner, R. & Keane, M. (1998) *Youth Matters: Evidence-based Practice for the Care of Young People in Hospital*. Action for Sick Children, London.

Warham, J. (1998) Transferring to an adult unit. *Cascade*, **27**, 10–11.

Webster, C. Simpson, D., MacDonald, R., Abbas, A., Cieslik, M., Shildrick, T. & Simpson, M. (2004) *Poor Transitions, Social Exclusion and Young Adults*. The Policy Press, Bristol. Accessed at http://www.jrf.org.uk/sites/files/jrf/1861347340.pdf on 6/11/09.

Wilby, P. (2009) Young at heart, the choice of the next children's commissioner has been mired in controversy, but what legacy does the incumbent, Sir Al Aynsley-Green, leave his successor? *Education Guardian*, 3 November 2009, pp. 1–2.

Young Minds (2009) *The YoungMinds Children and Young People's Manifesto*. Accessed at http://www.youngminds.org.uk/young-people/YoungMinds%20Manifesto%20Oct09.pdf on 20/9/2010.

Web sites

Action for Sick Children www.actionforsickchildren.org

Association for Young People's Health www.youngpeopleshealth.org.uk

Brook Advisory Organisation www.brook.org.uk

Child Poverty Action Group www.cpag.org.uk

National Society for the Protection of Cruelty to Children (NSPCC) www.nspcc.org.uk

Teenage Cancer Trust www.teenagecancertrust.org

Young People in Focus www.youngpeopleinfocus.org.uk

Walk the Talk www.walk-the-talk.org.uk

Suggested further readings

Coleman, J., Hendry, L.B. & Kloep, M. (eds) (2007) *Adolescence and Health*. John Wiley & Sons, Chichester.

DCSF (2007) *Integrated Working Exemplar: Teenage Sexual Health and Pregnancy, INTEGRATED Working to Improve Outcomes for Children and Young People*. Department for Children, Schools and Families, London. Accessed at http://www.dcsf.gov.uk/every childmatters/resources-and-practice/IG00258/ on 25/11/09.

Rogstad, K.E. (2007) Confidentiality versus child protection for young people accessing sexual health services: "To report or not to report, that is the question". *Journal of Family Planning and Reproductive Health*, **33** (1), 7–9.

Viner, R. & Barker, M. (2005) Young people's health: The need for action. *British Medical Journal*, **330** (16 April), 901–903.

Web sites

Association for Young People's Health www.youngpeopleshealth.org.uk

Young People in Focus www.youngpeopleinfocus.org.uk

11 MILLION www.11million.org.uk

10 Ethical and Legal Aspects of Working with Children and Young People with Emotional and Psychiatric Health Needs

Tim McDougall

Introduction

This chapter is structured in three parts. First is a discussion of the role of the nurse in supporting children and young people with mental health problems. Second is a focus on the processes of engagement, assessment and treatment in order to illustrate the range of moral and ethical issues that arise. Third is a summary of recent changes to the Mental Health Act, the Mental Capacity Act and the Children Act as they affect children and young people with mental disorders.

SECTION ONE

What do we mean by children and young people's mental health?

The terms *mental health* and *mental health problems* are often used interchangeably and this can be misleading. Mental health, or emotional health and well-being as it is increasingly known in children's services, is used to refer to psychological building blocks such as emotional resilience, good self-esteem and the skills to resolve conflict and cope in the face of stress and adversity. All chil-

dren should have the opportunity to develop good emotional health, and this is fundamental to their overall health and well-being. In comparison, the terms *mental health problems* and *mental disorders* refer to problems that require resolution. Mental health problems are often not serious and many are transient in nature. Whilst they can interfere with a child's development and functioning, they are distinguished from mental disorders as being less severe, complex or persistent in nature. Mental health problems and disorders manifest in children's behaviour, how they feel and what they tell us.

Background

There are over 11 million children under 18 living in England, and as many as 1 million will have a mental health problem serious enough to require specialist help (Green *et al.* 2005). This is in addition to many more young people with significant mental health needs, including children in need, looked-after children and disabled children, all of whom are at heightened risk of developing mental health problems and disorders (Department for Education and Skills 2007). Rates of mental disorder rise steeply during late

Ethical and Philosophical Aspects of Nursing Children, First Edition. Edited by Gosia M. Brykczyńska and Joan Simons.
© 2011 Blackwell Publishing Ltd. Published 2011 by Blackwell Publishing Ltd.

adolescence and early adulthood. Of the 7 million young people aged between 16 and 25 in the UK, as many as 1 million will have a mood or anxiety disorder, and 13,000 will have a psychotic disorder (YoungMinds 2006).

Epidemiological research has been confirmed by the voices of service users. The Princes Trust recently interviewed 2000 young people aged between 16 and 25 across Great Britain. Nearly half told researchers they felt regularly stressed, over a quarter reported that they were often or always down or depressed and 1 in 10 insisted that life was meaningless (Princes Trust 2009). The most hopeless attitudes were found among those not in education, employment or training. Young people in this group were significantly less happy and lacked confidence in every aspect of their lives. A recent report on child well-being published by UNICEF (2007) suggested that out of 21 economically advanced nations across the developed world, the UK has the unhappiest children.

These issues should concern each and every one of us. They show all too clearly that many of our nations' children are unhappy and hopeless. The emotional health and well-being of children and young people should be of major concern to leaders since the future prosperity of our country and its inhabitants depends crucially on the future health and welfare of our children. However, this basic moral endeavour has been a difficult case to make to policy makers.

Investing early to save later

The emotional health and well-being of children and young people is now a key plank of policy and strategy in all four countries of the UK (Leighton 2006; McDougall 2006). Internationally, governments are becoming increasingly aware that there are numerous reasons to invest now for the future economy and prosperity of their respective countries. The last two decades has witnessed a growing interest in universal and targeted programmes to prevent poor outcomes for children and families. Treatment at an earlier stage is likely to be more effective and less costly than that which will be needed over a lifetime if the opportunity for early intervention is missed (Layard 2004; Policy Research Bureau 2007). Research and outcome studies prove clearly that untreated mental health

problems place children and young people on developmental trajectories towards educational failure, family dysfunction, poor physical health, crime and antisocial behaviour. Many unresolved mental health problems in childhood persist into adulthood, disrupting personal development, social functioning and economic well-being. Moreover, there is the moral obligation to do all that is possible to help facilitate the positive development of all children.

Recent reports have attempted to quantify the costs of untreated mental health problems to our society. A compelling report jointly published by Action for Children and the New Economic Foundation (2009) suggests that failure to tackle the psychosocial problems that combine to produce negative outcomes for young people may cost the UK economy as much as £4 trillion over 20 years. The report called *Backing the Future* goes on to suggest that savings to the UK economy through interventions to prevent poverty, family breakdown, social exclusion and mental disorder may be as high as £486 billion over two decades. In the current financial climate, it is more important than ever for services to get it right first time for children and young people. The King's Fund (2009) has projected that the cost of mental health services will increase from £22.5 billion in 2007 to at least £32.6 billion by 2026. If we add loss of earnings and the costs that fall to other agencies, this figure will be even higher.

What are child and adolescent mental health services?

Usually referred to by its acronym CAMHS, child and adolescent mental health services refers to a network of universal, targeted and specialist services that are collectively designed to meet the emotional and psychological needs of children and young people. However, the term *CAMHS* is used in a variety of different ways and this often causes confusion. This can be in the minds of service commissioners and managers, individual professionals (including nurses) and the general public. Although various attempts have been made to clarify what CAMHS means in practice, debate continues within the professions and services and consensus about what the term means has not been reached (McDougall 2006). For the purposes of this chapter,

CAMHS is used in two ways. First, it refers to service provision that leads to an improvement in the emotional health and well-being of children and young people, whether provided by specialist teams or by professionals whose responsibility for the mental health of children and young people is only one part of their role. Here, the terms *primary*, *universal*, *mainstream* CAMHS are used to refer to a comprehensive range of multi-agency mental health services. Second, where the term *specialist CAMHS* is used, this refers to individuals or teams whose core business is to work with children and young people with complex, severe or persistent mental disorders.

The most influential strategic document to set the context in which CAMHS in the UK have evolved was the NHS Health Advisory Service (HAS) report, *Together We Stand* (NHS Health Advisory Service 1995). This introduced the now widely applied tiered model of service delivery, explored the commissioning, role and management of CAMHS and recommended a coordinated, tiered approach to service commissioning and delivery. Within this framework, CAMHS are described according to a four-tier framework, with each tier characterised by increasingly specialised levels of care and treatment (see Figure 10.1 adapted from McDougall 2006).

Frontline professionals in Tier 1 primary, universal or mainstream services share responsibility for the development of children and young people's emotional health and psychological well-being. School nurses, health visitors and nurses on paediatric wards are amongst those primary care professionals with whom children and young people have most contact. For Tier 1 professionals, CAMHS is not their core business and they do not usually have expertise in relation to children's mental health. However, like all professionals charged with the care and welfare of children, primary care workers share joint responsibility for safeguarding and promoting mental health and psychological well-being. They also help prevent mental health problems and disorders, and offer support for less complex mental health problems. Tier 1 professionals often encounter children and young people who have been traumatised, abused or bereaved, those who harm themselves or others and those with emotional and behavioural problems. Many nurses will be involved in helping children to develop self-esteem, emotional literacy and the skills to resolve conflict in non-destructive and pro-social ways.

CAMHS professionals working at Tier 2 provide training and consultation for Tier 1 colleagues and practice as part of a multi-professional or multi-agency network rather than as part of a multidisciplinary team. Those working at both Tiers 1 and 2 must be able to access specialist CAMHS for children and young people with severe, complex or persistent mental disorders. This is for children and young people who require specialist assessment, treatment or management.

Tier 3 CAMHS are locality based multidisciplinary teams that include nurses, psychiatrists, psychologists, family therapists, social workers and creative therapists. Tier 3 CAMHS provide a range of assessment and treatment interventions. Sometimes young people have highly complex or treatment-resistive mental disorders. Tier 4 CAMHS are defined as highly specialised CAMHS and include in-patient child and adolescent units, specialised outpatient services and forensic CAMHS, as well as multi-agency services such as home-based treatment services, community support teams and crisis teams (see Figure 10.1).

Engaging children, young people and families

Nurses in CAMHS usually practice holistically (Armstrong 2006; Woolley 2006). This means they see the young person as a whole and recognise that their needs, as well as those of their family, are broad and varied. This insight is enabled by nurses' well-developed communication skills and ability to engage, creatively and flexibly, with the young person and their family in a number of different ways. This is not to say that all nurses have the same philosophical, theoretical and therapeutic approach to their work. Indeed, the background and training of nurses working in specialist CAMHS is broad and varied (McDougall 2006; Dogra & Leighton 2009). Most specialist CAMHS nurses have qualifications in psychotherapeutic interventions, including psychodynamic, cognitive behavioural and family therapy training. The therapeutic approach they adopt is based on the developmental needs of the child, the evidence base and the views and choices of the service user.

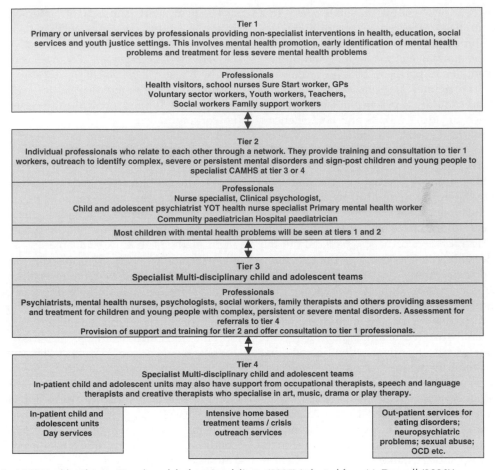

Figure 10.1   NHS Health Advisory Tiered model of service delivery (1995) (adapted from McDougall (2006)).

When working with children and young people with mental health problems, a holistic assessment is the foundation on which successful treatment can be built and therapeutic change can grow and develop. The purpose of any assessment is to assess the child's difficulties within the context of their normal developmental milestones and experiences of everyday living. This is so that a whole picture of the young person and an understanding of their needs can be established. This does not necessarily mean that the nurse must be clear about the cause of the problems, and indeed this is rarely a straight-forward matter. Some argue that it is not necessary to understand causes and we should instead focus on solutions. Whatever their theoretical orientation, the nurse must strive to understand what the present difficulties feel like for the child and their parents or carers, and embark on a common understanding and journey towards providing help and support.

SECTION TWO

What kind of assessment?

There are many different ways of undertaking an assessment. Deciding which approach to use will depend on the developmental status of the child, the evidence base for use and the specific wishes of the child, their family or carers. Most of us have heard the question, 'how do you eat an elephant?', and the answer is of course 'in small bites'. This approach applies to the assessment of a child or young person with mental health problems where there may be many needs to consider and numerous interventions to perform. Like all professionals, nurses have neither all the questions nor all the answers, and should not practice in isolation. It is the combined breadth of skills and competencies provided by the CAMHS multidisciplinary team which makes the whole greater than the sum of its parts (Ryan & McDougall 2009).

Rather than a one-off activity or nursing task, assessment should be thought of as an ongoing, fluid and dynamic process. It evolves as information is generated, appraised and understood within the wider formulation of needs. Not only is the nurse undertaking their assessment, but the young person and their parents or carers will be testing the nurse for trustworthiness, knowledge and understanding (Lewer 2006). It is therefore vital for the nurse to facilitate a climate of support where the whole family will feel heard and understood. It is important also for the nurse to demonstrate that they understand the young person and their family across the breadth of their development and in the immediate context of their relationships, expectations and environments (Farrell 2000). Any hopes and fears must be discussed, explored and understood, and expertise should be shared. To facilitate this, the nurse should make it clear that there is more than one way of viewing the young person's problems.

The nursing assessment not only acts as a medium for gathering information, but also allows for a relationship to develop and forms the basis for a collaborative alliance between the nurse and the child and family. This trusting relationship enables the nurse to consider which problems are amenable to change and is a therapeutic space to work with the child and their family to achieve this (Barker 1997). The nurse's primary task in the assessment process is to draw together all the fragmented pieces of information that have previously been disparate or uncoordinated (Lewer 2006). This usually involves contacting other professionals for further information, and issues in relation to consent and information should always be explored.

The expertise and professional experience of a nurse influences the nature and quality of their assessment and subsequent intervention. For example, a nurse consultant working with children who have attention-deficit hyperactive disorder (ADHD) will be expected to complete a more thorough, holistic assessment to inform a planned treatment programme than a teacher or youth worker with limited mental health experience who is working in a universal or primary care setting. However, all nurses who are assessing children and young people for mental health problems should have a basic understanding of normal child development, range of mental disorders of childhood and be aware of the range of risk and protective factors for mental health problems in general.

Nurses should be aware of the different assessment methods that are available and how to use them (Scahill & Ort 1995). Core skills include good communication and negotiation skills, active listening skills and the ability to identify barriers to change such as parental mental health problems, alcohol or substance misuse and domestic violence. Specific skills include an ability to assess the child for risk of suicide (de Wilde et al. 2001) and to identify coexisting mental health or developmental problems (Stock et al. 2001). With the rapidly developing range of National Institute for Health and Clinical Excellence (NICE) guidelines on the assessment and management of a range of psychological conditions, nurses and other health professionals can access a growing evidence base of interventions to inform competent assessments.

What information should nurses collect?

As noted above, assessment entails obtaining information from several sources. Notwithstanding issues of age, capacity and consent which are discussed later, this should always include the child or young person themselves, as well as their parents, siblings and teachers. It is not unusual for children to be shy or guarded when being questioned about their thoughts and feelings in front of parents. It can therefore be helpful to see them individually as well as with their families wherever possible, particularly when assessing teenagers who are in the transition from dependence to independence.

The nursing assessment should include the presenting concerns of the family or carers, the child's motor and cognitive development, family history and social development, physical health and school performance. A thorough nursing assessment should comprise a family interview, parent or carer interview and a child interview. A range of assessment methods may be used including interviews, observation, rating scales and consultation with other professionals. In addition, nurses may use creative or non-verbal therapeutic interventions using play, music or art materials if assessing infants or younger children (Boyd-Webb 2002).

In summary, a comprehensive nursing assessment should aim to:

- Identify the child's problems including duration, intensity and frequency
- Identify their effects on everyday life and functioning
- Identify any intrinsic, family and environmental factors which trigger and maintain the problem
- Analyse the relationship between different variables
- Identify specific risk factors
- Assess the child's and family's capacity to participate in treatment
- Begin to establish a therapeutic relationship with the child and their family or carers

Assessing family needs

CAMHS nurses should not work in isolation from parents or carers. It is parents or carers who usually know their child best and a holistic assessment should incorporate the opportunity for them to describe their concerns. The duration of the child's difficulties and what parents or carers have tried to do to alleviate some of the problems is important information which should always be considered. The parental interview should collect information about:

- The main concerns of parents or carers
- Attempts by them to resolve the child's problems
- Impact of the problems on the family system
- Parental communication
- Sibling relationships

The purpose of taking a detailed family history is to provide an understanding of family functioning and to assess strengths and barriers to change. It should identify:

- Who is in the family and who lives at home
- The nature of contact, if any, with absent parents
- Family relationships and communication style
- The coping style of the family
- Family support systems
- Significant life events

Developmental assessment

A comprehensive account of childhood development is an important aspect of overall assessment. This is particularly important when assessing developmental disorders such as ADHD or autism spectrum disorders where information about early years is crucial. The developmental assessment should include an account of the following factors:

- Maternal health during pregnancy
- Post-natal history (including birth complications, birth weight, neonatal complications)
- Use of medication during pregnancy (including drugs and alcohol)
- Developmental milestones (including motor development, attachment, growth and temperament)
- Speech and language development
- Early medical history

With the consent of the child and parents, it can also be helpful to contact school or college to gather information about academic, behavioural, developmental and social functioning. Information obtained through interview may be supplemented by standardised rating scales, for example, the Conner's Teacher Questionnaire (Conners 1989) and the Strengths and Difficulties Questionnaire Teacher Report (Goodman 1997) which help provide information about the child's functioning in school. If necessary, more detailed information can be sought from speech and language therapists, educational psychologists, paediatricians and voluntary agencies to add important information in relation to the child's overall presentation.

SECTION THREE

Children and young people with mental health problems – legal issues

During the last few years, there have been several recent changes to the law affecting children and young people receiving treatment for mental health problems. This part of the chapter summarises human rights legislation, and changes to the Mental Health Act, Mental Capacity Act and Children Act as they affect children and young people. Consent to treatment, competence and capacity decisions and recent guidance on the *zone of parental control* are also discussed.

Human rights

The European Convention on Human Rights (ECHR), the United Nations Convention on the Rights of the Child (UNCRC) and the Human Rights Act (HRA) 1998 provide the overarching human rights framework. The ECHR became operational in 1953 and was the first legally binding international instrument to incorporate the full range of human rights. It was intended to give binding effect to the guarantee of various rights and freedoms contained in the UN Declaration on Human Rights. The UNCRC establishes a range of civil, political, socio-economic and cultural rights that apply to all children and young people. There are two guiding principles that nurses who work with children and young people must always take into account in their day-to-day work. First, the best interests and views of the child should always be considered. Second, decisions in relation to children and young people must be made in a manner consistent with the evolving capacities of the child.

Human rights law has led to an increasing recognition that children and young people have rights and entitlements and can often make decisions for themselves. This means that as they grow up towards independence, the views and wishes of young people should be given greater weight than those of their parents in the decision-making process. The HRA (1998) became operational in 2000. This requires public authorities, organisations and professionals to take into account human rights in their day-to-day work with children and young people.

Children Act (1989)

The Children Act was passed in 1989 and became operational in 1991. The principles of the Act are to support parents or carers in childcare matters and to allow them to reinforce their position of autonomy in the care of children at the same time as protecting them from significant harm. The Children Act 2004 complements the 1989 Act by requiring agencies to work more collaboratively together and to safeguard and promote the well-being of children and young people.

Consent

Consent to medical treatment by or for children can be complex and requires a balance between preserving the principle of legal autonomy for children, whilst providing protection to safeguard their physical and mental health. Medical treatment for the purposes of this chapter includes psychiatric, psychological and psychotherapeutic interventions including creative therapy using art, music, drama or play. Before examining, treating or caring for a child, consent must be given. In order for consent to be valid, the child or young person must be capable of consenting, the consent must be freely given and the child or young person involved must be given appropriate information. Ensuring that these conditions are present is both a legal and ethical obligation for the health-care team.

Children under 16

Children under 16 who fully understand the nature of treatment can provide consent. Judges in a 1985 court case ruled that the parental right to determine whether or not their minor child below the age of 16 will have medical treatment terminates if and when the child achieves sufficient understanding and intelligence to enable him or her to understand fully what is proposed. This became known popularly as the test of *Gillick competence* and the effect was to allow a Gillick competent child under the age of 16 a right to consent to treatment without the necessity to obtain parental consent (Harbour 2008).

Young people aged 16 or 17

Young people aged 16 and 17 are presumed to have competence to consent for themselves. If they do not consent to their informal admission to hospital for the treatment of mental disorder, a 16 or 17 year old cannot be admitted to hospital for such treatment on the basis of consent from someone with parental responsibility for them. This change is brought in by section 43 of the Mental Health Act 2007 which amends section 131 of the Mental Health Act 1983. This means that where a young person aged 16 or 17, who has the capacity to make a decision on their health care, decides that they do not want to consent to treatment for mental disorder, the young person cannot be admitted to hospital for that treatment unless they meet the conditions to be detained under the Mental Health Act 1983 as amended, even if a person with parental responsibility is prepared to consent. It also means that where a young person aged 16 or 17, who has the capacity to make a decision on their health care, consents to being admitted to hospital for treatment of a mental disorder they should be treated as an informal patient in accordance with section 131 of the Mental Health Act 1983 as amended even if a person with parental responsibility is refusing consent (NIMHE 2009).

Treatment without consent

Treatment without consent using the common law can only be given in emergencies. This is when immediate action is needed to either save life, protect them from serious harm or prevent a serious and immediate danger to the public. In such cases, the treatment must be reasonable and limited to whatever appears necessary to resolve the emergency. The Children Act (1989) refers to circumstances where a child can refuse to be assessed, examined or treated. The provisions state that, not withstanding any court direction, a child with sufficient understanding to make an informed treatment decision can refuse to be assessed, examined or treated. However, in rare circumstances the court can override such a refusal if it is deemed to compromise the best interests of the child.

How do nurses evaluate competence and capacity?

Evaluating competency is an essential part of the assessment process prior to the provision of any assessment or treatment for children and young people. Children's competence is determined by their maturity and understanding rather than their fixed chronological age. This means that they may be competent to make one treatment decision but not another. When assessing a child or young person's ability to consent to treatment, nurses need to be aware of the differing tests that can be applied. In general a child or young person with competence or capacity should be able to:

- Understand in broad terms what the treatment is, what it is for and why it is being proposed;
- Understand the principal benefits, risks and alternatives to the treatment being proposed;
- Understand the likely consequences of not receiving the treatment being proposed;
- Retain the above information for long enough to make and informed decision;
- Make a choice that is free from external pressure and secondary gain.

A person can be said to lack capacity if they are incapable of understanding or retaining information relevant to making the treatment choice, or if they are incapable of using this information to arrive at a choice. Where children are incapable of consenting to treatment themselves, the consent of their parents or those with parental responsibility must be obtained except in emergencies. It may be appropriate to involve a court to intervene where parents refuse to consent for treatment (considered by a physician to be necessary) to be given to their child, or where there are child protection concerns that have a negative impact on parental ability to act in the best interests of their child.

Involving parents in treatment decisions

Whatever their age, children and young people must be given the opportunity to be involved, as far as is practicable in the circumstances, in planning, developing and reviewing their own treatment and care. The involvement of carers, family members and other people who have an interest in the child's welfare should also be encouraged unless there are particular reasons to the contrary, and their views taken seriously. Even when it is not necessary to obtain the consent of the child or young person's parents, it is good practice to involve them. However, this should always be with the expressed permission of the child or young person.

Wherever the care and treatment of a child is being considered the person or persons with parental responsibility must be identified, and their views sought as appropriate.

If the child is subject to a care order the local authority and parents share responsibility for the child, subject to the local authority's power to limit the exercise of such responsibility by the parents in order to safeguard the child's welfare. Where more than one person has parental responsibility for a child, each of them may act alone, and without the other, in meeting that responsibility. This means that, for example, professionals can lawfully provide treatment to the child with the authority of one parent, even though both parents have parental responsibility. A person who does not have parental responsibility for a child but has care of the child may do what is reasonable under the circumstances to safeguard or promote the child's welfare. This provision will, for example, allow professionals to act in emergencies (NIMHE 2009).

Confidentiality

The moral right to confidentiality enjoyed by adults applies to children and young people. The decisions of Gillick competent children and young people with capacity about the use and disclosure of information they have provided in confidence should be respected in the same way as adults. However, this right to confidentiality can be qualified or limited in certain circumstances. For example, where child abuse is suspected or where public interest may justify disclosure.

Mental Health Act 1983

The Mental Health Act 1983 was amended in 2007 and its guiding principles apply to people of all ages. Treatment for children and young people with mental disorder is regulated by the Mental Health Act when the young person is detained in hospital or, for some treatments, when the young person or their parents agree that they should receive treatment in hospital. Young people can also be treated for a mental disorder in the community using a community treatment order, and this is also regulated by the Mental Health Act.

One of the most important amendments affecting children and young people is provided by Section 31 of the Mental Health Act 2007. This states that young people requiring hospital treatment for mental disorder should only be admitted to environments that are suitable for their age, subject to their needs. The Act places a duty on hospital managers to provide an age-appropriate environment, and to consult a person with expertise and knowledge of working with children and young people in deciding whether such an environment is age appropriate. This person will usually be a Tier 3 or Tier 4 CAMHS professional.

In exceptional circumstances, the Act allows flexibility for young people under 18 to be placed on an adult mental health ward. This is where the need for urgent treatment outweighs the need for the young person to be admitted to an adolescent ward, and that placing the young person on an adolescent ward is likely to jeopardise the safety and welfare of other children or young people. Discrete accommodation within an adult mental health ward for a young person aged 16 or 17 is permissible, but only if this is deemed to be the most appropriate placement, and CAMHS support, safeguarding measures and age-appropriate facilities are made available.

Supervised community treatment

Supervised community treatment (SCT) allows a person with a mental disorder to receive their care and treatment in the community rather than in hospital. Whilst there is no lower age limit for SCT, the number of young people whose clinical and family circumstances make them suitable to move from being detained in hospital to having SCT in the community is likely to be low.

Electroconvulsive therapy

The amended Mental Health Act states that no child or young person under the age of 18 may be given electroconvulsive therapy (ECT) without the approval of a second opinion appointed doctor (SOAD), unless it is an emergency, even if they consent to it. Children and young people who are not detained under the Act but who may require ECT are eligible for access to an independent mental health advocate to represent their needs to hospital managers and mental health tribunals.

Zone of parental control

Parental responsibility is defined in the Children Act (1989) as all the rights, duties, powers, responsibilities and authority which by law a parent has in relation to a child and his property. In some circumstances those with parental responsibilities can authorise the child or young person's admission to hospital and/or consent to treatment. It is therefore important that nurses who are working with children and young people are able to identify who has parental responsibilities.

The concept of the *zone of parental control* (ZPC) was introduced by the updated Mental Health Act Code of Practice. This states that in certain circumstances, parents can consent on behalf of their child if a decision is said to fall within the ZPC. There are no clear rules on what may fall within the ZPC and each decision needs to be considered in the light of the particular circumstances of the case. Factors such as the potential impact that the decision will have on the child or young person, their age and maturity, the nature of the treatment being considered and whether the child or young person is objecting to the treatment will all have to be considered before it can be decided whether the decision falls inside or outside the zone (NIMHE 2009). In assisting practitioners to decide whether a decision falls within the ZPC, the Code poses the following questions:

- Is this a decision that a parent would usually be expected to make, having regard to what is considered to be within the realms of normal parenting and human rights?
- Are there any indicators that the parent might not act in the best interests of their child or young person?
- The less confident the professional that the answer to these questions is 'yes', the more likely it will be that the decision in question falls outside the zone of parental control.

Mental Capacity Act 2005

The Mental Capacity Act 2005 came into force in October 2007 and provides the legal framework for adults who lack capacity to make decisions themselves. The main provisions of the Act apply to 16 and 17 year olds. There are several guiding principles in the Mental Capacity Act:

- A person must be assumed to have capacity unless it is established that they lack capacity;
- A person is not to be treated as unable to make a decision unless all practicable steps to help them do so have been taken without success;
- A person is not to be treated as unable to make a decision merely because they are likely to make an unwise decision;
- An act done or decision made using the Act must be done or made in the person's best interests.

Having capacity to make a decision means having the ability to understand information, weigh this information up and come to an informed decision. People are said to lack capacity if they cannot do one or more of the four following things:

1. Understand information that is given to them
2. Retain information for long enough to be able to make the decision
3. Use the information to make the decision
4. Verbally or non-verbally communicate their decision

When assessing the young person's best interests, the person providing care or treatment must consult those involved in the young person's care and anyone else interested in their welfare which may include parents. Care should be taken not to unlawfully breach the young person's right to confidentiality. In the event that there are disagreements about the care, treatment or welfare of a young person aged 16 or 17 who lacks capacity, the case may be heard in the family courts or the Court of Protection.

Advocacy

Nurses are often required to advocate on behalf of children and young people with mental health problems. This may involve helping them to navigate the mental health system, access independent and confidential information or to access representation and support. Advocacy by nurses on behalf of children and young people can occur at a range of different levels. This may be through representing the views of the child or young person at a review or case conference, informing them of their rights or making their voice heard throughout the care and treatment process (McDougall 2006). It is not always appropriate or possible for nurses to advocate on behalf of a particular child or adolescent. For example, the young person may have a complaint that they do not want the nurse to know about or the complaint may be about the nurse themselves. Independent advocacy services can also help children and young people to understand their rights, make complaints about their care, treatment or detention and provide confidential advice. In 2002, the Department of Health published national standards for the provision of children's advocacy services (Department of Health 2002). Advocacy is not only a legal nicety it is also an ethical consideration. In partnership with the child or young person, the nurse is obliged to ensure that the child's or adolescent's voice is heard.

Conclusion

There is a growing evidence base showing that strategies for mental health promotion, prevention of mental ill health and early intervention can offset the development of mental health problems and disorders in later childhood, adolescence and early adulthood. Failure to interrupt the negative developmental trajectories of children places a future burden on the economy through long-term demands on adult mental health services, social services, general health services and the criminal justice system. Growing awareness and interest of politicians has generated a suite of universal, public health and prevention strategies. Preventing child mental health problems requires a comprehensive, integrated effort involving children and young people, families and local communities, schools and the media. No single approach is likely to be effective in addressing what is a large-scale universal concern.

Investment and growth in both mental health and paediatric nursing has offered opportunities for nurses to extend their role in the field of child and adolescent mental health services, and make a major contribution to the care and treatment of children and young people with mental health problems. Nurses in CAMHS usually practice holistically and recognise that the needs of young people and their families are broad-based and varied. This insight is enabled by nurse's well-developed communication skills and ability to engage, creatively and flexibly, with the young person and their family in a number of different ways.

It is important that nurses who work with children and young people are clear about the legal and ethical frameworks within which they work. Appropriate to their area of practice, they should be familiar with human rights legislation, children's law and both the Mental Health Act and Mental Capacity Act in order to deliver competent, legal and ethical care. Any intervention in the life of a child or young person should be considered in the context of benefits and risks. Any intervention should be the least restrictive available, and be least likely to expose children to additional risks such as stigma or disruption to family, social and educational functioning.

Reflective scenario

Rahella is a 15-year-old Somali girl who has arrived in the UK as an unaccompanied refugee. Both her parents and older brother were recently killed by rebels and she was forced to flee her country with her surviving brother, Haris. The two children initially travelled alone, but were later picked up and separated by human traffickers in the Netherlands. Rahella has been detained by the UK Border Agency and has been placed in a secure detention centre. On reception to the centre, Rahella tells the admitting officer that she wants to go to sleep and never wake up.

The local child and adolescent mental health services are contacted and asked to see Rahella. The nurse specialist who assesses Rahella finds her anxious, tearful and suicidal. Rahella has hardly eaten or slept in several days and is worried about the welfare of her younger brother. Rahella states that she wishes to go to heaven to be with her family. She tells the nurse that she is constantly troubled by flashbacks of soldiers with guns and hears loud bangs. Rahella reluctantly agrees to be admitted to hospital and the nurse arranges for Rahella to be transferred to the local adolescent mental health unit. It takes several days before Rahella feels safe enough to discuss her experiences of trauma and abuse. She learns that her brother has been detained in Belgium and that plans are underway with Social Services to reunite the children with an aunt in Yemen.

In time, Rahella is able to use cognitive behavioural strategies to cope with flashbacks and feelings of anxiety. She slowly begins to work through the loss of her parents and brother with one of the nurses. She later asks about making contact with her friends in Somalia and is keen to continue with her education and train to be a teacher. Six months later she is reunited with Haris who has also been receiving help from the Belgian authorities. Both children eventually travel to Yemen to live with their aunt and uncle.

Questions

1. What is the legal authority for Rahella's admission to hospital?
2. How would you engage Rahella? How would you go about prioritising her many needs?
3. How will you identify Rahella's cultural needs?
4. How would you plan Rahella's assessment? Who else would you need to involve?
5. How would you plan Rahella's treatment? What would be the short, medium and long-term goals? Which of these would you be able to help meet?
6. How would you address issues of parental responsibility?
7. As a nurse working with Rahella, what would your own needs be? How would you address these?
8. How can services for refugee and asylum-seeking children be improved?

References

Armstrong, M. (2006) Self harm, young people and nursing. In: *Child and Adolescent Mental Health Nursing* (ed. T. McDougall). Blackwell, London.

Barker, P. (1997) *Assessment in Psychiatric and Mental Health Nursing. In Search of the Whole Person.* Stanley Thornes, Cheltenham.

Boyd-Webb, N. (2002) *Helping Bereaved Children: A Handbook for Practitioners*, 2nd edn. Guilford Press, New York.

Conners, C. (1989) *Conners Adolescent Self Report Rating Scale Manual.* Multi-Health System, New York.

Department for Education and Skills (2007) *Care Matters: Time for Change*, HMSO, London.

Dogra, N. & Leighton, S. (2009) *Nursing in Child and Adolescent Mental Health.* McGraw-Hill, Maidenhead.

Farrell, E. (2000) *Lost for Words: The Psychoanalysis of Anorexia and Bulimia.* Other Press, New York.

Goodman, R. (1997) The strengths and difficulties questionnaire: A research note. *Journal of Child Psychology and Psychiatry*, **38** (5), 581–586.

Green, H., McGinnity, A., Meltzer, H., Ford, T. & Goodman, R. (2005) *Mental Health of Children and Young People in Great Britain.* ONS, London.

Harbour, A. (2008) *Children with Mental Disorder and the Law.* Jessica Kingsley, London.

Layard, R. (2004) *Mental Health: Britain's Biggest Social Problem. Prime Minister's Strategy Unit.* HMSO, London.

Leighton, S. (2006) Nursing children and young people with emotional disorders. In: *Child and Adolescent Mental Health Nursing* (ed. T. McDougall). Blackwell, London.

Lewer, L. (2006) Nursing young people with eating disorders. In: *Child and Adolescent Mental Health Nursing* (ed. T. McDougall). Blackwell, London.

McDougall, T. (2006) *Child and Adolescent Mental Health Nursing.* Blackwell, London.

NHS Health Advisory Service (1995) *Together We Stand: The Commissioning, Role and Management of Child and Adolescent Mental Health Services.* HMSO, London.

NIMHE (2009) *The Legal Aspects of the Care and Treatment of Children and Young People with Mental Disorder: A Guide for Professionals.* National Institute for Mental Health in England, London.

NEF/Action for Children (2009) *Backing the Future.* New Economics Foundation/Action for Children, London.

Policy Research Bureau (2007) *Interventions for Children at Risk of Developing Antisocial Personality Disorder: Report to the Department of Health and Prime Minister's Strategy Unit.* Policy Research Bureau, London.

Princes Trust (2009) *The Princes Trust YouGov Youth Index.* Princes Trust, London.

Ryan, N. & McDougall, T. (2009) *Nursing Children and Young People with ADHD.* Routledge, London.

Scahill, L. & Ort, S. (1995) Selection and use of clinical rating instruments in child psychiatric nursing. *Journal of Child & Adolescent Psychiatric Nursing*, **8** (3), 33–34.

Stock, S., Werry, J. & McClellan, J. (2001) Pharmacological treatment of paediatric anxiety. In: *Anxiety Disorders in Children and Adolescents: Research, Assessment and Intervention* (eds W. Silverman & P. Treffers). Cambridge University Press, London.

UNICEF (2007) *An Overview of Child Wellbeing in Rich Countries: A Comprehensive Assessment of the Lives and Well-Being of Children and Adolescents in the Economically Advanced Nations.* United Nations Children's Fund, Florence.

de Wilde, E., Kienhorst, I. & Diekstra, R. (2001) Suicidal behaviour in adolescents. In: *The Depressed Child and Adolescent* (ed. I. Goodyer), 2nd edn. Cambridge University Press, London.

Woolley, E. (2006) Treatment interventions for children and young people with mental health problems. In: *Child and Adolescent Mental Health Nursing* (ed. T. McDougall). Blackwell, London.

YoungMinds (2006) *A Call to Action: Commissioning Mental Health Services for 16 to 25 Year Olds.* Young Minds, London.

Suggested further readings

Dwivedi, K. & Harper, P. (2004) *Promoting the Emotional Wellbeing of Children and Adolescents and Preventing Their Mental Ill Health: A Handbook.* Jessica Kingsley, London.

Jackson, C., Hill, K. & Lavis, P. (2008) *Child and Adolescent Mental Health Today: A Handbook.* Mental Health Foundation/Pavilion/YoungMinds, London.

Vostanis, P. (2007) *Mental Health Interventions and Services for Vulnerable Children and Young People.* Jessica Kingsley, London.

Part III

Ethical Issues in the Acute Care Setting

If you went to hospital what would you like a nurse to do to help you get better?

Be kind and helpful.   (Girl 10yrs)

Get some toys and Lego, ice cream and my DS with R4.   (Boy aged 8yrs)

Say that everything is ok (comfort me), look after me and talk about all the good things that will happen when I come out of hospital.   (Girl 11yrs)

I would want them to talk to me to try and distract me. I would want them to give me something to take away the pain (ice cream).   (Girl 14yrs)

Tell me what's going on and do regular check ups and be kind.   (Girl 11yrs)

My Nurse

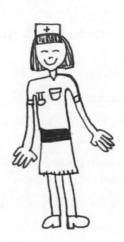

Girls aged 12yrs

11 Children's Experience of Hospitalisation and Their Participation in Health-Care Decision-Making

Imelda Coyne

Introduction

The purpose of this chapter is to critically appraise the current position concerning care of children in hospital based on research evidence. The focus will be on children and young people's experience of hospitalisation and their participation in health-care decision-making. The care of hospitalised children raises many ethical and philosophical issues which challenges us to adopt a more ethical approach to nursing children. The effects of hospitalisation on the child and the family unit raise issues associated with trust, respect, privacy, autonomy and self-determination. The role which children play in their health-care provision will be explored in relation to parents' and health-care professionals' roles. As more research is conducted directly with children, we are becoming increasingly aware that children often desire a more active role in their care and in the communication process. The different views held on children's capacity to participate are linked to principles such as beneficence, paternalism, informed consent and children's best interest. Children's experiences of communication interactions and participation in decision-making in the

health-care setting will be explored. This will illustrate how children's rights may be overlooked or denied which raises moral and ethical issues. As will be seen later, sometimes children's rights to information and participation may be denied or curtailed by adults, and this approach is sometimes justified by recourse to the principle of beneficence and protecting the child. We need to be aware that in children's health care, particularly, tensions can exist between beneficence and respect for autonomy because of parents' legal responsibility for their children's welfare. Likewise health-care professionals must operate from a professional code which requires them to respect parents' roles whilst also supporting children's rights to participation. I will also explore in this chapter, parents' and health-care professionals' respective roles in minimising the effects of hospitalisation and facilitating children's participation in health-care matters. The chapter will conclude with a summary of the key issues against a philosophical and ethical background. Some recommendations for future practice will be outlined, which you may find useful to consider in your clinical practice and interactions with sick children.

Ethical and Philosophical Aspects of Nursing Children, First Edition. Edited by Gosia M. Brykczyńska and Joan Simons.
© 2011 Blackwell Publishing Ltd. Published 2011 by Blackwell Publishing Ltd.

Care of children in hospital

Hospitalisation remains a stressful experience for many children[1] despite unrestricted parent participation and considerable improvements in hospital environments. Separation from family and loved ones can be the greatest stressor for children during hospitalisation, particularly children younger than 5 years of age. Reflecting this, parental involvement in the hospitalised child's care has been advocated since the publication of the Platt Report (Ministry of Health C.H.S.C. 1959). Parents are now encouraged to stay with their children and participate in the delivery of their child's care. Over a period of time, about three decades, the terminology changed from parent involvement to partnership in care to care-by-parent and finally to family-centred care (Coyne 1996; Power & Franck 2008). Although the terminology changed, it is questionable as to whether commensurate change has occurred in clinical practice (Coyne & Cowley 2007). Family-centred care is now promoted widely within paediatric health services as a particular method of delivering care. It is an approach to care that involves the parents, the child and the health professional working together in the delivery of the child's care. It is a framework that recognises that families have a very important role in their hospitalised child's care. It is widely believed that children benefit from the continuous presence of their parents and that it has a positive effect on the child's well-being during hospitalisation. Though the family-centred care philosophy is integral to understanding the child's experience of hospitalisation, it is not the focus here as it is addressed in more detail in the next chapter.

Although a wealth of knowledge exists on adults' experiences of hospitalisation, there remains a deficit of data on children's own perceptions of hospitalisation. Traditionally, the adults' view of children's perspectives has been sought, with parents generally acting as proxies for children. However, adult proxies' views of children's experiences may differ quite markedly from children's

own views and in some situations may be flawed or inaccurate. Hence researchers are increasingly recognising the importance of directly recording children's own perspectives (Oldfield & Fowler 2004; Greig et al. 2007; Coad et al. 2008; Coyne et al. 2009) which would contribute towards a better understanding of children's experiences and needs. This is particularly important for sick children because their views may not be heard due to illness, developmental status, limited communication abilities or professional attitudes. Children's experiences of hospitalisation will now be discussed and where possible direct quotes from children will be used to illustrate the data and to reflect the ethical stance which is that children's voices be prioritised.

Children's experiences of hospitalisation

Effects of hospitalisation

The crisis of childhood illness and hospitalisation can be a very stressful and traumatic time for all involved. More than 50 years ago, classic studies highlighted the adverse effects of hospitalisation and identified the potential long-term negative effects post hospitalisation for children and their families (Robertson 1958a, b; Wolfer & Visintainer 1975; McClowry 1988). Concerns about pain, mutilation, immobility, separation from significant others, loss of control and disruption have all been reported by hospitalised children as potentially stressful (Timmerman 1983; Stevens 1986; McClowry 1988; Barnes et al. 1990; Bossert 1994; Thompson 1994). As a result, significant changes have occurred in health-care provision for children over the decades. Health professionals are now more aware of the impact of hospitalisation for children and significant efforts have been made to implement interventions that reduce the adverse aspects of hospitalisation for children and their relatives. Such strategies include: family-centred care policy, preadmission programmes, child-friendly décor and environment, child-sized furniture and equipment, provision of playrooms and play specialists and resident school teachers.

However, despite these improvements, recent research indicates that hospitalised children continue to find hospitalisation stressful and have similar

---

[1]   For the purposes of this chapter, children are taken to include anyone under the age of 18, in accordance with the UN Convention on the Rights of the Child. To avoid cumbersome repetition, where the words *children* or *child* appear, this includes young people.

concerns and fears reported two decades ago (Battrick & Glasper 2004; Coyne 2006b; Coyne & Conlon 2007). Battrick & Glasper (2004) used questionnaires to obtain children's views and reported that 11–16 year olds ($n = 13$) felt the ward did not cater for their age group, expressed dissatisfaction with level of privacy and disliked the food and noisy ward, whilst the 4–10 year olds ($n = 12$) expressed fears about the operation. Coyne (2006b) interviewed children aged 7–14 years ($n = 11$) from four paediatric wards in two hospitals in England. Eight of the eleven children had chronic conditions (asthma, orthopaedic, skin conditions) and three had acute conditions. The children reported concerns and fears about the hospitalisation which include: separation from family and friends, unfamiliar people and environment, unfamiliar investigations/treatments and loss of self-determination. Similar findings were reported by children aged 7–16 years ($n = 17$) from three hospitals (two children's hospitals and one district general hospital) in Ireland (Coyne & Conlon 2007). Seven of the children had chronic conditions (renal, epilepsy, orthopaedic conditions) and ten were acute admissions. Children with both acute and chronic illness reported feeling anxious about the unfamiliar setting and fearful of intrusive procedures, injections and blood tests and the possibility of pain.

Although these studies may be limited by small samples, similar concerns and fears were expressed by children from larger samples in other countries (Polkki et al. 2003; Wikstrom 2005; Lindeke et al. 2006). In Sweden, children's drawings ($n = 22$) revealed feelings of anxiety about procedures, longing for family life and powerlessness (Wikstrom 2005). In Finland, children ($n = 52$) aged 8–12 years who had undergone surgery expressed fears about the operation, anaesthesia, injections and needle sticks, recovery after surgery and staying in hospital (Polkki et al. 2003). Lindeke et al. (2006) asked American children ($n = 120$) to describe the best and worst things about their hospitalisation. Pain and discomfort were cited the most frequently as the worst aspects of hospitalisation whilst play activities and good relationships with hospital staff were valued by children of all ages. These findings clearly indicate that separation from significant others is not the only factor to consider in children's experiences of hospitalisation. The effects of hospitalisation will now be examined in more detail within four main areas: the ward environ-

ment, treatments and procedures, knowing health professionals and loss of self-determination.

Children's views on the ward environment

Hospitals can be frightening and alien environments for many children whether it be the child's first admission or one in a series of admissions. Children's wards are often busy environments with many people (e.g. nurses, doctors, patients, families, teacher, play therapist, social worker, support worker, volunteers, ward clerks, cleaners, kitchen staff, etc.) congregating in a confined area and all focused on different activities. It can be potentially threatening and disorientating for children to be exposed to such a busy environment peopled by strangers. As one child said:

> I was afraid of the traffic. You know all people going up and down, up and down and then they might have something dangerous in their hands trying to sort something out and then you know you might accidentally bang into them and you'd hurt everybody and yourself.
>
> (Girl aged 9)
>
> … don't actually mind staying in hospital as long as I know that I'm safe.
>
> (Boy age 9)

The labelling of constant throughput of staff as *ward traffic* illustrates the busyness of the ward from a child's perspective. The characteristics of the hospital environment can strongly influence children's reactions to being hospitalised. Children have reported feeling anxious about the unfamiliar environment and that they particularly dislike hot *stuffy* wards, high noise levels, bright lights, lack of privacy and inadequate play facilities (Coyne 2006b; Coyne & Conlon 2007) which has also been reported in other studies (Boyd & Hunsberger 1998). Children often experience difficulty sleeping due to poor ventilation, bright lights and the noise created by phones ringing, nurses talking and babies and children crying. Sick children prefer peace and quiet rather than a chaotic environment (Forsner et al. 2005).

Older children and particularly adolescents dislike the lack of privacy and often complain about the ward décor being too *babyish* and that play facilities and toys are geared towards younger children (Coyne 2006b) which has also been reported elsewhere (Boylan 2004; Hutton 2005). For example:

> I don't like is hearing babies crying as it keeps me awake and then there are times when I can't watch some things on T.V. because the other kids in the room are too young to watch what I want to watch and that's annoying. So it would be better if I had my own room.
>
> (Boy aged 14)

Compared to the past, hospital environments have become more child-centred in that hospital décor having motifs/drawings on the walls and wards are usually decorated in bright colours, cartoon characters or bright images on curtains and floor surfaces. However, the environment and facilities may not be suitable for children of all ages in that the *disneyesque* themes may only be appreciated by children younger than 7 years old. Similar dislikes about the ward environment have been reported in recent research with children (n = 255) from three hospitals in England (Curtis *et al*. 2007). The children aged 7 and older viewed the decoration of hospital spaces and facilities for recreation, as geared towards very young children. They universally disliked the clown motifs in all three sites with even the older children regarding them as frightening which is an interesting finding considering the trend towards employing clowns to provide humour and diversion on certain wards in England. The children also disliked dull, dirty, disordered and crowded spaces.

Children's fears of treatments and procedures

Children perceive intrusive procedures, blood tests and pain as particularly threatening and very stressful (Boyd & Hunsberger 1998; Carter 2002; Polkki *et al*. 2003; Coyne 2006b). In interviews with six hospitalised children, aged 10–13 years, with various chronic conditions, they reported fears of invasive procedures, injections, surgery, fear of death, loss of independence and loss of control (Boyd & Hunsberger 1998). Polkki *et al*., interviewed Finnish children (n = 52) aged 8–12 years who had undergone surgery, and 75% of the children had experienced fear of operations, anaesthesia, injections and needle sticks, recovery after surgery and staying in hospital. In Coyne's study (2006b),

the children expressed dislike and fears about the pain associated with injections, blood tests and intrusive procedures. When the children described the treatment or investigations, they used terms such as: 'pushing in', 'drilling in', 'going through me', 'opening up', 'taking out' and 'losing'. These terms indicated feelings of intrusion and loss which implies that children may see invasive medical procedures as the same invasion of privacy and bodily space. Some children did not like being examined by doctors as illustrated by this comment:

> They just have to hurt you, they can't get out of the room without hurting you. They just feel around you and poke you, first the doctor professor does it and then they do it, the students always hurt you, they have cold hands.
>
> (Boy age 9)

The children who required surgical treatment felt worried and scared about the surgical process involved such as having to wear a theatre gown, the journey to theatre, waiting in theatre, having the operation and waking up in pain. As one boy explained:

> Scared at the thought of hospital that I was going to need an operation … like if I was going to get slit open. Nobody told me what would happen in surgery but I have seen it on films so I know that's what happens so I was afraid of that mainly. I didn't know what it was going to be like … any of it … I thought it would be scary.
>
> (Boy age 12)

Some children recalled previous experiences of pain and were worried about experiencing pain again. Similar findings were reported by children in another study where 55 children from three hospitals in Ireland were interviewed about their experiences of hospitalisation (Coyne *et al*. 2006). The children talked about suffering pain at some point in the hospitalisation, which caused upset, distress, suffering and restricted movement. Some children's pain experience was not helped because of the difficulty they experienced in receiving attention from nurses and doctors for their pain. They complained about having to wait for medication for pain relief and having to *shout* for painkillers. Some children had to endure blood tests and cannulations without the necessary preparatory cream called EMLA (a local anaesthetic cream) because the health professional chose not to use the cream. The children described their feelings of pain during blood tests as stabbing and stinging and psychological feelings as worry, fear, anxiousness, nervousness and feeling *rotten*. For example:

> Well I was shocked because like I thought they would have told me, and like I'm real bad for getting cannulas in so I always ask them for the cream, you know the cream. Yea, but they never gave it to me, they never gave it to me then. I didn't want to bother the nurse.
>
> (Girl age 13)

In other studies, children have reported feeling unprepared for procedures and lacking information on aspects of the hospitalisation (Smith & Callery 2005; Alderson 2008; Howells & Lopez 2008). Children need information so that they can understand their illness, be involved in their care, prepare themselves for procedures and direct their actions towards *getting well* again. In the absence of information some children drew upon their experiences and knowledge of television programmes which led to misconceptions and increased anxieties. They appear to obtain information from a variety of sources including parents, nurses and doctors, observing other children on the ward, books from the local library, medical television programmes and past experiences. Similar informational deficits and strategies have been reported by children aged 7–11 years ($n = 9$) awaiting planned surgery to meet their information needs (Smith & Callery 2005).

Children's experiences of loss of self-determination

In Coyne's study (2006b), the children experienced some loss of self-determination over meeting personal needs in that they appeared to lack control over matters such as wakening time, sleeping time, obtaining food and drinks and using facilities on the ward. The children talked about needing permission or of getting permission to perform activities such as getting up, dressing, getting food, using the bathroom, bringing in personal effects,

asking questions and leaving the ward. They prefaced their comments with 'allowed to do' which indicated the issue of control. The children reported having to sleep at a certain time and being woken at a certain time. The children had to *fit in* with the ward routines and this appeared to cause feelings of frustration and powerlessness for some children, particularly adolescents:

> I'd be like 'yuck' it's seven in the morning and I am waking up to a load of doctors at the end of my bed … so that was kind of scary and I'd be there asleep and suddenly somebody would wake you up and all of a sudden there are loads of people standing at the end of the bed looking at me. I hadn't a clue who they were.
>
> (Girl aged 16)

It is generally accepted that the experience of illness itself causes disruption to children's sense of well-being and consequently hospitalisation may represent a threat to children's independence, usual self-caring abilities and self-control. Indeed research has found that adolescents want to be involved in care and decisions so that they can exercise some control over what is happening to them in hospital (Lansdown 1994). Moreover, concern about loss of control, and feelings of dependence have been reported by hospitalised children as potentially stressful and of particular significance for hospitalised adolescents (Britto *et al.* 2004). There is a growing body of research which demonstrates positive benefits to empowering children and adolescents in their own health care. Recent studies suggest that using children and young people's views in the development and evaluation of services can have a significant influence on health outcomes (Boylan 2004; Curtis *et al.* 2004; Alderson 2008; Coad *et al.* 2008). Children's participation in information exchange and decision-making will be discussed in more depth later in this chapter.

Summary

As demonstrated earlier, children dislike wards that have high noise levels, excessive heat, poor ventilation, bright lights, dull décor, lack of privacy and inadequate play equipment and facilities. They experience sleep disturbances and dislike hospital food. Sleep and nutrition are essential components of health. Hence sleep deprivation and inadequate nutrition is detrimental to the child's psychological health and will impair recovery. Clearly some aspects of hospital environments create stress and anxieties for children and hinder their coping strategies and, therefore, are not always optimum for children's welfare. Children are a particularly vulnerable group of patients because they may not voice their concerns and hence may have unmet needs which is unethical. Children prefer hospitals to be clean, tidy, bright, colourful, spacious and welcoming, comfortable and quiet (Curtis *et al.* 2007). Children seek order and security in an environment that is alien to them, so décor should be kept simple, clean and areas clearly signposted. The constant throughput of staff could be controlled by ensuring quiet times are scheduled during the day and professionals minimise loud interactions in spaces occupied by children. Dim lights and coordination of activities could reduce the disruption at night-time and promote children's efforts to obtain rest and sleep. Nurses should encourage children to bring in familiar items from home to personalise their bed space. Such simple actions can have a significant effect on a child's overall experience in hospital.

Unfortunately, many children's ward facilities and play facilities are geared towards younger children and current service provision does not meet adolescents' needs adequately (RCPCH 2003). Young children as well as adolescents value personal space and privacy, so their preferences should be accommodated where possible bearing in mind that some children may prefer single cubicles whilst others prefer sharing bed space for the contact with peers. Despite growing awareness of adolescents' requirements, there appears to be a lack of commitment to providing appropriate resources. Many of the unsatisfactory environmental issues could be minimised by hospital and ward managers. They have a moral responsibility to ensure that children's surroundings are adequate and advocate for improvements when shortfalls are identified.

Hospital safety reports tend to focus on structural aspects of safety and fail to recognise the psychological impact of adverse environments on children's well-being. As the child's advocate, nurses need to recognise the negative effect of adverse surroundings on children's welfare, see the ward environment from the child's perspective and take active measures to remedy any deficits. The impact of the hospital environment on patients' recovery from illness is receiving increasing attention and has led to identifying ways to promote well-being. Music and pet therapy are interventions that promote hospitalised children's well-being, which suggests that such therapies should be considered for children's care (Barrera *et al.* 2002; Longhi & Pickett 2008). There is now more interest in soliciting children's views on hospital décor, environments and hospital services (Curtis *et al.* 2007; Coad & Coad 2008; Eisen *et al.* 2008) which should lead to health-care environments and spaces tailored to children's preferences rather than what adults assume children like.

As seen earlier, many children feel anxious and unprepared for hospitalisation which is unethical considering that we know that preparation helps reduce anxieties and promotes coping. Research indicates that children who are prepared for surgery and hospitalisation recover more quickly and have decreased anxiety and fewer emotional problems, such as separation anxiety and sleep disturbances, than those who are not prepared (Claar *et al.* 2002; Brewer *et al.* 2006; Justus *et al.* 2006). Nurses need to be aware that familiarity with the hospital and/or routines will not necessarily eliminate or decrease a child's reaction to hospitalisation, especially if events and procedures have not been explained beforehand. It is also very likely that when children have had bad experiences of hospitals in the past, those memories resurface and influence their reactions even if further experiences are more positive. In consideration of children's range of fears about hospitalisation, it is important that preparatory procedures and preadmission programmes be freely available and always offered to children and parents. There are numerous ways to prepare children prior to procedures and surgery such as: hospital tours, videos, role play, books, leaflets, computer games and toys (O'Connor-Von 2000). There is a danger with the current emphasis on cost efficiency and speedy throughput of patients that children's needs for preparation may be overlooked. Therefore, better efforts need to be made by health-care professionals to prepare children and lack of time or resources should not be used as an excuse.

Since children's reactions to hospitalisation may vary according to circumstances, a more individualised approach needs to be used in developing interventions that will reduce children's worries and strengthen their coping strategies. Health-care professionals need to be sensitive to the emotional and informational needs of children. Information should not be forced on children who are disinterested as information limiting is an effective coping behaviour for some children (Thompson 1994). Ideally, they should use questioning, listening and clarifying to gain the perspective of each child. Children are more likely to be less distressed if their views are listened to and adults respond to their concerns with compassion and sensitivity.

As discussed earlier, injections, blood tests, intrusive procedures and investigations are obvious sources of stress for hospitalised children. Performing blood tests without adequate preparation or pain relief seems to be a frequent occurrence according to hospitalised children which implies a lack of consideration of how threatening and painful blood tests/injections can be for many children. In an American study with 120 hospitalised children aged 4–20 years, the children identified pain as the most troublesome aspect of hospitalisation (Lindeke *et al.* 2006). There is a growing body of evidence which suggests that nurses may misinterpret children's expressions of pain, underestimate children's pain and provide inadequate pain relief (Byrne *et al.* 2001; Carter 2002; Simons & Robertson 2002). Likewise, junior doctors due to inexperience may perform cannulations without using appropriate pain relief or pain control strategies. Such evidence indicates the relatively powerless position children can occupy when it comes to conveying their needs to *more powerful* adults, and how children's rights are not always upheld with regard to pain relief. Performing potentially painful procedures without adequate pain relief and leaving children experiencing pain is morally wrong and should not occur. Such practice does not adhere to the principle of beneficence and non-maleficence. These findings indicate the critical importance of sufficient pain relief, age-appropriate explana-

tions and use of relaxation techniques prior to and throughout invasive procedures on children. There are several pain control techniques that can be taught relatively quickly by play specialists to other health-care professionals that could make a substantial difference to the care of children (Lawes *et al.* 2007).

Along with parents' presence, knowing the health-care professionals as human beings helps considerably in reducing anxieties and ameliorating the adverse aspects of hospitalisation (Coyne 2003; Lindeke *et al.* 2006; Coyne & Conlon 2007). Children appreciate and value relationships with health-care professionals where they show interest, reassurance, kindness, gentleness, humour and comfort (Dixon-Woods *et al.* 2002; Pelander & Leino-Kilpi 2004; Schmidt *et al.* 2007). Adolescents (*n* = 155) with chronic illnesses rated the interpersonal aspects of care, such as honesty and respect, as key determinants of quality for them (Britto *et al.* 2004). Health-care professionals can use a variety of actions to develop a trusting relationship such as: chatting informally, seeing the child as an individual, respecting the child's views, sharing some personal information about oneself, establishing common interests and using humour. These actions demonstrate respect for children as individuals and are fundamental to a child's positive experience of hospitalisation (Coyne 2007; Pelander & Leino-Kilpi 2004). Health-care professionals can either enhance a child's coping abilities or cause additional stressors if they are unsupportive and insensitive to children's needs (Boyd & Hunsberger 1998). We need to remember that interventions designed to reduce children's stress during hospitalisation are not only likely to decrease their stress at the time, but they are also likely to influence how future experiences are appraised and managed (LaMontagne 2000).

Health-care professionals may not be aware of other events that are stressful for children such as disruption to normal routines and loss of self-determination. Loss of self-determination may exacerbate some children's fears and anxieties about hospitalisation. School-age children may find the loss of control particularly difficult since adolescence is a time when children are relatively self-sufficient and increasingly striving for independence. Encouraging children's autonomy is an important element of fostering self-esteem in children of any age. Most wards purport to deliver care according to the child's usual routine but this may be difficult to achieve on a busy ward with 20 or more patients. Hence nurses could help by eliciting children's preferences when making decisions about their care so that they feel that they have some control over events in hospital and where possible to accommodate children's individual preferences. It should be customary practice for children to be involved in planning their care as this will help alleviate or at least minimise fears and anxieties. Loss of self-determination may encourage learned helplessness rather than develop autonomy and negatively influence children's adjustment to their illness and overall welfare. This leads us to the next section on children's right to be heard and their experiences of participation in decision-making.

Children's right to be heard

The importance of children's right to be heard in matters that affect their lives has been established both at a national level in England (BMA 2001; DoH 2003), Ireland (Department of Health and Children 2000a, b) and also at the international level (UN 1989; American Academy of Pediatrics Committee on Bioethics 1995; RCPCH Ethics Advisory Committee 2000). There has been a significant increase in the level of activity by almost all organisations in the last 5 years to facilitate children and young people's participation in matters that affect their lives (Oldfield & Fowler 2004). Consultation with children is now a key policy issue that is recognised and actively promoted by many non-government and voluntary organisations such as Action for Sick Children, Barnardo's, Carnegie Young People Initiative, National Youth Agency, National Children's Bureau and Save the Children. There appears to be growing acceptance of children's right to be heard and the right to participate in decision-making. The European Convention on the Exercise of Children's Rights (Council of Europe 1996) recommended that in all actions concerning children, the best interests of the child should be the primary consideration. In England, the appointment of a Children's Taskforce, Children's Ombudsman and the Children's National Service Framework (NSF) are significant initiatives designed to encourage

children and young people's active participation. The Children's NSF for Children, Young People and Maternity Services – Standards for Hospital Services (DoH 2003) explicitly states that hospital services should be child-centred and that children should be consulted and involved in all aspects of their care. The report states that:

Children and young people should receive care that is integrated and co-ordinated around their particular needs, and the needs of their family. They, and their parents, should be treated with respect, and should be given support and information to enable them to understand and cope with illness or injury, and the treatment needed. They should be encouraged to be active partners in decisions about their health and care, and, where possible, be able to exercise choice.

(DoH 2003:9)

These reports emphasise the importance of children's voices being heard in the health-care system from a rights perspective but also because it has considerable benefits for children particularly. The benefits of participation generally include: better provision of information; having an opportunity to express feelings; developing confidence, competence and self-esteem; increasing skills in decision-making; increased compliance and take-up of service, developing civic skills and encouraging participation in wider society (Cohen & Emanuel 1998). Research suggests that children's participation in health-care matters results in increased adherence (de Winter et al. 2002), increased locus of control (Tieffenberg et al. 2000), decreased fears and concerns, feeling valued (Angst & Deatrick 1996), understanding of illness (Coyne et al. 2006) and satisfaction with health care (Freed et al. 1998). The converse of the above is seen in relation to non-participation of children. Children are at risk of being unable to evaluate options and make informed decisions if they are not given the opportunities to participate and learn such skills. Lack of involvement may have adverse consequences such as increased fears and anxieties, reduced self-esteem, depersonalisation and feeling unprepared for surgery (Runeson et al. 2002; Coyne 2006a, 2008; Coyne et al. 2006). Clearly children's participation in their own health care appears to have health-promoting value.

Children's participation in health-care matters

Although there is increasing support for the principle of children's participation, the actual implementation of this principle in health-care settings is questionable. Despite the huge increase in consultation by children's organisations, research has found that children's voices remain generally excluded and they were less likely to be involved in service delivery or policy setting (Hill *et al.* 2004; Oldfield & Fowler 2004). The National Youth Agency (NYA) and the British Youth Council (BYC) surveyed statutory and voluntary sector organisations in England ($n = 849$) in order to establish the extent to which children are involved in public decision-making (Oldfield & Fowler 2004). They found that the level of participation was greatest in organisations that had a specific remit to work with children but was more limited in health and criminal organisations. Sloper & Lightfoot (2003) commented on how little information is available on children's involvement in health-care treatment services although more information is available about children's involvement in local government. The evidence suggests that children are rarely consulted as partners in the planning and delivery of health services.

Research on children's medical encounters in clinics reported that children, even the older children, were routinely excluded from discussions and granted limited autonomy (Shiminski-Maher 1993; Van Dulmen 1998; Carter 2002). Likewise, observational studies of patient–professional interactions have revealed that children are often relegated to a non-participant status in consultations with information giving directed at the parent as opposed to the child (Tates & Meeuwesen 2001; Wassmer *et al.* 2004; Savage & Callery 2007). Similarly, research conducted with children in hospitals indicate that children have varying experiences of being consulted and involved in their care and that children often experience less than optimal communication (Carter 2002; Runeson *et al.* 2002; Beresford & Sloper 2003; Curtis *et al.* 2004; Hallstrom & Elander 2004; Coyne 2006a; Coyne *et al.* 2006). Information may be kept from children by both parents and health-care professionals because of the traditional view of the child as incompetent and being in need of protection.

Sharing information and sharing decisions are not synonymous; they are separate goals within the consultation, with information sharing being prerequisite to shared decision-making (Ong *et al.* 1995; Tates *et al.* 2002a). It is difficult to see how children can grow as autonomous decision-makers if withheld information hinders their ability to contribute to the decision-making process. Thus, having the relevant information is as important as being allowed to participate.

Children's participation in decision-making

It appears that children would like to be involved in decisions that concern them and their health care. In a summary of 59 separate health reports from voluntary bodies and statutory organisations, Boylan concluded that children and teenagers wanted the right to participate in decisions about their treatment rather than being passive recipients of care (Boylan 2004). However, the evidence suggests that children are rarely involved in the decision-making process and that parents' and health professionals' actions are major contributory factors in facilitating or hindering children's efforts to participate. In Sweden, Runeson *et al.* (2000) interviewed 26 children aged 6–17 years and found that in most cases the children's wishes were ignored or not elicited. Using the same sample, Runeson *et al.* (2002) observed interactions between parents ($n = 21$), children ($n = 24$) and nurses in relation to consultations and decision-making and reported that parents did not always support their children in difficult situations and that health-care staff frequently informed children without eliciting their views or presenting alternatives. Using the same data sample again, Hallstrom & Elander (2004) explored how decisions were made and found that children and parents made few decisions themselves and even if they disagreed with the decision made, few decisions were reconsidered.

Similar findings have been reported in a qualitative study of children's experiences of participation in consultations and decision-making in Ireland. Coyne *et al.* (2006) interviewed 55 children aged 7–18 years from three hospitals and reported that most of the children appeared to occupy a marginal position in health-care interactions, with discussions largely carried out between parents and health professionals. The children actively sought participation in health-care encounters, but were hindered by factors that included: fear of causing *trouble* by asking questions, lacking time with health professionals, difficulty contacting health professionals, being ignored, being disbelieved, health professionals not listening, not knowing health professionals, difficulty understanding medical terminology, being sick and parents' actions. Although there were many factors that appeared to obstruct children's participation, the key factors were health professionals' communication styles and behaviours.

Using the critical incident technique, Runeson *et al.* asked 92 Swedish health professionals (81 nurses, 8 doctors, 2 play therapists and 1 psychologist) to write about a situation in which a child (0–15 years) was allowed or not allowed to participate in decision-making (Runeson *et al.* 2001). They found that several factors influence whether children's voices were heard such as: child's protest, child's age and maturity, role of parents, attitudes of staff, time factor and alternative solutions to the problem. In England, Coyne (2006a) explored children's (*n* = 11), their parents' (*n* = 10) and nurses' (*n* = 12) views on children's participation in care and decision-making and found that children's own opinions and views were underused and they had varying experiences of being involved in treatment decisions. This is not to say that children did not have a voice as their views may have been mediated through the parents or other family members. However, the data from children indicated that they felt that they were not listened to and that health professionals did not generally actively seek their views. Likewise, parents felt that children should be involved in the decision-making process thereby enhancing and promoting children's self-esteem and positive self-regard, which would consequently enhance their overall welfare. However, nurses appeared to hold varying and discrepant views on the involvement of children in decisions, and for some nurses, the child's involvement seemed to be dependent on the child's cognitive maturity and being defined as a rational subject.

Miller (2001) found that although nurses (*n* = 8) viewed children's involvement as an integral part of their role, they found it as the most challenging part because of issues related to truth telling (truth could be frightening and damaging) and consent (balance between free will and persuasion). Doctors may not support children's participation in consultations for a variety of reasons such as: uncertainty about children's competence to understand or participate, lack of conviction of benefit for children, not agreeing with the children's wishes, loss of power and control, having their decisions questioned, lack of time, busy wards and lack of communication skills (Coyne 2008). It appears that doctors have traditionally seen child patients as *incompetent* and thus of subordinate status, and research on doctor–parent–child communication has found that doctors are more inclined to involve older children more directly in the consultation process (Mendelsohn *et al.* 1999; Tates & Meeuwesen 2001; Tates *et al.* 2002a, b). Thus doctors' behaviour may be influenced by their assumptions about children's immaturity. Or, alternatively, they may lack appropriate communication skills and also lack knowledge of children's communicative abilities (Beresford & Sloper 2003). Honeycutt *et al.* (2005) found that younger doctors were more likely to report using a participatory decision-making style with both children and their parents than older physicians. Today most medical schools provide training in patient-provider communication and interviewing skills. Therefore, a deficit in educational theory or communication skills cannot fully explain why doctors have problems facilitating children's participation. Perhaps doctors resist children's participation in decision-making because their power status is threatened, they lack the skills to deal with empowered children and they lack conviction that it is beneficial for children.

But others would argue that along with health professionals' beliefs and agendas, the organisational and legal setting needs to be taken into account (Tates *et al.* 2002a, b, c; Gabe *et al.* 2004). Doctors often experience difficulty reconciling opposing objectives: on the one hand, children are seen as immature and in need of protection and on the other, they have a right to be heard (BMA 2001). Gabe *et al.* (2004) point out that poor standard accommodation in the public health system (e.g. restricted space on wards), time pressures, and tight time slots result in hurried consultations. Communicating with young children cannot be rushed, and if time is an issue, perhaps some doctors choose to communicate with the parents. Tates *et al.* (2002a) argue that past research has not fully explored how the interaction between parent–doctor–child in the medical encounter can influence the active participation of the child. They analysed 105 videos of doctor–parent–child medical encounters in the Netherlands and found that in most consultations both doctors and parents displayed non-supportive behaviours towards children's participation. They observed that although doctors seemed to be orientated towards facilitating children's participation, they were often constrained by the parents' presence and demands for inclusion. Consequently, Tates *et al.* (2002c) argue that previous research on doctor–patient interactions has failed to consider how parents may influence health professionals' behaviour.

These are important findings as parents may exert influence in the parent–child–professional communication interaction. In research with children, they reported how their parent(s) inhibited their attempts to participate by various actions, for example, answering questions on their behalf, telling them to stay quiet, reprimanding them for interrupting discussions and withholding information (Coyne *et al.* 2006). Perhaps parents' actions may reflect their genuine need to protect their children's well-being and thus were well intentioned. But this does not fully explain why some parents overrule their children or silence them in front of health professionals. There may be different reasons why parents do not support their children's participation. Parents may struggle to balance their requirements for information with their child's needs for inclusion and active participation. Gore *et al.* (2005) found that parents (*n* = 31) had clearly defined unmet information needs which forced them into more active roles in the decision-making process than they desired. Equally, parents because of their own parenting, culture or social class may be socialised to a role which values obedience to professionals. Parents may themselves feel unequal to the authority of the health professionals, particularly doctors, and therefore may feel more comfortable adopting a subordinate position. Parents may have been discouraged from participation in their childhood and consequently may apply the same parenting style to their children. Gabe *et al.* (2004) suggest that the extent to which children are encouraged by their parents to take responsibility for decision-making (in the home) will influence the children's willingness to

take an active part in the consultation and their subsequent compliance with whatever is decided.

Acting in the child's best interest?

Clearly adults hold different philosophical beliefs which influence their behaviour towards children's participation in decision-making. Participation in decision-making in childhood is especially problematic because the management of the three-way relationship (parent, child, health professional) is complicated by issues of development and instincts for protection on the part of adults involved. Some parents and health professionals may have difficulty supporting children's participation because they feel children should be protected from potentially distressing information and the burden of decision-making. As the child's guardians, parents hold significant responsibility to ensure that their child's best interests are the primary consideration in all matters. Likewise, health professionals have a professional duty to ensure that the child's best interests are upheld. Acting in the child's best interest is founded on the ethical principle of beneficence which means to do good for another. Whilst the best interest principle is inherently beneficial for children, some argue that this thinking has the potential to deny children the right to be involved in health-care decisions (Bricher 2000; Young *et al.* 2003; Kilkelly & Donnelly 2006) and has the potential to be abused by adults who wish to override the wishes and feelings of children (Lansdown 1994). These are important concerns as the more one is in a position to make decisions for children, to speak on their behalf, the more one is able to silence their voices (Lee 2001).

Liberationists hold the belief that since children have equal rights as human beings they should be involved as much as possible in the decision-making process. However, the liberationist thinking could potentially endanger the long-tem best interests of the child by abandoning them to their own devices without informed adult support. Acknowledging children's rights to be heard could be interpreted by some adults as giving children sole responsibility for making decisions or overestimating desired level of autonomy (Britto *et al.* 2007). Children may be forced to exert self-determination before they have the cognitive ability to recognise the implications of their actions which may lead to them making decisions which they could regret later. Sometimes, adults make bad decisions on behalf of children and have to live with the consequences. But some would argue that it is unfair for children to be placed in such a position when decisions are about health-care matters that could have long-term implications. A *free-for-all* approach to children's participation may be harmful in that they could be placed in situations without adequate safeguards. It is important, therefore, that acknowledging children's rights to be heard is not seen as giving them sole responsibility for making decisions. Research has found that even when children are deemed capable of making health-care choices, they often need support for their decisions from family members and the health-care team and favour shared decision-making (Coyne *et al.* 2006; Zwaanswijk *et al.* 2007).

Support for shared (collaborative) decision-making

Children may want to participate in discussions about their care so that their voices are heard in relation to their needs rather than have full responsibility for decision-making (Boylan 2004). Alternatively, children's preferences for participation may vary according to the situation, their illness, their age and the type of decision (Garth *et al.* 2009). Hence, children's participation need not be total or complete; it may involve only selected aspects which implies that parents and health-care professionals need to be aware of the preferred style of the child and be adaptive enough to respond appropriately and be supportive. Likewise, parents often need the support and guidance of health professionals so that they can support themselves and their children in the decision-making process. Parents can experience difficulties participating in decision-making on their children's behalf and some prefer a collaborative role instead of an active decision-making role (Hallstrom *et al.* 2002; Gore *et al.* 2005). The pragmatic approach recognises that decision-making should be a shared collaborative process that respects each participant's contribution. Taking such an approach guards against the danger that professionals might relinquish their professional

responsibilities so that decision-making becomes an unwelcome burden for children and parents or they feel unsupported by practitioners.

Conclusion

As mentioned in the introduction, children are a vulnerable group entitled to special care and assistance because they have limited autonomy and are dependent upon others for physical care, emotional care and protection. They are dependent upon adults to advocate for them until they have the verbal and cognitive ability to give voice to their needs. Young hospitalised children are particularly vulnerable because of their illness, their limited understanding and because they have so little control over what is happening to them. Furthermore, children are vulnerable because they often lack the necessary coping mechanisms to help them negotiate the adverse aspects of hospitalisation.

To ensure that children's needs are met appropriately, it is extremely important that children are listened to and their views taken into account. Children want to be included in health-care interactions, to know what to expect about their care and to be respected as having opinions about their care and treatment. When children are provided with information and consulted about their care, they feel happy, reassured and treated as a person with rights. They feel prepared and less anxious about undergoing operations and treatment. When children are not involved in communication interactions or decisions about their care, they feel vulnerable, powerless and depersonalised. It appears, however, that the practice of speaking with children, listening to them and involving them in the decision-making process is not widespread among health professionals. Lack of consultation allied with an imposed subordinate role may adversely affect the physical and emotional welfare of the child. Children's perceptions of their personal value are important because research suggests that there is a relationship between self-worth and medical outcomes (Prilleltensky *et al.* 2001).

Increasing numbers of children with chronic illnesses are now surviving into adulthood and coping with conditions that require lifelong management. Therefore, children, and particularly adolescents, need to learn how to manage their own health condition over time; supporting children to acquire knowledge of their illness and to develop decision-making skills is therefore essential for their long-term welfare and health promotion. Restricting young children's participation in decision-making may lead to children being unprepared for the transition to adult services and consequently unprepared for the responsibility for their illness management (DoH 2006; Kirk 2008). Considering the health-promoting value of children's participation, it is important that adults respect children's views and help them contribute their views and preferences to health-care interactions.

Health professionals need to begin to view the involvement of children in decision-making as a moral issue since this is a child's right as a human being. Children have a right to have their opinion and wishes heard and respected and have a right to involvement in decisions about their care in hospital. Health professionals need to allow children to be involved so that through experience the child may develop competence in evaluating options and making informed decisions. This does not mean that all sick children, irrespective of circumstances, should be pressurised to get involved in decisions about their care or to have sole responsibility for decision-making. Children's participation should be viewed as a process that evolves over time and involves shared responsibility or negotiation of responsibility throughout childhood. Decisions should be seen as existing on a continuum ranging from everyday decisions to major decisions, with most decisions consisting of everyday decisions about ongoing care that children could easily participate in.

As discussed earlier, hospitalisation can be stressful for children and their parents and can result in considerable disruption to families. Children tell us that they value safe, secure, comfortable wards; knowing the health-care professionals as persons; being prepared for procedures; receiving information; having pain relief; being allowed to express their views and being heard; being able to have some choices over everyday matters whilst hospitalised and having a role in shared decision-making. Health-care professionals, particularly children's nurses, need to recognise how children's vulnerabilities may be exacerbated by the hospital system and identify strategies that will reduce the adverse aspects of the ward environment and demonstrate respect for children's autonomy and rights.

Good communication between health-care professionals and children is linked to increased understanding of illness and treatment which in turn leads to decreased stress for children and provides the foundation for quality care. It is important that children's views are sought, heard and valued, and their preferences accommodated where possible to ensure that services are responsive to their needs. Listening to and being with the child and family will help establish doctors' and nurses' humaneness and normality as human beings. Children experience less anxieties when they form a trusting relationship with the health-care staff. Listening to, interacting with the child as an individual, using kind and gentle words and being there as a caring human presence for children (and parents) are all actions which children really appreciate and which promote well-being. These are simple actions which are nevertheless fundamental to a child's positive experience of hospitalisation and overall well-being. Compassion, understanding, respect and caring are fundamental ethics in any human relationship. Seeing these qualities as integral to children's nurses' role will result in better quality of care and better outcomes for hospitalised children.

This chapter has discussed children's experience of hospitalisation and their participation in health-care decision-making. It is clear that the concepts of autonomy, trust, respect, privacy, autonomy and self-determination are essential concepts that overlap in the health care of the child. These concepts are closely connected with child–professional relationships, regulation of information, communication interactions, lack of preparation, inadequate facilities, and unsuitable ward environments. It is imperative that health-care professionals on an individual and organisational level reflect on practice to identify areas where children's rights are not upheld. To act in a manner that respects children's rights requires new approaches and skills as well as a clear understanding of how children's rights can be advanced in the hospital setting. Health-care professionals need to recognise that children are social beings and active social actors, and they should value the contribution that children make to their care. The challenge is to work *with* children rather than *for* them or *on* them.

Reflective scenario

Just a few days ago, Isobel Morgan, a bright and articulate girl aged 11, was diagnosed with cancer. She appears interested in what is happening to her but at times can be quiet during discussions around treatment decisions. Her parents are very concerned and are asking a lot of questions. They are keen to have discussions with the doctor away from Isobel as they do not want her to hear potentially distressing information. They want to filter the information she receives because in this way they can protect her from undue distress. You are aware that they have Isobel's best interest at heart, but at the same time you are worried that Isobel's right for information and preferences for participation may be overlooked.

Questions

1. What are the ethical standards for information sharing for children and adolescents?
2. What role ought parents to play in involving their child in communication and decision-making?
3. Should parents' preferences for information sharing be respected even if it differs from their child's desires?
4. How can Isobel's needs be taken into account when parents act as a barrier to information sharing?

References

Alderson, P. (2008) *Young Children's Rights: Exploring Beliefs, Principles and Practice*. Jessica Kingsley, London.

American Academy of Pediatrics Committee on Bioethics (1995) Informed consent, parental permission, and assent in pediatric practice. *Pediatrics*, **95**, 314–317.

Angst, D.B. & Deatrick J.A. (1996) Involvement in health care decisions: Parents and children with chronic illness. *Journal of Family Nursing*, **2**, 174–194.

Barnes, C.M., Bandak, A.G. & Beardslee, C.I. (1990) Content analysis of 186 descriptive case studies of hospitalised children. *Maternal-Child Nursing Journal*, **19**, 281–296.

Barrera, M.E., Rykov, H.M. & Doyle, L.S. (2002) The effects of interactive music therapy on hospitalized children with cancer: A pilot study. *Psycho-Oncology*, **11**, 379–388.

Battrick, C. & Glasper, E.A. (2004) The views of children and their families on being in hospital. *British Journal of Nursing*, **13**, 328–338.

Beresford, B.A. & Sloper, P. (2003) Chronically ill adolescents' experiences of communicating with doctors: A qualitative study. *Journal of Adolescent Health*, **33**, 172–179.

BMA (2001) *Consent, Rights and Choices in Health Care for Children and Young People*. British Medical Association, London.

Bossert, E. (1994) Stress appraisals of hospitalized school-age children. *Children's Health Care*, **23**, 33–49.

Boyd, J.R. & Hunsberger, M. (1998) Chronically ill children coping with repeated hospitalizations: Their perceptions and suggested interventions. *Journal of Pediatric Nursing*, **13**, 330–342.

Boylan, P. (2004) *Children's Voices Project: Feedback from Children and Young People about Their Experience and Expectations of Healthcare*, pp. 1–37. Commission for Health Improvement, UK.

Brewer, S., Gleditsch, S.L., Syblik, D., Tietjens, M.E. & Vacik, H.W. (2006) Pediatric anxiety: Child life intervention in day surgery. *Journal of Pediatric Nursing*, **12**, 13–22.

Bricher, G. (2000) Children in hospital: Issues of power and vulnerability. *Pediatric Nursing*, **26**, 33–39.

Britto, M.T., DeVellis, R.F., Hornung, R.W., DeFriese, G.H., Atherton, H.D. & Slap, G.B. (2004) Health care preferences and priorities of adolescents with chronic illnesses. *Pediatrics*, **114**, 1272–1280.

Britto, M.T., Slap, G.B., DeVellis, B.M., *et al.* (2007) Specialists understanding of the health care preferences of chronically ill adolescents. *Journal of Adolescent Health*, **40**, 334–341.

Byrne, A., Morton, J. & Salmon, P. (2001) Defending against patients' pain: A qualitative analysis of nurses' responses to children's postoperative pain. *Journal of Psychosomatic Research*, **50**, 69–76.

Carter, B. (2002) Chronic pain in childhood and the medical encounter: Professional ventriloquism and hidden voices. *Qualitative Health Research*, **12**, 28–41.

Claar, P.L., Walker, L.S. & Smith, C.A. (2002) The influence of appraisals in understanding children's experiences with medical procedures. *Journal of Pediatric Psychology*, **27**, 553–563.

Coad, J. & Coad, N. (2008) Children and young people's preference of thematic design and colour for their hospital environment. *Journal of Child Health Care*, **12**, 33–48.

Coad, J., Flay, J., Aspinall, M., Bilverstone, B., Coxhead, E. & Hones, B. (2008) Evaluating the impact of involving young people in developing children's services in an acute hospital trust. *Journal of Clinical Nursing*, **17**, 3115–3122.

Cohen, J. & Emanuel, J. (1998) *Positive Participation: Consulting and Involving Young People in Health-related Work: A Planning and Training Resource*. Health Education Authority, London.

Council of Europe (1996) European convention on the exercise of children's rights. In: *European Treaty Series/160*, 25 January 1996, Strasburg.

Coyne, I.T. (1996) Parent participation: A concept analysis. *Journal of Advanced Nursing*, **23**, 733–740.

Coyne, I.T. (2003) *A grounded theory of disrupted lives: Children, parents, and nurses in the children's ward*. Unpublished PhD thesis, King's College University of London, London.

Coyne, I. (2006a) Consultation with children in hospital: Children, parents' and nurses' perspectives. *Journal of Clinical Nursing*, **15**, 61–71.

Coyne, I.T. (2006b) Children's experiences of hospitalisation. *Journal of Child Health Care*, **10**, 326–336.

Coyne, I.T. (2007) Critical engagement with practice: Being a human caring presence for children and their parents. *Journal of Children's and Young People's Nursing*, **1**, 298.

Coyne, I.T. (2008) Children's participation in consultations and decision-making at health service level: A critical review of the literature. *International Journal of Nursing Studies*, **45**, 1682–1689.

Coyne, I.T. & Conlon, J. (2007) Children's and young people's views of hospitalisation: 'It's a scary place'. *Journal of Children's and Young People's Nursing*, **1**, 16–21.

Coyne, I.T. & Cowley, S. (2007) Challenging the philosophy of partnership with parents: A grounded theory study. *International Journal of Nursing Studies*, **44**, 893–904.

Coyne, I.T., Hayes, E., Gallagher, P. & Regan, G. (2006) *Giving Children a Voice: Investigation of Children's Experiences of Participation in Consultation and Decision-making in Irish Hospitals*. Office of the Minister for Children, Dublin.

Coyne, I., Hayes, E. & Gallagher, P. (2009) Inclusion of hospitalized children in healthcare research: Ethical, practical and organisational challenges. *Childhood*, **16**, 413–429.

Curtis, K., Liabo, K., Roberts, H. & Barker, M. (2004) Consulted but not heard: A qualitative study of young people's views of their local health service. *Health Expectations*, **7**, 149–156.

Curtis, P., James, A. & Birch, J. (2007) Space to care: Children's perceptions of spatial aspects of hospitals. *Full Research Report. ESRC End of Award Report, RES-000-23-0765*, pp. 1–25. ESRC, Swindon, http://www.cscy.group.shef.ac.uk/research/spacetocare.htm

Department of Health and Children (2000a) *The National Children's Strategy: Our Children – Their Lives*. Department of Health and Children, Dublin.

Department of Health and Children (2000b) *Report of the Public Consultation for the National Children's Strategy*. Department of Health and Children, Dublin.

DoH (2003) *Getting the Right Start: The National Service Framework for Children, Young People and Maternity Services – Standards for Hospital Services*. Department of Health, London.

DoH (2006) *Transition: Getting It Right for Young People, Improving the Transition of People with Long Term Conditions from Children to Adult Services*. Department of Health, London.

Dixon-Woods, M., Anwar, Z., Young, B. & Brooke, A. (2002) Lay evaluation of services for child with asthma. *Health and Social Care in the Community*, **10**, 503–511.

Eisen, S.J., Ulrich, R.S., Shepley, M.M., Varni, J.W. & Sherman, S. (2008) The stress reducing effects of art in pediatric health care: Art preferences of healthy children and hospitalised children. *Journal of Child Health Care*, **12**, 173–190.

Forsner, M., Jansson, L. & Soerlie, V. (2005) Being ill as narrated by children aged 11–18 years. *Journal of Child Health Care*, **9**, 314–323.

Freed, L.H., Ellen, J.M., Irwin, C.E. & Millstein, S.G. (1998) Determinants of adolescent satisfaction with health care providers and intentions to keep follow-up appointments. *Journal of Adolescent Health*, **22**, 475–479.

Gabe, J., Olumide, G. & Bury, M. (2004) 'It takes three to tango': A framework for understanding patient partnership in paediatric clinics. *Social Science & Medicine*, **59**, 1071–1079.

Garth, B., Murphy, G.C. & Reddihough, D.S. (2009) Perceptions of participation: Child patients with a disability in the doctor-patient-child partnership. *Patient Education and Counseling*, **74**, 45–52.

Gore, C., Johnson, R.J., Caress, A.L., Woodcock, A. & Custovic, A. (2005) The information needs and preferred roles in treatment decision-making of parents caring for infants with atopic dermatitis: A qualitative study. *Allergy*, **60**, 938–943.

Greig, A., Taylor, J. & MacKay, T. (2007) *Doing Research with Children*. Sage, Los Angeles.

Hallstrom, I. & Elander, G. (2004) Decision making during hospitalization: Parents' and children's involvement. *Journal of Clinical Nursing*, **13**, 367–375.

Hallstrom, I., Runeson, I. & Elander, G. (2002) An observational study of the level at which parents participate in decisions during their child's hospitalization. *Nursing Ethics*, **9**, 202–214.

Hill, M., Davis, J., Prout, A. & Tisdall, K. (2004) Moving the participation agenda forward. *Children & Society*, **18**, 77–96.

Honeycutt, C., Sleath, B., Bush, P.J., Campbell, W. & Tudor, G. (2005) Physician use of a participatory decision-making style with children with ADHD and their parents. *Patient Education and Counseling*, **57**, 327–332.

Howells, R. & Lopez, T. (2008) Better communication with children and parents. *Paediatrics and Child Health*, **18**, 381–385.

Hutton, A. (2005) Consumer perspectives in adolescent ward design. *Journal of Clinical Nursing*, **14**, 537–545.

Justus, R., Wyles, D., Wilson, J., Rode, D., Walther, V. & Lim-Sulit, N. (2006) Preparing children and families for surgery: Mount Sinai's multidisciplinary perspective. *Pediatric Nursing*, **32**, 35–43.

Kilkelly, U. & Donnelly, M. (2006) *The Child's Right to be Heard in the Healthcare Setting: Perspectives of Children, Parents and Health Professionals*. Office of the Minister for Children, Dublin.

Kirk, S. (2008) Transitions in the lives of young people with complex healthcare needs. *Child: Care, Health and Development*, **34**, 567–575.

LaMontagne, L. (2000) Children's coping with surgery: A process-oriented perspective. *Journal of Pediatric Nursing*, **15**, 307–312.

Lansdown, G. (1994) Children's rights. In: *Children's Childhoods Observed and Experienced* (ed. B. Mayall), pp. 33–44. Falmer Press, London.

Lawes, C., Sawyer, L., Amos, S., Kandiah, M., Pearce, L. & Symons, J. (2007) Impact of an education programme for staff working with children undergoing painful procedures. *Paediatric Nursing*, **20**, 33–37.

Lee, N. (2001) *Childhood and Society: Growing Up in an Age of Uncertainty*. Open University Press, Buckingham.

Lindeke, L., Nakai, M. & Johnson, L. (2006) Capturing children's voices for quality improvement. *American Journal of Maternal Child Nursing*, **31**, 290–297.

Longhi, E. & Pickett, N. (2008) Music and well-being in long-term hospitalised children. *Psychology of Music*, **36**, 247–256.

McClowry, S.G. (1988) A review of the literature pertaining to the psychosocial responses of school-aged children to hospitalization. *Journal of Pediatric Nursing*, **3**, 296–311.

Mendelsohn, J.S., Quinn, M.T. & McNabb, W.L. (1999) Interview strategies commonly used by pediatricians. *Archives of Pediatrics & Adolescent Medicine*, **153**, 154–157.

Miller, S. (2001) Facilitating decision-making in young people. *Paediatric Nursing*, **13**, 31–35.

Ministry of Health C.H.S.C. (1959) The welfare of children in hospital. In *Chairman: Sir H. Platt*. HMSO, London.

O'Connor-Von, S. (2000) Preparing children for surgery – An integrative research review. *AORN Journal*, **71**, 334–343.

Oldfield, C. & Fowler, C. (2004) *Mapping Children and Young People's Participation in England*. Department for Education and Skills, Nottingham.

Ong, L.M.L., de Haes, J.C.J.M., Hoos, A.M. & Lammes, F.B. (1995) Doctor-patient communication: A review of the literature. *Social Science & Medicine*, **40**, 903–918.

Pelander, T. & Leino-Kilpi, H. (2004) Quality in pediatric nursing care: Children's expectations. *Issues in Comprehensive Pediatric Nursing*, **27**, 139–151.

Polkki, T., Pietila, A. & Vehilainen-Julkunen, K. (2003) Experiences of fears in surgical paediatric patients. *Sairaanoitaja*, **76**, 18–21.

Power, N. & Franck, L. (2008) Parent participation in the care of hospitalized children: A systematic review. *Journal of Clinical Nursing*, **62**, 622–641.

Prilleltensky, I., Nelson, G. & Peirson, L. (2001) The role of power and control in children's lives: An ecological analysis of pathways toward wellness, resilience and problems. *Journal of Community and Applied Social Psychology*, **11**, 143–158.

Robertson, J. (1958a) *Going to Hospital with Mother*. Tavistock, London.

Robertson, J. (1958b) *Young Children in Hospital*. Tavistock, London.

RCPCH (2003) *Bridging the Gap: Health Care for Adolescents*. Royal College of Paediatrics and Child Health, London.

RCPCH Ethics Advisory Committee (2000) Guidelines for the ethical conduct of medical research involving children. *Archives of Disease in Childhood*, **82**, 117–182.

Runeson, I., Elander, G., Hermeren, G. & Kristensson-Hallstrom, I. (2000) Children's consent to treatment: Using a scale to assess degrees of self-determination. *Pediatric Nursing*, **26**, 16–22.

Runeson, I., Enskar, K., Elander, G. & Hermeren, G. (2001) Professionals' perceptions of children's participation in decision making in healthcare. *Journal of Clinical Nursing*, **10**, 70–78.

Runeson, I., Hallstrom, I., Elander, G. & Hermeren, G. (2002) Children's participation in the decision-making process during hospitalisation: An observational study. *Nursing Ethics*, **9**, 583–598.

Savage, E. & Callery, P. (2007) Clinic consultations with children and parents on the dietary management of cystic fibrosis. *Social Science & Medicine*, **64**, 363–374.

Schmidt, C., Bernaix, L., Koski, A., Weese, J., Chiapetta, M. & Sandrik, K. (2007) Hospitalized children's perceptions of nurses and nurse behaviors. *MCN. The American Journal of Maternal Child Nursing Administration Quarterly*, **32**, 336–342.

Shiminski-Maher, T. (1993) Physician-patient-parent communication problems. *Pediatric Neurosurgery*, **19**, 104–108.

Simons, J. & Robertson, E. (2002) Poor communication and knowledge deficits: Obstacles to effective management of children's postoperative pain. *Journal of Advanced Nursing*, **40**, 78–86.

Sloper, P. & Lightfoot, J. (2003) Involving disabled and chronically ill children and young people in healthcare service development. *Child Care, Health and Development*, **29**, 15–20.

Smith, L. & Callery, P. (2005) Children's accounts of their preoperative information needs. *Journal of Clinical Nursing*, **14**, 230–238.

Stevens, M. (1986) Adolescents' perception of stressful events during hospitalisation. *Journal of Pediatric Nursing*, **1**, 303–313.

Tates, K. & Meeuwesen, L. (2001) Doctor-parent-child communication: A review of the literature. *Social Science and Medicine*, **52**, 839–851.

Tates, K., Elbers, E., Meeuwesen, L. & Bensing, J. (2002a) Doctor-parent-child relationships: A "pas de trois". *Patient Education and Counseling*, **48**, 5.

Tates, K., Meeuwesen, L., Bensing, J. & Elbers, E. (2002b) Joking or decision-making? Affective and instrumental behaviour in doctor-parent-child communication. *Psychology and Health*, **17**, 281–295.

Tates, K., Meeuwesen, L., Elbers, E. & Bensing, J. (2002c) I've come for his throat': Roles and identities in doctor-parent-child communication. *Child Care Health and Development*, **28**, 109–116.

Thompson, M.L. (1994) Information-seeking coping and anxiety in school-age children anticipating surgery. *Children's Health Care*, **23**, 87–97.

Tieffenberg, J., Wood, E., Alonso, A., Tossutti, M. & Vincente, M. (2000) A randomized trail of ACINDES: A child centered training model for children with chronic illnesses (asthma and epilepsy). *Journal of Urban Health*, **77**, 280–297.

Timmerman, R.R. (1983) Preoperative fears of older children. *AORN Journal*, **38**, 827–834.

UN (1989) *Convention on the Rights of the Child*. United Nations, Geneva.

Van Dulmen, A.M. (1998) Children's contributions to pediatric outpatient encounters. *Pediatrics*, **102**, 563–568.

Wassmer, E., Minnaar, G., Atkinson, M., Gupta, E., Yuen, S. & Rylance, G. (2004) How do paediatricians communicate with children and parents? *Acta Paediatrica*, **93**, 1501–1506.

Wikstrom, B.-M. (2005) Communicating via expressive arts: The natural medium of self-expression for hospitalised children. *Pediatric Nursing*, **31**, 480–485.

de Winter, M., Baerveldt, C. & Kooistra, J. (2002) Enabling children: Participation as a new perspective on child-health promotion. *Child Care Health and Development*, **28**, 109–116.

Wolfer, J.A. & Visintainer, M.A. (1975) Pediatric surgical patients' and parents' stress responses and adjustment. *Nursing Research*, **24**, 244–255.

Young, B., Dixon-Woods, M., Windridge, K.C. & Heney, D. (2003) Managing communication with young people who have a life threatening chronic illness: A qualitative study of patients and parents. *British Medical Journal*, **326**, 305–309.

Zwaanswijk, M., Tates, K., van Dulmen, S., Hoogerbrugge, P., Kamps, W. & Bensing, J. (2007) Young patients', parents', and survivors' communication preferences in paediatric oncology: Results of online focus groups. *BMC Pediatrics*, **7**, 35.

Suggested further readings

Alderson, P. (2008) *Young Children's Rights: Exploring Beliefs, Principles and Practice*, 2nd edn. Jessica Kingsley, London.

Boylan, P. (2004) *Children's Voices Project: Feedback from Children and Young People about their Experience and Expectations of Healthcare*, pp. 1–37. Commission for Health Improvement, UK.

Cavet, J. & Sloper, P. (2005) *Children and Young People's Views on Health and Health Services: A Review of the Evidence*, pp. 1–83. National Children's Bureau, London.

Web sites

Every Child Matters – UK Government www.everychild-matters.gov.uk/**participation**/

UNICEF www.unicef.org/crc/files/**Participation**

RCPCH (Royal College of Paediatrics and Child Health) www.**rcpch**.ac.uk/page.aspx?id_Content=862

12 The Ethics of Family-Centred Care for Hospitalised Children

Linda Shields

Introduction

Family-centred care (FCC) is a well-known concept. Or is it? If one visits just about every children's hospital, child health facility, paediatric health centre and, of late, many adult health services, in just about every country, one will find policy documents, standards, guidelines, all espousing FCC. A trawl through web sites of 15 children's hospitals in several English-speaking countries showed that FCC was well known in 13 of them. Policy documents from paediatric health services in non-English-speaking countries will find similar results. Many will agree that FCC is widely recognised and used. But do we really know what FCC is? How is it defined? What does it mean for families? For health professionals? Is it the best model for use with children and their families? Is there an alternative? Does it work in different cultures? And is it ethical for us to continue to use the term so widely if we cannot answer the previous questions adequately? This chapter defines FCC, gives a brief history of its evolution and then examines it using several theories of ethics. The end result is more questions than answers, and a plea for more debate and discussion over a widely applied model for which no real evidence exists.

What is family-centred care?

The Institute for Family-Centered Care (IFCC) (2009) in the US defines FCC as

> ... an innovative approach to the planning, delivery, and evaluation of health care that is grounded in mutually beneficial partnerships among health care patients, families, and providers. Patient- and family-centered care applies to patients of all ages, and it may be practiced in any health care setting.

They describe four main concepts which comprise FCC: dignity and respect, information sharing, participation and collaboration.

However, while the above describes what FCC is about, it lacks a clear delineation of what FCC really is. These are descriptive definitions, useful in their own right, but they are superficial and one is left in some doubt as to what FCC is, what it means and how it works. From an Aristotelian perspective, these definitions do not contain the essential nature of FCC, in other words, they are *nominal* definitions. In contrast, a *real* definition gives the *real nature* of the thing being defined (Wolfram 1995). To meet these problems, a more complete definition has been coined, one that includes meaning rather than description, and leaves one in no doubt as to what FCC really means when it is applied:

> Family-centered care is a way of caring for children and their families within health services which ensures that care is planned around the whole family, not just the individual child/ person, and in which all the family members are recognized as care recipients.
>
> (Shields *et al.* 2006:318)

In the UK, many authors have written about FCC, but the most cogent to date have been Lynda Smith, Valerie Coleman and Maureen Bradshaw (Smith *et al.* 2002), who describe effective FCC as a continuum of care from all nurses, delivered to all done by the family. They give fine examples of how FCC can work in practice, and describe negotiation and effective communication between parents, children and nurses as the cornerstone for the successful implementation of FCC models.

Historical background

FCC grew out of the work of researchers and theorists working in the UK and US in the middle of the twentieth century. The first specialist children's hospitals opened in France (1802), Vienna (1837) and London (1852) (Shields & Nixon 1998), and largely catered for children of the poor, as most wealthy patients of all ages were cared for at home. Prior to World War I, there was an emphasis on the emotional needs of the child. Before the 1920s, nurses practiced a form of care that took full account of the child's social and psychological needs (Wood 1888; Yapp 1915). However, by the 1920s, this had changed to a more industrialised environment, and hospitals became unhappy places for children (Jolley 2007; Jolley & Shields 2008). Ward routines suited the staff rather than the patients, and parents relinquished responsibility for their child to the hospital staff (Shields & Nixon 1998). In some places, parents were excluded completely from visiting their children. Nurses and doctors genuinely believed that this was beneficial to the child rather than having them

upset when their parents went home at the end of visiting hours (Shields & Nixon 1998).

Nursing between 1920 and the end of World War II was characterised by the fight against infectious diseases and cross-infection in hospitals. Parents were excluded for fear of them spreading infection (Aubuchon 1958). Antibiotics were yet to come, and contagious diseases were well known. Hospital staff worked in fear of an outbreak of infectious disease which would spread amongst patients, which might force the hospital to close, and thereby malign its reputation (Lomax 1996). In the absence of antibiotics, order, discipline and asepsis were matched against the spread of infection, and, perhaps necessarily for the time, were given higher priority than the emotional needs of either children or parents.

The years between 1920 and 1970 saw some attempts at change which would allow mothers to stay with their children. Sir James Spence in Newcastle-upon-Tyne in England established the first mother-and-child unit in 1927 (Spence 1947; Robertson 1962), admitting breastfeeding mothers with their infants. In the US, Renee Spitz (1945) used the term *hospitalism* to denote a decline in the health of a child due to long confinement in a hospital. Some described the traumatic effects of surgery on children and alleviation of such effects by involving the mother (Levy 1945; Powers 1948; Stevens 1949). Bowlby begins his groundbreaking work about mother–child separation in the 1940s with the publication of his study of *44 juvenile thieves* (Bowlby 1944a, b) which demonstrated that children separated from their mothers for long periods before the age of 5 years could develop psychopathology later. This was a time when a hospital admission for a child could be as long as a week for a minor procedure, and several years for chronic and long-term conditions (Shields & Nixon 1998). Research from New Zealand showed that infection rates did not increase if parents stayed with their hospitalised infants (Pickerill & Pickerill 1945, 1946), and psychiatrists began to trace conditions in adults to the childhood experience of hospitalisation (Pearson 1941). Psychologists turned their attention to the phenomenon of child–parent separation caused by wartime evacuations (Burlingham & Freud 1942), and to other forms of separation such as that which took place when children were admitted to hospital (Robertson &

Bowlby 1952; Illingworth 1956). However, it was the cataclysmic events of World War II which provided the catalyst for change in public opinion which facilitated the eventual implementation of FCC. Childhood and parenting as concepts were changed as, in many European countries, children were evacuated to country areas and away from their parents for extended periods (Isaacs 1941), while millions were orphaned and made homeless (Shields & Bryan 2002). Jolley (2007) believes that this led to a redefining of the parent–child relationship, and new perceptions about the need for increased involvement of parents in the health care of their children.

The winds of change speeded up in the 1950s. A *Citizen's Committee on Children of New York City*, in 1955, questioned the citing of infection as a reason to restrict parents from visiting their children (Faust 1953; Fleury *et al*. 1954; Citizen's Committee on Children of New York City 1955). The most important event in the development of FCC, though, was the setting up, by the British government, of a select committee of parliament to examine the way children were cared for in hospital. The report of this committee came to be known as the *Platt Report* (Ministry of Health 1959) (after Sir Harry Platt who chaired the committee). It had 55 recommendations, but the most far-reaching were that the mother be admitted with her child, that accommodation for the parent be provided by and in the hospital and that school and play facilities be provided. The Platt Report is still widely quoted today. Across the world, lobby groups consisting of parents and health professionals grew up. For many years, changes in hospitals where children were nursed continued slowly, and these lobby organisations supported the changes and acted as *watchdogs*. They now focus on the health and well-being of all children and families, not just those in hospital.

Over subsequent years, and with consideration of the role played by parents and family, models of care of children in hospitals have been developed, such as *care-by-parent* where a family of a sick child moves into a purpose-built unit constructed like a home and where care is given to the sick child (Goodband & Jennings 1992). This works well with children with long-term conditions, but is costly to set up, and in these times of short hospital stays has become somewhat redundant. *Partnership-in-care*

(Casey 1995) was developed in the UK to provide a way to incorporate parents into the care planning and delivery of care around a sick child, and *negotiated care* was an extension of this (Smith 1995) where parents and staff negotiated about who was to do what care for a sick child in hospital. These were useful models to promote the involvement of parents, and were based on the assumption that parents know their child best and are needed by the child when he or she is most vulnerable, such as during an illness.

Family-centred care

FCC followed from these models of care which involved parents. At first, it was a rather nebulous concept, as health professionals, largely nurses, tried to grapple with the ideal way to include parents in decision making and care planning. Some important work was done in Canada with parents of children with disabilities (King *et al*. 1997), and in other work, the elements of FCC, as defined by the Association for the Care of Children's Health, were as follows:

(1) Recognizing that the family is the constant in a child's life, whereas service systems and personnel within those systems fluctuate

(2) Facilitating parent/professional collaboration at all levels of health care

(3) Recognizing family strengths and individuality, and respecting different methods of coping

(4) Sharing unbiased and complete information with parents about their child's care on an ongoing basis in an appropriate and supportive manner

(5) Encouraging and facilitating parent-to-parent support

(6) Understanding and incorporating the developmental needs of infants, children, adolescents and their families into health care systems

(7) Implementing appropriate policies and programs that are comprehensive and provide emotional and financial support to meet the needs of families

(8) Assuring that the design of the health care delivery system is flexible, accessible, and responsive to family needs (Bruce & Ritchie 1997:215).

The IFCC (2009) in the US was founded in 1992, and now states its purpose as to provide 'leadership to advance the understanding and practice of patient- and family-centered care'. It is an internet-based organisation focusing entirely on FCC, providing a very good reference point for parents, children and health professionals. It has a wide range of resources, including validated research tools and supporting information for consumers of health care. It also has an educational focus, and runs many conferences and workshops. Their web site is worth a visit: http://www.familycentered care.org/

In summary, FCC has evolved through a series of developments from allowing mothers to stay with their breastfed infants, through various levels of involvement for parents, to FCC as we know it today. Such development has been sociological, psychological, managerial and philosophical. Currently, FCC is a well-known concept, bandied around in most health-care facilities across the world, though the lack of rigorous research (Shields *et al.* 2007) about it must lead one to ask if it is fully understood. We must be somewhat critical of its ubiquity, ask if there is anything wrong with this model and if it presents ethical issues which need to be addressed.

Debate and contention about family-centred care

Health professionals around the world are using FCC widely, in practice, education and research. However, there is some debate over its applicability. Darbyshire (1994) has suggested that better insight is needed into what constitutes the parent–nurse relationship, and what are real experiences for parents of hospitalised children. He conducted a phenomenological study of parents who lived in hospital with their children in a large Scottish children's hospital in 1987–88, and described parenting a child in hospital as *parenting in public* and the nurses caring for them as *nursing in public* (Darbyshire 1994:17). Some parents felt that they were being imposed upon to stay with their children, and that the nurses expected them to contribute to their child's care. They moved into a mode described by Darbyshire as *defensive parenting*, felt they were in danger of being a nuisance to the nursing staff and consequently would modify their parenting style while the child was in hospital to meet what they thought was expected of them by the nurses (rather than what they thought their child needed). When nurses assessed parents for participation in their child's care, they drew their conclusions from parents' responses to their interpretation and explanation of situations. This created a climate where parents who were not demonstrative in their care and love for their child may have been misinterpreted as not being able to fully participate in the care.

Darbyshire's (1994) work encapsulated the feelings of parents and nurses, and provided reference points for both clinical work and further research. His work has shown that while parents are an accepted part of the hospital scene in many children's wards, they are sometimes not comfortable about staying and participating in care. Sometimes this is because of factors such as other children who need care, or because they may feel judged by the staff. He suggested that FCC is an ideal that, because of human nature, cannot be reached.

Imelda Coyne (1995a, b, 1996, 2008) has been equally contentious about the use of FCC. In a 1995 literature review about parental participation in care, she described wide variations in the amount of care that parents were willing to undertake, that confusion existed over parents' roles and their expectations and a lack of role definition for both parents of hospitalised children and nurses caring for them. In another study, Coyne (1996) used concept analysis to explore the meanings of parent participation in British literature. She found that the descriptions usually comprised negotiation, control, willingness, competence and authority, but in the main, was poorly defined. She recommended that major rethinking needed to occur before FCC would be fully understood or utilised.

In 1995, using phenomenology and a sample of 18 parents, Coyne (1995b) examined parents' views of partnership in care. All viewed their participation as necessary for the child's well-being, a non-negotiable part of parenthood. Nurses were seen as too busy to provide consistent care. Sixteen parents had other siblings cared for by friends, neighbours or family, and worried about those children. Parents were prepared to learn more complex care, but only when necessary, preferring to leave it to the nurses because of the anxiety it caused.

Information, communication and negotiation were the most important part of ensuring successful partnerships with the nurses.

By 2008, little had changed. Coyne (2008) found in a grounded theory study of 12 nurses from paediatric wards in two English hospitals that parents were socialised into the roles in the wards as perceived for them by the nurses, rather than allowing the parents themselves to determine their level of participation. The nurses used inclusionary and exclusionary tactics to implement this socialisation, and were rewarded or punished to reinforce the nurses' demands about their participation. Parents had to fall into line, had no other option but to participate in the care of their child at the level demanded by the nurses and were expected to behave properly according to the nurses' lights. Coyne (2008) summarised the situation as parents being used for managerial efficiency rather than as active consumers of care for their child. Such findings, though an extreme example of the unethical use of the erroneous application of FCC principles, are reminiscent of earlier Swedish studies (Kristensson-Hallström & Elander 1997; Hallström & Runeson 2001) which found that parents had to use strategies to ensure they have the support they require and these include (a) relinquishing all care to the staff, (b) trying to retain a measure of control over their child and (c) insisting that they know what is best for their child. Strategies used by parents to ensure their needs were met included avoiding making themselves a nuisance to the nurses, being positive towards the staff, asking questions, ensuring they were as prepared as possible for whatever might happen during the child's admission and informing the staff about their expectations.

One of the main ethical principles of applying any model of care, in any setting, is the use of rigorous evidence to substantiate its use, and herein lies a problem for any health facility which espouses a policy of FCC. There is no rigorous evidence that it makes any difference at all to the way care is delivered. A Cochrane systematic review of the literature (Shields *et al.* 2007) has found no studies that could be included to demonstrate the effectiveness of FCC. In this same review, a summary of qualitative studies (Shields *et al.* 2006) provided some tantalising

reports that FCC may be of benefit, but without level one evidence it is not possible to know if it really works or not. It may make a difference, it may make the health service experience for children and families better than if there was no such policy in place, but we do not know. Coyne's (2008) work, in particular, must make us query whether or not we should be trying to implement FCC, and perhaps Darbyshire (1994) is right – it may be a great ideal, but almost impossible to implement effectively.

Children's rights to health care

Children have the right to fair and equitable access to good health and health care. This was enshrined in the United Nations (UN) Declaration of the Rights of the Child in 1959 and more latterly, such tenets were included in the 1989 UN Convention on the Rights of the Child. From an ethical stance, this would seem self-evident, and something that should be in place everywhere, regardless of the country and culture. FCC would seem an ideal way to promote the rights of children to receive the highest level of health possible, for few children are without family of some kind, and it is often through the family that children access health care. However, we have to examine if this is so, and we do this using a series of ethical theories and constructs.

Philosophy and ethics of family-centred care

Beauchamp and Childress paradigm

We can examine FCC using the Beauchamp & Childress (2005) paradigm of respect for autonomy, beneficence, non-maleficence, justice and context. A family being cared for in a health service can only act autonomously if (a) the health professional allows them to be, and (b) if they want to. Coyne (2008) has bleakly demonstrated that health professionals may not always be very good at recognising parents' claim to autonomy over their child, and Bradshaw (2002) points out that depending on a range of factors, parents may not want to have to choose and make autonomous decisions around their child's care. Autonomy can be questioned in relation to FCC. The family (patient) may be said to have autonomy, but there is also the autonomy of the health professional to take into account. That is, there may be a conflict between uncompromised family autonomy and the ability of the health professionals to operate. A respect for autonomy of both the giver(s) and receiver(s) of care is required, and this perhaps may limit the autonomy of either.

Models of FCC are beneficent, that is, their intent is to deliver good, and the good of the patient is primary but only if they are implemented properly; otherwise, as Darbyshire (1994) and Coyne (1995a, b, 2008) have demonstrated, they can create situations where communication between parent and health professional breaks down, rendering the potential good ineffective despite the good intention inferred when one says one is working within a model of FCC. According to the Beauchamp and Childress paradigm, a practice or policy should avoid causing harm, that is, it must be non-maleficent. Can we say that about FCC? If FCC is implemented effectively, is it the most moral way to deliver health care to children? As we have no level one evidence of its effectiveness (Shields *et al.* 2007), we cannot make an informed decision about whether or not it should be used. The little evidence that exists suggests that it is a wonderful ideal on paper, but almost impossible to implement. This suggests that the next factor of the paradigm, justice, cannot be met either. It cannot be just to continue to try to implement a model of care that not only has unknown results (Shields *et al.* 2006) about its application, but also is showing more and more to be ineffective (Coyne 2008). However, in philosophy and ethics, justice is a complex concept. There may be different elements of justice involved. It may be just to encourage family involvement if the family unit is considered to be a moral *patient*, as it is with the child as an individual. There are many definitions and characteristics of justice within ethical theories. Johnstone (1999) suggests that two of these are most pertinent to the nursing of patients (in our case, families). Justice as fairness, that is, 'one acts justly toward a person when that person has given what is due or owed' (p. 42), is the first. She describes it as when a person receives something that he or she deserves. By definition for

all nurses, patients being nursed deserve the best care that the nurse can give, and for our purposes, this translates to families. Therefore, the receipt of good nursing care is just, and an injustice occurs when the care is not good. Johnstone's (1999) second applicable type of justice within nursing is distributive justice, in other words, an 'equal distribution of benefits and burdens' (p. 43). All persons are required to receive benefits, harms and responsibilities equally. However, this can be contradicted and inequalities can be acceptable only if the least well off achieve a level of well-being to match that of their better-off counterparts. Johnstone's example of an abrogation of distributive justice in nursing is the continued poor status and low pay of nurses when compared with other professions of equal educational standing. For our argument about FCC, distributive justice would hold that all families are entitled to the best care available, and for it to be judged *best*, FCC would have to be applied according to the particular needs of every individual family.

Virtue ethics

The *Stanford Encyclopedia of Philosophy* (Hursthouse 2007) defines virtue ethics as a form of ethics 'that emphasizes the virtues, or moral character', in other words, focuses on good motives and character as well as good actions. A virtuous act is one done predominantly from the desire to do what is good and right, and not from self-interest. There are several forms of virtue. Aristotelian philosophy would recognise that in health service provision, the virtue of *practical wisdom* (phronesis), the core or primary virtue in Aristotelian virtue theory, with the conjunction of intellectual virtue, moral virtue and expertise, is most relevant. Can FCC be examined from such a position? To do so, one must explore the good in FCC. Is there an inherent good in FCC, or should it be viewed more on its results, that is, the family's well-being (if it is applied successfully), or lack of well-being if it is not? If the family did not receive care from a health service through use of the FCC model, would they be missing out on a good which would make their lives happier, or better, if they had received their care that way? Do health professionals who deliver FCC provide it because it is a good, or do they have other motives for doing so? Is it possible that health professionals try to deliver FCC because they feel they have a duty to do so (a deontological approach), because they know they are under scrutiny of the family members (as in Darbyshire's (1994) *nursing in public*) or because they feel good themselves through the sense of accomplishment of having done the job well? If it is not possible for a truly virtuous person to act in a truly virtuous way, is the difficulty of being virtuous what is making it so difficult for FCC to be implemented properly?

Deontology

Deontology is a branch of ethical thought in which one's choice of action is guided by what one ought to do. (*Deontology* comes from the Greek for duty (*deon*) and science (or study) of (*logos*) (Alexander & Moore 2008).) Under this branch of ethical reasoning, one acts in a certain way because one is guided by what is perceived to be one's duty. From a religious perspective, it is one's duty to follow the tenets of the Ten Commandments, or the teachings of Mohammed, etc. Regardless of religion, deontological moral guides tell us what our moral duties are.

A truly deontological action follows one's moral duty, but may take little notice of possible consequences. An action, of itself and regardless of consequences, is assessed as inherently right or wrong (Crisp 1995). Kant was the main philosopher in whose work deontological ethics was developed, and he saw duty as something that is done for its own sake, and not for its consequences (Kant 1972). However, he warned that by doing such actions one must not be benefiting oneself over others; rather, we should act only on the premise that the action will be acceptable to anyone, and the action must be based on a subjectively valid principle, one that would be the operating principle for all similar actions. Roughly, Kant's ethics are exemplified in the biblical maxim 'do unto others as you would have them do unto you'. Such an outlook could be said to be why FCC has been so widely accepted in health services. It sounds lovely, and anyone would wish it to be done to them when their child is ill.

So while a person will be said to be acting morally when following one's duty, is it right when *following one's duty* is given as the reason for undertaking something that while done according to one's duty has a bad outcome? For example, nurses in Nazi Germany firmly believed they had a duty to kill children with disabilities as they were *useless feeders* and *life unworthy of life* (propaganda terms used at the time), and a burden on the State. Less extreme examples in health services could be a nurse who acts in a certain way because that is the way it has always been done, believing such to be his or her duty, with little regard for evidence about the action. Over time, nurses have learned to question such actions, and to seek evidence for everything one does when delivering care to patients. One problem with this is that sometimes, despite detailed searching, evidence of effectiveness of aspects of nursing care may not exist, or at least has not been generated as yet. FCC is a very good example of this. While there is much written about FCC, hard evidence to show whether or not it works is not yet available (Shields *et al*. 2007).

This brings up several questions which can be examined from a deontological viewpoint. Why do health professionals continue to cite FCC as the best way to deliver care to children and families? Is it because they feel a moral duty to employ a method which has been enshrined in the health services' policy documents (which it often has)? Do they feel it a duty to try to implement FCC because that is what has been done for many years? As can be seen from the example from Nazi Germany, blindly following one's duty can have negative consequences. Because of the paucity of evidence about the use of FCC, it has to be asked if the duty to employ FCC, which, after all, sounds good, nevertheless results in negative consequences for the family and patients. If Coyne's (2008) work on parental involvement in the care of hospitalised children is any guide, then the duty to employ FCC methods is having negative consequences on the parents and children, but it is enshrined in health service dogma and policy and it is seen as one's duty to say that one is following it when delivering care. While this may be true, the fact that a policy has some negative consequences does not show that it is not the best policy available to us. The argument needs to show that the consequences are so bad that the policy should be abandoned.

Consequentialism is often seen as the antithesis of deontological ethics (Alexander & Moore 2008). Much argument occurs over this philosophy (Griffin 1995) with some critics saying that this ethical theory requires that the only right action is one that maximises the best consequences for all of those affected. If we examine FCC from this perspective, it gives some insight into why FFC is so problematic in practice. If a health service prescribes FCC in its policy documents, those trying to adhere to it may be acting absolutely, in other words, 'if it says I must do this, then I will'. Because they may not fully grasp the complexities of the FCC model, they have difficulty applying it, but because the policy says they must and the consequence of not applying it is that they go against the written policies of the service, they go ahead and are seen to be adhering to the policy.

Utilitarianism

Utilitarianism as a construct was most famously developed by Jeremy Bentham in the eighteenth century, John Stuart Mill in the nineteenth and Henry Sidgwick in the early twentieth century (Sinnott-Armstrong 2008). In a very brief summary of its main tenet, it prescribes 'the greatest good for the greatest number of those affected'. There exists a range of types of utilitarianism, with many seemingly contradicting each other. However, they are all underpinned by the principle that an act or state of affairs should give pleasure, not pain, and an act is morally right if it maximises pleasure/happiness and decreases pain or suffering (Sinnott-Armstrong 2008). One branch of this school of thought is *act utilitarianism* in which if one is presented with a choice, one must consider the consequences of what the alternatives will generate, and then choose that action from which the most pleasure or happiness will be derived. Another is *rule utilitarianism* where a set of happiness-maximising rules can be used to determine the moral good of an act, and one would examine what would happen if that set of rules was consistently followed, thereby maximising the good, or if, on balance, the set of rules produces more happiness than if the rules were not followed. Act utilitarianism, therefore, determines moral action on a case-by-case basis, whereas rule utilitarianism

uses a generalised determination. However, each can be applied to a case. Argument suggests that rule utilitarianism collapses into act utilitarianism because the rules are rules of thumb (Johnstone 1999; Sinnott-Armstrong 2008). As an example, a rule utilitarian might argue that some form or type of killing another is always wrong, regardless of the circumstances, as it generally brings unhappiness, or pain; whereas an act utilitarian might say that killing another is morally right if one is being attacked by a psychopathic killer because it will remove the killer from being able to kill again, as well as saving one's own life, that is, the good is, on balance, greater than the bad of killing another. If the situation is one that is likely to arise more than once, a rule utilitarian will make a rule to cover this; otherwise a rule utilitarian will be obliged to make a decision on the case as a single act.

As utilitarianism evolved, *consequentialism*, which is a branch of utilitarian philosophy, has arisen (Sinnott-Armstrong 2008). In any action, to judge its rightness or wrongness, consideration must be given to its consequences rather than just the balance between its positive and negative consequences. This brings the questions of what are good or bad consequences, who judges them as such and who benefits. Preference utilitarianism holds that one's preferences for autonomy and individual preferences have an intrinsic good which should be considered in any weighing of moral action (Johnstone 1999). Such an approach is considered plausible by Johnstone (1999) as, she says, 'all we have to do is ask people what they prefer. And where their preferences are at odds with ethical conduct, we have no obligation to respect them' (Johnstone 1999:58). This approach has some serious flaws such as how it judges the right and wrong and value of actions determined, and who has the guiding hand in such decisions.

The implementation of FCC suffers from this, such as in who judges the right and wrong of an approach such as involving a parent in the care of his or her child, and who makes the decision to include them. Is it the place of the health professional, or should a parent be the one who decides when and where to become involved in care (and this would assume that parents had the knowledge to know what involvement is appropriate given the child's illness or condition, ward environment, etc.)? This may explain the difficulties health professionals face when trying to apply FCC as a care model. Involvement of the family occurs across a continuum, from the parents undertaking almost all the care to handing all care of the child over to the health professional. The greatest good for that particular family has to be determined by exploring their preferences, but if such preferences are at odds with those of the health professionals, the balance between good and bad can be obscured.

Health professionals could be using rule utilitarianism when insisting that parents be involved in care of their sick child. FCC is believed to be the common rule by which care should be given, and it is thought to produce the greatest good for the family. However, the health professionals should, perhaps, weigh each case on its individual preferences and merit. Until we get all this right, the ethics of imposing FCC on families and health services must be questioned.

Conclusion

There is little evidence that applying a model based on FCC principles works, although, as described previously, many paediatric health services in many countries have it enshrined in policy. It is also being used more and more widely in adult health services (Mitchell *et al.* 2009). On balance, we must ask if it is morally right to continue to use something for which we have little real evidence. Perhaps the breakdown of effective implementation of FCC occurs because the ethical constructs which underpin it have not been sufficiently examined and debated. Unless this is done, and unless the ethical and theoretical underpinnings of any model are secure, it is ethically untenable to continue to apply it when caring for children and their families. It is time for two things – to begin a rigorous debate about FCC, and to examine other models of care, ready to replace FCC if it is found wanting.

Reflective scenario

You are a newly graduated nurse, working in the children's ward in a large rural hospital. Alex, aged 4, with cystic fibrosis has come into hospital for his routine chest physio and antibiotic treatment. You know that Alex's mother, Cathy, has twin babies at home and her husband, Phil works two jobs. Cathy believes in the healing power of crystals, despite being told by Alex's doctors and nurses that there is no scientific evidence that they work. Cathy has to leave Alex in the ward and go home to help Phil and feed the twins, but is confident because you are on and she knows you and Alex get on well.

Cathy has put a crystal on a chain around Alex's neck and asks you to make sure it is put back on after his bath. You agree, happy to do so as you know it makes Cathy happy (but you also know the crystal is useless).

As you are bathing Alex, the nurse in charge of the ward sees the crystal and takes it away, saying 'load of nonsense!'

1. Can you apply the principles of FCC to help this family?
2. Where do the principles of the Beauchamp and Childress paradigm fit here?
3. What do the concepts of obedience and autonomy mean in this situation for this young nurse?

References

Alexander, L. & Moore, M. (2008) Deontological ethics. In: *The Stanford Encyclopedia of Philosophy (Fall 2008 Edition)* (ed. E.N. Zalta). Stanford University, Stanford. Available from http://plato.stanford.edu/archives/fall2008/entries/ethics-deontological/ (accessed 16 March 2009).

Aubuchon, M. (1958) To stay or not to stay – Parents are the question. *Hospital Progress*, **39**, 170–177.

Beauchamp, T.L. & Childress, J.F. (2005) *Principals of Biomedical Ethics*, 5th edn. Oxford University Press, Oxford.

Bowlby, J. (1944a) Forty-four juvenile thieves: Their characters and home life (i). *International Journal of Psychoanalysis*, **25**, 19–53.

Bowlby, J. (1944b) Forty-four juvenile thieves: Their characters and home life (ii). *International Journal of Psychoanalysis*, **25**, 107–127.

Bradshaw, M. (2002) Implications and challenges of family-centred care. In: *Family-centred Care* (eds L. Smith, V. Coleman & M. Bradshaw). Palgrave, Basingstoke.

Bruce, B. & Ritchie, J. (1997) Nurses' practices and perceptions of family-centred care. *Journal of Pediatric Nursing*, **12** (4), 214–222.

Burlingham, D. & Freud, A. (1942) *Young Children in War-time*. Allen & Unwin Ltd., London.

Casey, A. (1995) Partnership nursing: Influences on involvement of informal carers. *Journal of Advanced Nursing*, **22**, 1058–1062.

Citizen's Committee on Children of New York City (1955) Liberal visiting policies for children's hospitals. *Journal of Pediatrics*, **46**, 710–716.

Coyne, I.T. (1995a) Parental participation in care: A critical review of the literature. *Journal of Advanced Nursing*, **21**, 716–722.

Coyne, I.T. (1995b) Partnership in care: Parents' views of participation in their hospitalized children's care. *Journal of Clinical Nursing*, **4**, 71–79.

Coyne, I.T. (1996) Parent participation: A concept analysis. *Journal of Advanced Nursing*, **23**, 733–740.

Coyne, I. (2008) Disruption of parent participation: Nurses' strategies to manage parents on children's wards. *Journal of Clinical Nursing*, **17** (23), 3150–3158.

Crisp, R. (1995) Deontological ethics. In: *The Oxford Companion to Philosophy* (ed. T. Honderich). Oxford University Press, Oxford.

Darbyshire, P. (1994) *Living with a Sick Child in Hospital: The Experiences of Parents and Nurses*. Chapman & Hall, London.

Faust, O.A. (1953) Stop scaring the children. *Modern Hospital*, **80** (94), 96.

Fleury, S., Dymterko, S. & Lemoine, H. (1954) Visiting in the pediatric department. *The Canadian Nurse*, **50**, 292–294.

Goodband, S. & Jennings, K. (1992) Parent care: A US experience in Indianapolis. In: *Caring for Children in Hospital: Parents and Nurses in Partnership* (ed. J. Cleary). Scutari Press, London.

Griffin, J.P. (1995) Consequentialism. In: *The Oxford Companion to Philosophy* (ed. T. Honderich). Oxford University Press, Oxford.

Hallström, I. & Runeson, I. (2001) Needs of parents of hospitalised children. *Theoria*, **10**, 20–27.

Hursthouse, R. (2007) Virtue ethics. In: *Stanford Encyclopedia of Philosophy (Fall 2008 Edition)* (ed. E.N. Zalta). Stanford University, Stanford. Available from http://plato.stanford.edu/entries/ethics-virtue (accessed 5 February 2009).

Illingworth, R.S. (1956) Young children in hospital. *Nursing Times*, 03/02/1956, 112–115.

IFCC (2009) About us. Institute for Family-Centered Care, Bethesda. Available from http://www.familycentered care.org/about/index.html (accessed 16 March 2009).

Isaacs, S. (1941) *The Cambridge Evacuation Survey: A Wartime Study in Social Welfare and Education*. Methuen & Co., London.

Johnstone, M.-J. (1999) *Bioethics: A Nursing Perspective*, 4th edn. Churchill Livingstone, Sydney.

Jolley, J. (2007) Separation and psychological trauma: A paradox examined. *Pediatric Nursing*, **19**, 22–25.

Jolley, J. & Shields, L. (2008) The evolution of family centered care. *Journal of Pediatric Nursing*, **24** (2), 164–170. DOI: 10.1016/j.pedn.2008.03.010.

Kant, I. (1972) *The Moral Law* (translated by H.J. Patton). Hutchinson University Press, London.

King, G.A., Rosenbaum, P.L. & King, S.M. (1997) Evaluating family-centred service using a measure of parents' perceptions. *Child: Care, Health, Development*, **23** (1), 47–62.

Kristensson-Hallström, I. & Elander, G. (1997) Parents' experience of hospitalization: Different strategies for feeling secure. *Pediatric Nursing*, **23**, 361–376.

Levy, D.M. (1945) Child patients may suffer psychic trauma after surgery. *Modern Hospital*, **65**, 51–52.

Lomax, E.M.R. (1996) *Small and Special: The Development of Hospitals for Children in Victorian Britain*. Wellcome Institute for the History of Medicine, London.

Ministry of Health (1959) *The Report of the Committee on the Welfare of Children in Hospital (the Platt Report)*. HMSO, London.

Mitchell, M., Chaboyer, W., Burmeister, E. & Foster, M. (2009) The positive effects of a nursing intervention on family-centred-care in adult critical care. *American Journal of Critical Care*, **18**, 543–552.

Pearson, G.H.J. (1941) Effect of operative procedures on the emotional life of the child. *American Journal of Diseases of Children*, **62**, 716–729.

Pickerill, H.P. & Pickerill, C.M. (1945) Elimination of cross-infection. *British Medical Journal*, **1**, 159–160.

Pickerill, C.M. & Pickerill, H.P. (1946) Keeping mother and baby together. *British Medical Journal*, **2**, 337.

Powers, G.F. (1948) Humanizing hospital experiences: Presidential address. *American Journal of Diseases of Children*, **76**, 365–379.

Robertson, J. (1962) *Hospitals and Children: A Parents' Eye View*. Victor Gollancz, London.

Robertson, J. & Bowlby, J. (1952) Responses of young children to separation from their mothers. *Courrier Centre International de l'enfance*, **2**, 131–142.

Shields, L. & Bryan, B. (2002) The effects of war on children: The children of Europe after World War 2. *International Nursing Review*, **49**, 87–98.

Shields, L. & Nixon, J. (1998) I want my Mummy –
Changes in the care of children in hospital. *Collegian*, **5**
(2), 16–19.

Shields, L., Pratt, J. & Hunter, J. (2006) Family centred
care: A review of qualitative studies. *Journal of Clinical
Nursing*, **15**, 1317–1323.

Shields, L., Pratt, J., Davis, L.M. & Hunter, J. (2007)
Family-centred care for children in hospital. *Cochrane
Database of Systematic Reviews*, Issue 1. Art. No.:
CD004811. DOI: 10.1002/14651858.CD004811.pub2.

Sinnott-Armstrong, W. (2008) "Consequentialism." In: *The
Stanford Encyclopedia of Philosophy (Fall 2008 Edition)*
(ed. E.N. Zalta). Stanford University, Stanford. Available
from   http://plato.stanford.edu/archives/fall2008/
entries/consequentialism/ (accessed 16 March 2009).

Smith, F. (1995) *Children's Nursing in Practice: The
Nottingham model*. Blackwell Science, Oxford.

Smith, L., Coleman, V. & Bradshaw, M. (2002) *Family-
centred Care*. Palgrave, Basingstoke.

Spence, J.C. (1947) The care of children in hospital. *British
Medical Journal*, **1** (4490), 125–130.

Spitz, R.A. (1945) Hospitalism: An inquiry into the genesis of psychiatric conditions in early childhood.
Psychoanalytic Study of the Child, **1**, 53–74.

Stevens, M. (1949) Visitors are welcome on the pediatric
ward. *American Journal of Nursing*, **49**, 233–235.

United Nations (1959) *United Nations Declaration of the
Rights of the Child*. United Nations, New York.

United Nations (1989) *United Nations Convention on the
Rights of the Child*. United Nations, New York.

Wolfram, S. (1995) Definition. In: *The Oxford Companion to
Philosophy* (ed. T. Honderich), pp. 181–182. Oxford
University Press, Oxford.

Wood, C. (1888) The training of nurses for sick children.
Nursing Record, **1**, 507–510.

Yapp, C.S. (1915) *Children's Nursing: Lectures to Probationers*.
Poor Law Publications, London.

Suggested further readings

Institute for Family-Centered Care (2010) http://www.
familycenteredcare.org/

Taleb, N.N. (2007) *The Black Swan: The Impact of the Highly
Improbable*. Penguin, London.

Van Hooft, S., Gillam L. & Byrnes, M. (1995) *Facts and
Values: An Introduction to Critical Thinking for Nurses*.
MacLennan & Petty, Sydney.

13 Above All Else do No Harm: An Ethical Evaluation of Paediatric Nurses Management of Children's Pain

Joan Simons

Introduction

Pain is a critical, ethical issue because of its capacity to dehumanise the human person (Lisson 1987). Acute pain is one of the most common adverse stimuli experienced by children, occurring as a result of injury, illness and necessary medical procedures (American Pain Society 2001).

For many years, the body of research on children's pain lagged behind that of studies on adult pain. However, more recently we have reached a situation where there is sufficient evidence-based knowledge to deliver good quality, effective pain management to children. Despite this improving situation, evidence shows pain in children is still often inadequately assessed and treated. In 2005, the International Association for the Study of Pain, Special Interest Group produced a position statement on *Pain in Childhood*, stating that pain relief is a human right (International Association for the Study of Pain 2005). Children undergo pain from the many procedures and investigations used by doctors and nurses to investigate and treat disease. Children remember pain, and may avoid future medical care because of painful experiences in a hospital or clinic. This chapter will review the evidence on the management of children's pain through the use of Beauchamp and Childress' ethical principles (2008) of non-maleficence, justice, autonomy and finally beneficence.

Two facts about pain assessment and management are uncontroversial – first, health-care professionals have an ethical obligation to relieve pain experienced by their patients, and second, this obligation has been largely neglected (Blacksher 2001).

Non-maleficence, to do no harm

Jameton (1984) states that for nurses it is more important to avoid doing harm than it is to do good. The under-medication of children's pain is widely acknowledged (American Academy of Pediatrics 2001; Healthcare Commission 2004, 2007; Picker Institute 2005), but there is a lack of exploration of this phenomenon from an ethical perspective. When under-medication is raised as a moral concern, the underlying premise is that a patient may experience harm or not benefit from ineffective pain management practices. The harm amounts to moral negligence.

Untreated pain suffered early in life can have profound and long-lasting effects on social and

Ethical and Philosophical Aspects of Nursing Children, First Edition. Edited by Gosia M. Brykczyńska and Joan Simons.
© 2011 Blackwell Publishing Ltd. Published 2011 by Blackwell Publishing Ltd.

physical development (Fitzgerald & Beggs 2001), and can cause permanent changes in the nervous system that will affect future pain experiences and development. Hunter (2000) contends that nurses may justifiably be deemed morally negligent for failing to provide adequate pain relief, when a patient has a right to such. Pain is associated with increased anxiety, avoidance, somatic symptoms and – in the context of paediatric practice – increased parental stress. Insufficient knowledge among caregivers and inadequate application of knowledge contribute to the lack of effective pain management. The paediatric acute pain experience involves the interaction of physiological, psychological, behavioural, developmental and situational factors, therefore presenting a complex challenge for nurses to manage their pain effectively.

It is expected that nurses will use their professional judgement concerning the amount of analgesic administered to a patient. However, nurses tend to give the lower dose routinely and commonly do not actively pursue dosage increases from doctors, when there is evidence that pain relief is not being achieved (Carr & Thomas 1997).

It is nurses' professional and moral obligation to provide adequate medication to relieve unnecessary pain. However, it has been found that nurses still do not recognise the need for children's pain to be assessed and documented on a regular basis (Simons & Roberson 2002). Several studies provide evidence of nurses' lack of recognition and under-medication of children in pain: Jacob & Puntillo (1999) surveyed 260 nurses in a paediatric hospital in America on their perceptions of their practices in the assessment and management of pain in children, and found that nurses do not consistently assess pain in children, and pain management practices are not based on systematic assessment. In a study of nurses' ability to relieve children's pain, Van Hulle Vincent & Denyes (2004) found that 26% of children reporting pain received no analgesia, and of those children who received analgesia, 51% reported moderate to high levels of pain. In a study by Polkki et al. (2003) to describe children's experiences (aged 8–12 years) with postsurgical pain relieving methods, most children reported their worst pain to be moderate or severe, which indicates that pain management in hospitalised children was suboptimal; Glajchen & Bookbinder

(2001) assessed pain-related knowledge in a national survey in America. Although they found 1236 of nurses on average scored 56% of the items correctly, more than one third of the nurses either over- or underestimated what they knew. Those nurses who overestimate their competence but score low on pain management knowledge are unlikely to change their practice. Finally, Idvall (2004) found that in several important aspects of pain management, nurses assessed the quality of care to be lower than what was actually possible to do in clinical practice. Therefore, nurses demonstrated that they recognised that the quality of care they were delivering was less than they were capable of providing.

One may question why this lack of recognition and under-medication of children's pain occurs. Van Hulle Vincent (2005) found that nurses reported the greatest barriers to optimal pain management were inadequate or insufficient physician medication orders for pain. However, nurses only administered 38% of available morphine and 23% of available total analgesia. Van Hulle Vincent (2005) suggests nurses should be more aware of the limitations of relying on children's behavioural manifestations of pain. The study found that 49% of nurses relied on behavioural cues rather than the child's self-report of their pain, which suggests that children need to attract the attention of a nurse through their behavioural manifestations of their pain, rather than nurses approaching children to assess their pain.

Fine (2002) found that with regard to treatment of pain and other distressing symptoms, there seems to be an atypical measure of caution exercised by physicians compared with almost all other medical interventions. Nurses then add another layer of caution, thus making it less likely that the child will receive adequate analgesia, even if it is prescribed. Simons & Moseley (2008) studied nurses' administration of analgesia to 175 children in the first 24 hours post-operatively, and found that when analgesics were prescribed regularly children had a considerably greater chance of receiving the analgesic. On the other hand, when analgesics were prescribed prn (as required), meaning nurses had to judge the need for administering an analgesic, children only received 77% of the prescribed analgesics. De Rond et al. (2001) found that there is less of a discrepancy between prescription and administration of analgesics in adults, which may be explained by the larger therapeutic range in adults and consequently less fear for adult nurses of giving too much analgesia.

These anxieties and fears that prevent care and so cause breaches in ethics are not justified by our current science. One of the more vulnerable groups in paediatrics are the neonates who need intensive care. Franck (1997) suggests that critical care nurses are ethically obligated to make the pain of non-verbal infants visible to the healthcare team by clearly documenting the vital signs of pain and ensuring pain management is routinely discussed during patient rounds. Critical care nurses must also consider the effects of the nurses' actions on infants' lives beyond the neonatal unit, including the possible effects of pain on growth and development.

In summary, the lack of recognition of children's pain, the lack of documentation and the under-medication of children's pain amounts to the nurses' non-adherence to the principle of non-maleficence, that is, poor or inadequate pain management can result in harm to children.

Reflective scenario

Leo, aged 11 years, was admitted to the children's ward yesterday in sickle-cell crisis. Whilst recording his vital signs, his nurse Julie asks him if he is pain, to which he replies his pain is a 10. Leo has a morphine PCA running, which Julie thinks he is obsessed with. Julie checks to see if the pump is working and attempts to make Leo more comfortable. On finding no fault with the pump, she feels there is no need for further action. Perhaps Leo is bored.

- What else could Julie have done?
- Did Julie believe Leo?
- What are the possible consequences for Leo?

Justice

The ethical principle of justice may be defined as fairness, equality and non-discrimination (Harvey 1995). It involves distributing costs and

risks fairly, the notion that patients in similar positions should be treated in a similar manner. In order to uphold this principle, there is a need to explore what rights children have in relation to pain management.

Children have an ethical right to pain alleviation (Kankkunen *et al.* 2002). The American Academy of Pain Medicine (Emmanuel 2001) endorses the WHO declaration that pain relief is a human right. However, the reality today is that there has been little impetus or effort among agencies of influence to promote, no less uphold, an acceptable level of pain care among all groups of patients.

There are a number of well-known articles and policy documents that underpin children's rights to effective pain management (also see appendices in this book). Some examples of these moral imperatives are found in the UN Convention on the Rights of the Child (1991), The UK National Service Framework for Children and Families (DoH 2003, 2004).

UN Convention on the Rights of the Child

Children have a right to effective pain management

1. In all actions concerning children ... the best interests of the child shall be a primary consideration.
2. States Parties undertake to ensure the child such protection and care as is necessary for his or her well-being. ...

Article 12

1. States Parties shall assure to the child who is capable of forming his or her own views the right to express those views freely in all matters affecting the child, the views of the child being given full weight in accordance with the age and maturity of the child.

To uphold this article, there is a need for nurses to use age-appropriate validated pain-assessment tools with all children who may be in pain, and in particular to use a self-report tool (RCN 1999) for verbal children, giving children the opportunity to express their views on their pain.

The National Service Framework for Children and Families (DoH 2004) Standard 9 focuses on hospital policies for managing children's pain which should apply to all children in every hospital department, including newborns in neonatal units. Special focus should be given to children in A&E departments, post-operative pain, pain related to procedures and long-term pain as in cancer. They should be founded on the following principles:

- Children have a right to appropriate prevention, assessment and control of their pain.
- Clinical staff should receive training in the prevention, assessment and control of children's pain.
- Children can expect the management of pain to be a routine part of any treatment or procedure, in any part of the hospital. They can also expect to be involved as active partners in pain management.
- Pain should be assessed and reviewed in all children and monitored after all procedures.
- Protocols and procedures should support the safe use of pain-controlling medicines.
- Children's pain management should be demonstrated by regular audit.
- Trusts should support and coordinate activities and resources to ensure that children's pain is recognised and addressed.

Although the Framework has been in place since 2004, there is a real need still for many of the above principles to be applied in practice. One principle in particular would make a substantial difference, and that is if all paediatric units conducted regular audits of children's pain management. The results would demonstrate, through evidence, the quality of children's pain. Without such evidence, children's pain management can remain a low priority and largely invisible. Until such evidence is widely available, it is clear that in order to treat children's pain effectively, a thorough pain assessment is necessary, and a number of guides are available to do this, for example, from the RCN (1999, 2009) and the American Academy of Pediatrics (2001). Particular attention should be given to children

who cannot express their pain because of their level of speech or understanding, communication difficulties or their illness or disability. This includes babies, children with communication or learning difficulties and those with altered consciousness or serious illness.

In order to underpin pain management with fairness and equality, there is a need to consider pain as the fifth vital sign. The American Pain Society (Dennis 2004) and the American Joint Commission on Accreditation of Healthcare Organisations (Lanser & Gesell 2001) suggest that ratings of pain should be treated as a fifth vital sign. It is known that vital signs are taken seriously and if pain was assessed with the same zeal as other vital signs are, it would have a much better chance of being properly treated. Studies suggest that considering pain as the fifth vital sign is viewed as integral to a comprehensive pain management programme (Merboth & Barnason 2000; Gallo 2003). The Royal College of Anaesthetists (2003) also endorse pain as the fifth vital sign in their report on Pain Management Services Good Practice, in which it is stated that pain and its relief must be assessed and documented on a regular basis. Pain intensity should be regarded as a vital sign and along with response to treatment and side effects should be recorded as regularly as other vital signs such as pulse or blood pressure.

A recent study by Simons & Moseley (2009) explored the influences on nurses' documentation of children's pain post-operatively across two units. The study demonstrated the need for pain to be treated as the fifth vital sign and incorporating pain assessment into a vital sign observation chart. In one unit in the study, pain scores were recorded on 82% of children whereas 60% of children had their pain scores recorded in the second unit on a chart separate from the vital sign observation chart. The difference between the two units may be explained by Simons & MacDonald (2004), who found that nurses considered that the extra work in assessing and recording children's pain was an obstacle to delivering pain management. However, nurses routinely completed vital sign observations without considering this task as extra work. The alignment of pain-assessment scores with vital sign assessment on one unit may explain why the use of one chart facilitated nurses recording nearly one fifth more pain scores than when nurses were faced with a separate chart for pain scores as in another unit. It could be suggested that the inclusion of pain scores on the vital sign chart acted as an aide memoire to nurses on the paediatric unit, whereas the nurses at the paediatric hospital did not have this prompt to record pain scores.

It is accepted that children's pain can be difficult to recognise. Children may appear to sleep or play even when they have significant pain, so their pain is not easily identified. This recognition of the complexity in identifying children's pain further underpins the need to ask the child about their pain, thus giving them the opportunity to relay the most important information.

Children's pain must become a priority for all health-care professionals. There should be an expectation by children and their parents that pain will be assessed and managed, appropriate medications and resources for non-pharmacological management will be available and that pain will be assessed, prevented and treated. To meet these expectations, nurses must be knowledgeable and vigilant in relation to analgesic administration, have established good communication channels with the child's family and be aware of how environment and resources are managed and deployed and their effect on the physical and emotional well-being of the child.

Franck (1997) suggests that the adequacy of pain management is determined partly by the knowledge and skills of the health-care provider's personal and professional values. To avoid suffering along with patients, many health-care providers create a distance between themselves and the patient's pain. Carter (2004) promotes the use of pain narratives as a way of working with children in pain. It is suggested that a narrative approach to practice can help nurses to become more engaged with children's experience of pain, therefore preventing nurses from being distant and passive. Engaging with children in a more meaningful way, it is suggested, acknowledges our moral obligation to care for children in pain and overcomes the purely reductionist approach of measuring pain intensity. Such an approach has the potential to overcome the long-held belief that pain is not a priority, as nurses who are more engaged with children through the narrative approach are much more likely to deal with individual children's pain.

> **Reflective scenario**
>
> Ellie, aged 32, has just become a ward manager on an orthopaedic unit. She recognises that pain is an issue for most children after surgery and always allocates her more experienced nurses to the children who are having surgical procedures that day. She knows that these nurses are good at communication. There used to be a pain tool on the ward but it is not currently being used.
>
> - Is Ellie upholding the rights of all children on her ward?
> - Is she leading her team in the delivery of evidence-based care?
> - Are the practices in this scenario being fair to all children in pain?

Autonomy

Chadwick & Tadd (1992) define autonomy as determining one's own course of action in accordance with one's deliberations, values and aspirations. The ethical principle of autonomy involves respecting the decision-making capacities of autonomous persons, and enabling individuals to make reasoned informed choices. Lisson (1987) contends that pain is dehumanising and destroys autonomy. Pain which is caused or allowed to happen or to continue, as a result of human attitudes and practices, or as the result of human value judgements – in the absence of other modifying human values and priorities – becomes a matter of ethical concern and possibly constitutes moral misconduct. Nurses have been found to believe children have a fixed amount of pain requiring a fixed amount of analgesia. Twycross & Powls (2006) conducted a study where nurses were observed in their pain management practices. It was found that nurses did administer analgesia, but tended to wait until the child was in pain rather than give pre-emptive analgesia. Such practices deny the child their autonomy in being involved in their pain assessment and management. Blacksher (2001) suggests that unrelieved pain can impinge and ultimately erase a persons' autonomy, whereas providing pain relief can protect a person's dignity. Using a reductionist approach to pain denies children pain relief, whereas seeing each child as an individual (Carter 2004) would ensure each child in pain had their needs recognised and therefore increase the likelihood of effective pain management.

Pain is difficult to express for adults, and can be even worse for children, babies and parents. The subjectivity of the pain experience warrants specific communication skills on the part of nurses to elicit the right information necessary to inform the necessary treatment. Nurses do not trust the human voice of the parent or the child and need to make the subjective experience of pain real to themselves, which may mean disbelieving a child who says they are in pain. Holter (1988) stated that nurses have the ability to open channels of communication, free of power dimensions and thus, increase the parents' or patients' freedom for self-reflection and personal autonomy. Moreover, parents' knowledge of their infants normal behaviour and intuitive feelings about their level of discomfort make them second only to the child in being able to provide an accurate pain assessment.

Mill (2002) conducted a phenomenological study on parents' perceptions of children's pain and pain management perception. The findings highlighted parents' emotional turmoil in dealing with their children's pain, and the desire to *take* their child's pain. This study demonstrated the need for increased emotional parental support in coping with their children's pain, and the need for families to be encouraged to contribute to the assessment of children's pain.

Pain cues

It is recognised that nurses are more responsive to behavioural cues than verbal cues; nevertheless, self-report is accepted as the gold standard for children (Finley & McGrath 1998) who are of the appropriate age and developmental stage. Kortesluoma & Nikkonen (2004), who studied the pain experiences of 4–11-year-old hospitalised children, found that nurses assessed children's pain based on what they thought it was rather than following a validated pain-assessment tool.

Further evidence of nurses not using pain tools to assess children's pain was found by Simons & Mosely (2009). They found that older children in

their study had more pain, which could have been prevented if nurses asked them about their pain. It is more likely that nurses assumed that their lack of complaint of pain meant no pain, which may relate to nurses' level of education on pain management in children.

These findings of nurses relying on pain cues to trigger pain management are not new. Over 20 years ago, Burokas (1985) found that the factors which most influenced nurses' decisions to administer post-operative analgesia to children were vital signs, and type of surgery, followed by severity of pain, non-verbal behaviours, response to last medication and the age of the patient.

Reflective scenario

Lily, aged 16 years, with cerebral palsy, has had surgery on her ankle. Her Mum Jess is resident and provides most of Lily's care. Jess approaches Lily's nurse Kathryn to ask for analgesia, as Lily's restlessness and moaning is very out of character for Lily.

Kathryn check's Lily's prescription chart and states that Lily is not due anything for pain for 2 hours. Jess feels angry and frustrated with the nurse's reply and her apparent inability to deal with Lily's pain. She tries to comfort Lily.

- What else could Kathryn have done to manage Lily's pain?
- Whose autonomy was being undermined in this scenario?
- How could this situation have been prevented?

Beneficence

Justification for non-action becomes problematic when placed alongside the principle of beneficence, to do good.

Pain is an inherently subjective, multifactorial experience and should be assessed and treated as such. The Pain Society (2002) published recommendations for Nursing Practice in Pain Management and stipulated that one of the nursing skills necessary was the administration and interpretation of validated pain-assessment tools.

Treadwell *et al.* (2002) found that accurate pain assessment provides the foundation for the effective management of pain. Standards for the management of pain recommend the use of standard pain measures and well-documented, regular assessment as the first step in pain management. McArthur & Cunliffe (1998) state that it is imperative that pain assessment should become a routine integral part of a child's care.

It has been found that nurses' and parents' perceptions of pain management can be quite different (Simons *et al.* 2001) with nurses perceiving that parents are more involved than parents feel they are. The inclusion of parents in the care of their child's pain is recognised as beneficial to children and desired by parents (Greenberg *et al.* 1999). In a study by Simons & MacDonald (2006) where validated pain-assessment tools were introduced across a children's hospital, it was found that over a 12-month period the inclusion of parents increased by a quarter, whilst nurses' negative perceptions to the tools reduced and nurses found the tools easier to use. These simultaneous observations over time suggest that when nurses became more confident in using the pain-assessment tools, they felt more at ease in including parents in the assessment of their children's pain. There is a need therefore to explore the issue of nurses' confidence in the management of children's pain as a whole, in order to promote more holistic evidence-based pain management for children.

Miaskowski (2003) suggests that one of the fundamental barriers that impede the effective pain management for infants and children is the failure on the part of health-care professionals to incorporate valid and reliable pain-assessment tools for infants and preverbal children into clinical practice. The current situation where some nurses are not delivering evidence-based pain management runs contrary to the Nursing and Midwifery Council (NMC 2008) Standards of conduct, performance and ethics for nurses and midwives.

There are many sections of the NMC (2008) code that are particularly relevant to the ethical management of children's pain:

- As a professional, you are personally accountable for actions and omissions in your practice and must always be able to justify your decisions.

- Collaborate with those in your care.
- You must share with people, in a way they can understand, the information they want or need to know about their health.
- You must uphold people's rights to be fully involved in decisions about their care.
- Use the best available evidence.
- You must deliver care based on the best available evidence or best practice.
- Keep clear and accurate records.
- You must keep clear and accurate records of the discussions you have, the assessments you make, the treatment and medicines you give and how effective these have been.

If the above aspects of the NMC code could be linked to children's pain management audit, nurses might recognise the fundamental nature of the provision of evidence-based pain management practices for all children.

Rejeh *et al.* (2009) suggest that nurses are much closer to patients' pain and suffering than other health professionals, being aware of their ethical problems, and being able to reflect on them and discuss and learn from them will reduce the burden of the ethical challenges faced.

Conclusion

Having considered the ethical issues in relation to the management of children's pain, this chapter has utilised Beauchamp & Childress' (2008) four principles of medical ethics.

The primary moral and legal principle of non-maleficence – to do no harm – focused on the consequences of under-treatment or non-treatment of children's pain, which was followed by the ethical principles of justice and the well-documented rights of children to have their pain managed and not to be left in pain. The principle of *autonomy* focused on the need to involve both children and families in pain management, and finally the principle of beneficence explored the available evidence and support recommending evidence-based pain management for children.

I would like to end this chapter with a quote from Lisson (1987):

Few things a nurse does are more important than relieving pain.

Reflective scenario

Tommy was a 4-year-old boy recovering from serious abdominal surgery. He needed IV antibiotics, but his veins kept collapsing and the cannulas had to constantly be re-inserted. He would stand by his bed and visibly shake as a leaf whenever the time came for him to have his cannula re-inserted. The nurses kept complaining to the surgeon that the child needed better management and that the constant re-insertion of lines was not ethical (or practical). The surgeon replied that she did not want to give the child a central line or a more permanent line for fear of infection.

Points to consider:

1. How could the nursing team be seen to uphold the principle of beneficence in this scenario?
2. Is evidence-based practice being delivered?
3. The onus to act to reduce Tommy's pain lies with what health professionals in this scenario?

References

American Academy of Paediatrics (2001) The assessment and management of acute pain in infants, children and adolescents. *Pediatrics*, **108** (3), 793–797.

Beauchamp, T.L. & Childress, J. (2008) *Principles of Biomedical Ethics*, 6th edn. Oxford University Press, New York.

Blacksher, E. (2001) Hearing from pain: Using ethics to reframe, prevent, and resolve the problem of unrelieved pain. *Pain Medicine*, **2** (2), 169–175.

Burokas, L. (1985) Factors affecting nurses' decisions to medicate pediatric patients after surgery. *Heart and Lung*, **14** (4), 373–379.

Carr, E. & Thomas, V.J. (1997) Anticipating and experiencing post-operative pain: The patients perspective. *Journal of Clinical Nursing*, **6**, 191–201.

Carter, B. (2004) Pain narratives and narrative practitioners: A way of working "in Relation" with children experiencing pain. *Journal of Nursing Management*, **12** (3), 210–216.

Chadwick, R. & Tadd, W. (1992) *Ethics and Nursing Practice*. Macmillan, London.

Dennis, C.T. (2004) Progress and directions for the agenda for pain management. *American Pain Society Bulletin*, **14** (5), 3–13, URL (consulted 19 January 2009): http://www.ampainsoc.org/pub/bulletin/sept04/pres2.htm.

DoH (2003) *Getting the Right Start: National Service Framework for Children. Standard for Hospital Services*. Department of Health, London.

DoH (2004) *The National Service Framework for Children, Young People and Maternity Services*. Department of Health, London.

De Rond, M., De Wit, R. & van Dam, F. (2001) The implementation of a Pain Monitoring Programme for nurses in daily clinical practice: Results of a follow-up study in five hospitals. *Journal of Advanced Nursing*, **35**, 590–598.

Emmanuel, L. (2001) Ethics and pain management: An introductory overview. *Pain Medicine*, **2** (2), 112–116.

Fine, P.G. (2002) The ethical imperative to relieve pain at life's end. *Journal of Pain and Symptom Management*, **23** (4), 273–277.

Finley, G.A. & McGrath, P. (eds) (1998) *Measurement of Pain in Infants and Children, Progress in Pain Research and Management*. IASP Press, Seattle, Washington.

Fitzgerald, M. & Beggs, S. (2001) The neurobiology of pain: Developmental aspects. *The Neuroscientist*, **7** (3), 246–257.

Franck, L.S. (1997) The ethical imperative to treat pain in infants: Are we doing the best we can? *Critical Care Nurse*, **17** (5), 80–87.

Gallo, A. (2003) The fifth vital sign: Implementation of the neonatal infant pain scale. *Journal of Obstetric Gynaecological and Neonatal Nursing*, **32** (2), 199–206.

Glajchen, M. & Bookbinder, M. (2001) Knowledge and perceived competence of home care nurses in pain management: A national survey. *Journal of Pain and Symptom Management*, **21** (4), 307–316.

Greenberg, R.S., Billett, C., Zahurak, M. & Yaster, M. (1999) Videotape increases parental knowledge about paediatric pain management. *Anaesthetic Analgesia*, **89**, 899–903.

Harvey, H. (1995) Ethics and paediatric intensive care. *Intensive Critical Care Nursing*, **1**, 36–39.

Healthcare Commission (2004) *Patient Survey Report. Young Patients. Commission for Healthcare Audit and Inspection*. Healthcare Commission, London.

Healthcare Commission (2007) *Improving Services for Children in Hospital. Commission for Healthcare Audit and Inspection*. Healthcare Commission, London.

Hunter, S. (2000) Determination of moral negligence in the context of the undermedication of pain by nurses. *Nursing Ethics*, **7** (5), 379–391.

Holter, I. (1988) A foundation for the development of nursing theories. *Scholarly Inquiry for Nursing Practice. An International Journal*, **2**, 223–232.

Idvall, E. (2004) Quality of care in post-operative pain management: What is realistic in clinical practice? *Journal of Nursing Management*, **12** (3), 162–166.

International Association for the Study of Pain (2005) *Children's Pain Matters! Priority on Pain in Infants, Children and Adolescents. A Position Statement from the Special Interest Group*, Seattle, *Washington*. www.Childpain.org

Jacob, E. & Puntillo, K.A. (1999) A survey of nursing practice in the assessment and management of pain in children. *Pediatric Nursing*, **25** (3), 278–305.

Jameton, A. (1984) *Nursing Practice: The Ethical Issues*. Prentice Hall, Englewood, Chiff, New Jersey.

Kankkunen, P., Vehvilainen-Julkunen, K. & Pietila, A.M. (2002) Ethical issues in paediatric nontherapeutic pain research. *Nursing Ethics*, **9** (1), 80–91.

Kortesluoma, R.-L. & Nikkonen, M. (2004) 'I had this horrible pain': The sources and causes of pain experiences in 4–11-year-old hospitalized children. *Journal of Child Health Care*, **8** (3), 210–231.

Lanser, P. & Gesell, S. (2001) Pain management: The fifth vital sign. *Health Benchmarks*, **6** (6), 68–70.

Lisson, E.L. (1987) Ethical issues related to pain control. *Nursing Clinics of North America*, **22** (3), 649–659.

McArthur, E. & Cunliffe, M. (1998) Pain assessment and documentation – Making a difference. *Journal of Child Health Care*, **2** (4), 164–169.

Merboth, M.K. & Barnason, S. (2000) Managing pain: The fifth vital sign. *Nursing Clinics of North America*, **35** (2), 375–383.

Miaskowski, C. (2003) Identifying issues in the management of pain in infants and children. *Pain Management Nursing*, **4** (1), 1–2.

Mill, T. (2002) *Parents' perceptions of children's pain and pain management in hospital*. Unpublished Masters Thesis, RCN Institute, UK.

NMC (2008) *The Code. Standards of Conduct, Performance and Ethics for Nurses and Midwives*. Nursing and Midwifery Council, London.

The Pain Society (2002) *Recommendations for Nursing Practice in Pain Management. Nursing Focus in Pain Management Working Party of the Pain Society*. British Chapter of the International Association for the Study of Pain, London.

Picker Institute (2005) *Is the NHS Getting Better or Worse?* Picker Institute Europe, Oxford.

Polkki, T., Pietila, A. & Vehvilainen-Julkunen, K. (2003) Hospitalized children's descriptions of their experiences with postsurgical pain relieving methods. *International Journal of Nursing Studies*, **40** (1), 33–44.

Rejeh, N., Ahmadi, F., Mohamadi, E., Anoosheh, M. & Kazemnejad, A. (2009) Ethical challenges in pain management post-surgery. *Nursing Ethics*, **16** (2), 161–172.

The Royal College of Anaesthetists (2003) *Pain Management Services: Good Practice*. Royal College of Anaesthetists/The Pain Society, London.

RCN (1999) *The Recognition and Assessment of Acute Pain in Children. Clinical Practice Guidelines*. Royal College of Nursing, London.

RCN (2009) *The Recognition and Assessment of Acute Pain in Children*. Update of full guideline. Royal College of Nursing, London.

Simons, J., Franck, L.S. & Roberson, E. (2001) Parent involvement in children's pain care: Views of parents and nurses. *Journal of Advanced Nursing*, **36**, 591–599.

Simons, J. & Roberson, E. (2002) Poor communication and knowledge deficits: Obstacles to effective management of children's postoperative pain. *Journal of Advanced Nursing*, **40**, 78–86.

Simons, J.M. & MacDonald, L.M. (2004) Pain assessment tools: Children's nurses' views. *Journal of Child Health Care*, **8** (4) 264–278.

Simons, J.M. & MacDonald, L.M. (2006) Changing practice: Implementing validated paediatric pain assessment tools. *Journal of Child Health Care*, **10** (2), 160–176.

Simons, J. & Moseley, L. (2008) Post-operative pain: The impact of prescribing patterns on nurses' administration of analgesia. *Paediatric Nursing*, **20** (8), 14–19.

Simons, J. & Moseley, L. (2009) Influences on nurses' scoring of children's post-operative pain. *Journal of Child Health Care*, **13** (2), 101–115.

Treadwell, M., Franck, L. & Vichinsky, E. (2002) Using quality improvement strategies to enhance pediatric pain assessment. *International Journal for Quality in Health Care*, **14**, 39–47.

Twycross, A. & Powls, L. (2006) How do children's nurses make clinical decisions? Two preliminary studies. *Journal of Clinical Nursing*, **15**, 1324–1335.

United Nations Convention on the Rights of the Child (1991) *Office of the High Commissioner for Human Rights*. Accessed 06 August 2009: www.unicef.org/crc/.

Van Hulle Vincent, C. (2005) Nurses' knowledge, attitude and practices regarding children's pain. *American Journal of Maternal/Child Nursing*, **30** (3), 177–183.

Van Hulle Vincent, C. & Denyes, M.J. (2004) Relieving children's pain: Nurses' abilities and analgesic administration practices. *Journal of Pediatric Nursing*, **19** (1), 40–50.

Suggested further readings

Twycross, A., Dowden, S.J. & Bruce, E. (2009) *Managing Pain in Children. A Clinical Guide*. Wiley-Blackwell, Oxford.

www.iasp-pain.org

www.rcn.org.uk/development/practice/pain

14 Ethical Aspects in Children's and Young People's Cancer Care: Professional Views

Faith Gibson

Introduction

The care of children and young people (CYP) who have cancer has changed markedly over the last decade (Ablett 2002; Barnes 2005). The children's cancer nurse of today is facing challenges from both within the profession and society to provide clinical expertise in what is a complex and rapidly changing speciality. Developments in the medical treatment of childhood cancer mean that expected survival rates have never been better. Consequently, nurses caring for CYP with cancer have had to keep pace with and respond to advances in treatment as well as with technological and service developments (Gibson 2005). The nature of care provided in inpatients, outpatients and in community settings has changed over recent years, and will continue to do so, with an increasing number of CYP in all three settings requiring highly specialised care throughout their disease trajectory. For example, the speciality of palliative care has grown significantly with models of care for children (Goldman 1998) and adolescents in place (Edwards 2001). Services for teenagers and young adults are being described as the new clinical speciality (Kelly & Gibson 2008). In addition, long-term follow-up has become a major component of care as more children are surviving into adulthood (Stiller 1994; Gibson & Soanes 2001; Grinyer 2009; Ruccione 2009; DoH 2010).

Open communication about the illness and treatment is now regarded as the best policy for CYP. Mutual pretence and concealing information from children, a role shared by parents and health professionals in the past, and so sensitively described by Bluebond-Langner (1978), is now thought to be unhelpful. There is now general agreement that the sharing of cancer-related information leads to improved knowledge and understanding of the illness (Zwaanswijk et al. 2007). Shared information has the potential to enable CYP to feel more in control of their treatment and illness and to participate more fully in their care and decision-making. However, information that needs to be communicated is often very complex and can be quite uncertain and emotionally charged, setting the scene for miscommunication (Sobo 2004). There is clear evidence that CYP with cancer desire information about their illness and treatment (Ellis & Leventhal 1992; Last & van Veldhuizen 1996; Horstman & Bradding 2002; Gibson et al. 2005; Zwaanswijk et al. 2007; Ranmal et al. 2009). When Bluebond-Langner's work was conducted, the 5-year survival rate for childhood leukaemia was only 26%. Current figures suggest survival is now

Ethical and Philosophical Aspects of Nursing Children, First Edition. Edited by Gosia M. Brykczyńska and Joan Simons.
© 2011 Blackwell Publishing Ltd. Published 2011 by Blackwell Publishing Ltd.

80%, and for families there is now an expectation of cure despite the continuing arduous nature of the treatment. Survivorship can now be an outcome anticipated by many families, and hence questions about how to communicate effectively have become increasingly focused on supporting children with a chronic illness to live with and beyond cancer (Dixon-Woods *et al.* 2005).

Over the past several decades, changes have occurred that have altered the way that health care is both perceived and delivered. The availability of new health technologies, the increased consumer demand, limited resources in health care, reconfiguration of services and the improved professional skill and knowledge have all played their part in creating the complex and demanding workplace we work in today. On a daily basis, professionals face moral and ethical dilemmas alongside the rights and responsibilities of their daily practice. The children's and young people's cancer nurse is in a position to advocate for patients' rights and to identify and help resolve ethical conflicts (Forte 2002). This requires nurses to understand and apply ethical principles to practice, so that issues are considered from a more objective and less emotional viewpoint. The nurse is of course not working in isolation. Multi-professional working is the cornerstone of care delivery, within which professional roles should be clearly defined so that individual roles complement one another (Gibson 2009). Trust, respect and open communication are essential elements of an effective team, and are crucial when a team is faced with an ethical dilemma.

Professionals are not working alone and alongside children: young people and parents are essential members of an effective multi-professional team. Thus we talk about a triad, when we are referring to partnership working in our field: where partnership is both fluid and dynamic, with role boundaries between all three members of the triad changing over the course of a relationship (Bishop 2000). The perspective of CYP is strongly urged, and we have over the years witnessed greater inclusion of children in consultations. The empirical literature supports the position that many children, especially those who are veterans of illness, can produce coherent and rational views relevant to decisions about their care (Dixon-Woods *et al.* 2005). This literature also reveals that there is no straightforward association between

age and competence (Alderson 1993). Much of the new social studies literature has repeatedly argued to reposition children as competent and rational (Mayall 2002), therefore deserving of the right to make autonomous decisions. Children's and young people's ability and desire to be involved does of course vary. Respecting CYP means supporting them as far as they want to go, trying not to impose on them over-involvement or exclusion in decision-making (Alderson 1993). I would agree with Dixon-Woods and her colleagues (2005) that most decisions in our field are made informally and are negotiated within particular forms of social relations within which there are either shared decisions or situations where CYP and their parents defer to one another (Alderson 1993). Understanding this dyad, child/young person–parent roles, is essential for professionals to uphold the individuality of each partner and to respect their views and value their input into the multi-professional team.

Reams have been written on ethical and legal issues in child health, and in cancer care. It is certainly not the intention of this chapter to duplicate any of those influential and seminal pieces. Throughout this textbook, authors have drawn extensively on evidence to support their writings, much of which applies to the content of this chapter too. In order to contribute to the narrative that is embedded within this textbook, I have chosen to draw on the experience of those delivering direct cancer care. I have sought professional views to present a contemporary perspective on the challenges that they face, revealing experiences that might illuminate current ethical issues facing those working in children's and young people's cancer care today. My approach was to contact experienced individuals in the field by email to ask if they were able to contribute to this chapter by sharing what they thought were the main ethical challenges they face in day-to-day practice. The narrative that follows has been constructed around the central themes of our discussions through which I have woven relevant literature and some personal reflections. These themes can by no means account for all the ethical challenges we might face; they are a perspective on a point in time by a selected group of individuals. But what they do is highlight the complexity and varied nature of these challenges which, when viewed through the lens of ethical principles, help us see how we might use rules to inform our discussions and focus our debate, as well as gather and understand the perspectives of all those involved, in order to resolve an ethical dilemma. The professionals I spoke with are acknowledged at the end of this chapter.

Ethical issues frequently encountered

Topics consistently addressed by colleagues included informed consent, truth telling, refusing treatment, withdrawing treatment, futility of treatment and allocation of resources.

Informed consent

This it would seem is an area fraught with ethical issues. Almost all of the professionals I spoke with mentioned informed consent, their worries about the process and concerns that *true* consent was difficult to achieve: in some circumstances, with some age groups. Although the main focus for reflection was on consent for cancer therapies, and entering clinical trials, some professionals were equally concerned about consent for clinical interventions, such as venepuncture and passing a nasogastric tube. However, clinical care and clinical research differ, and vary depending on the context and level of risk (Jefford & Moore 2008). Despite these differences, seeking to incorporate the wishes or preferences of CYP in the decision-making process was seen to be important (the ethical principle of *autonomy*), but sometimes less than straightforward. There were situations where respect for others' rights to not always be involved in decisions, where decisions were deferred to parents, was felt to be appropriate. But then there were also situations where parents gave consent and children were subjected to necessary interventions, which were considered to be in their best interests (the ethical principle of *beneficence*), where consent from the child was sought but not gained. There were situations where, either because of a child/young person's clinical condition or because parents had chosen to withhold information from their child, CYP were excluded from decisions about their care. Finally, there were concerns that information was not shared, for example, in relation to fertility

and fertility preservation that influenced young people making an informed choice.

Despite the best intentions of professionals, the informed consent process may well be fraught with ethical issues (Dawson & Spencer 2005). Informed consent is a process that involves dialogue between the professional–child/young person–parent triad (Twycross *et al.* 2008). Many decisions made at the time of diagnosis, such as the choice of entering a clinical trial, choosing between different access devices, or what may be seen as more straightforward, the timing of oral care, often occur at a time of acute stress (Woodgate & Yanofsky 2010). There are known difficulties with learning and making decisions at times of stress that can be compounded by barriers such as language, knowledge, cultural differences and insufficient time (Abbe *et al.* 2006). Informed consent is not a *one-off* talk leading to a decision; some decisions may in fact take some time to reach, and on some occasions several days before everyone is satisfied that all elements have been covered. But time can be limited on some occasions, and in those circumstances stress levels can be even higher, affecting everyone's abilities to dialogue clearly and ensure information is being received as it was intended and understood. Implicit in the discussions I had with professionals were a number of themes: the need to involve the team; not to rely on age as a criterion; the need to make available to families, in stages if necessary, all the information they need to make informed choices; and the need for nurses to advocate for the families in their care.

A sequenced approach to consent has been advocated by parents, in relation to consent for a randomised clinical trial, which has been taught and tested by a team in the United States of America (Angiolollo *et al.* 2004; Eder *et al.* 2007; Yap *et al.* 2009). There is no reason why such an approach would not also be valuable in all clinical situations that consent is being sought. Sequencing information may well improve patient and family understanding of the important aspects of consent, where signing of a form signifies more than agreement to take part (Jefford & Moore 2008). Children, young people and their parents need information to make informed decisions, whether it is related to clinical care or research. Clearly, professionals were expressing their concerns about the process that remains complex in ensuring CYP are fully informed and that they can show that they understand what they are consenting to.

Truth telling

All professionals I spoke with signed up to the principle of truth telling, and advocated a policy of open communication in relation to diagnosis, treatment, progression of disease and honesty about the benefits of therapy. Upholding the principle of truth telling (the ethical principle of *veracity*) was less than straightforward, however, and examples were given of how professionals were sometimes troubled in their attempts to respect and on occasion challenge parents in their roles where they were clearly acting in what they thought was their child's best interest. Not telling has been associated with words such as evasion, paternalism, concealment, conspiracy of silence and nondisclosure (Hinds 2008). There were situations of parents withholding information from their child, irrespective of age, of parents withholding information from each other and professionals withholding information from families. Examples were recounted where parents did not want to use the word cancer or leukaemia with their child, and where they did not want to tell their child they were dying. Clearly, parents wanted to protect their child, but inadvertently they may well be preventing their child from coming to terms with a cancer diagnosis or their imminent death. Uncertainty is a major psychological burden for children with a serous illness because they are limited in their capacity to obtain information that could help and reassure them (Beale *et al.* 2005).

Not telling has been referred to as *corrosive* to the clinician–patient relationship (Hinds 2008). Colluding with parents, to ensure that information is withheld created tensions in clinical environments and was felt to influence relationships with CYP. Likewise, going against parents' wishes to tell young people over 16 years that they have cancer was felt to initially create tensions between parents and professionals. As we live in a multicultural society, professionals also shared examples of where they found it difficult to accept and work with certain practices, such as when fathers as the head of the household opt not to share the full information with their wife. There were also times

when professionals had some knowledge about a child's diagnosis or disease progression and where that was withheld from families because a medical consultant was not available to give that information or there was not enough time to speak with families when that information became available.

Differences in practices between children's and young people's cancer care were described. Those working with young children were in agreement that they would encourage parents to be truthful with their child, and they would respect parent's wishes unless asked directly by a child when they would be truthful. Those working with young people advocated being truthful with a young person, particularly those over 16 years irrespective of parent's views. Similarly, they respected young people's wishes; when although in one case a young man knew he was dying, he did not want his parents to know that he knew.

Truth telling was described as accepted by parents about 70% of the time, but it was in the remaining 30% of occasions that conflict between professionals and parents was a possibility professionals found daunting. Professionals expressed a responsibility to act in the child's best interests, to provide them with sufficient information to enable them to make an informed decision, describing a process of open communication that would allow them to do that. The truth is, according to Hinds (2008), regardless of truth telling or not telling, the care that we provide in oncology needs to be guided by patient preferences for information and for treatment. Tailoring cancer care information and viewing communication within the context of the family and other support systems was a key message from those I spoke with and is supported within the evidence of published literature (Eiser & Havermans 1992; Masera *et al.* 1997; Skeen & Webster 2004; Ranmal *et al.* 2009; Spinetta *et al.* 2009).

Refusing treatment

Many of the professionals gave examples of children, young people and parents refusing treatment. These experiences were described as the most difficult and challenging: where emotional responses to those decisions challenged professionals to remain objective. Situations were described where young children, who were offered further treatment following a relapse of their disease, refused treatment. There were examples where young women who were pregnant at the time of their diagnosis/relapse chose to delay therapy until their child was born. A young woman (21 years) who refused what she perceived to be radical surgery that would affect her body image severely refused an amputation and opted for less aggressive (and less effective) therapy. There was also a case of a young man (15 years) who refused therapy, and a separate case of parents who, when faced with a child's poor prognosis (neuroblastoma) or, in some cases, good long-term prognosis (leukaemia), refused treatment: clearly in those situations when there was a good prognosis, this was much more difficult for professionals to accept parents' decisions.

More problems arose where there was conflict between parents, either in cases of divorced or separated parents. There were cases of young single mothers, where other family members were involved, and there was a disagreement between family members. In many of these cases of conflict and divergence, open and inclusive discussion resulted in either a compromise or an agreement to change a decision. But where disagreement and conflict remained, cases were taken to court to seek an objective viewpoint outside of the clinical team that had become drawn into a relationship with the family. Professionals were keen to point out that involving the court should not be seen as a sign of failure, but more as a need for everyone involved to hear the views of an objective party so that all possible outcomes and consequences of decisions can be discussed.

Burdens and risks of treatment (Field & Behrman 2004), balanced against the percentage chance of cure, were clearly reflected in some of these stories. Many of the professionals spoke about taking into account the age of CYP, as well as their previous experience of cancer therapies. The rights of a minor and competence to consent, or in this case to refuse treatment, was the focus of our dialogue. Reflections on a recent case in the United Kingdom, of a 13-year-old (Hannah) who refused a heart transplant which was needed following treatment for leukaemia is an example of a young person exercising her legal rights on consent and treatment and illuminates the consent process in action (Cornock 2010). Competence, voluntariness of the decision and the information on which a person

has to base their decisions are the three guiding principles that underpin consent and refusal of treatment. All three principles are further illuminated in a case reported from the United States of America by Friebert & Kodish (2003). The right to decide in the latter case was less contentious as the young woman (Shelley) was 19 years old, and therefore defined as legally competent to make her own health-care decisions. Nonetheless, personal beliefs and value systems of the professionals providing care to the young woman were evident and were influenced by the curable nature of her ovarian tumour and the fact that she had a young child of her own. Both cases highlight the importance of enabling CYP to express their views and for professionals to respect CYP and their wishes: a clear message that was threaded through my discussions with professionals.

Withdrawing treatment

In those situations where a child has relapsed on therapy, where professionals state there is no more that can be done or where the effects of therapy have resulted in life-threatening effects and treatment must be stopped, there is potential conflict between those who share this information and those who receive it. Similar to other situations, professionals recounted stories of parents' acceptance that they understood it was *the end of the road* for them, and to go on with therapy would impact on their child's quality of life. But there were others who wanted more, irrespective of the fact that it would have an effect on their child's quality of life. There was quite a lot of discussion about timeliness of information and preparing families as well as we might for the trajectory of care that we might anticipate based on their prognosis or response to therapy. There was agreement that to decide to stop therapy was an extremely difficult one. Improved communication and explanation, increased honesty and trust were all described as essential in situations where recurrence, or further recurrence and *what happens next* were being discussed. Young people have reported the importance of being well informed and the careful weight they gave to the opinion and recommendations of health-care professionals and parents (Hinds *et al.* 2001). Further research by Hinds *et al.* (2005) supports the ability of children and adolescents between 10 and 20 years old with advanced cancer to participate in end-of-life decision-making. Key issues are the duration and quality of remaining life, and the rights of the child to careful, compassionate management from the health-care team (Masera *et al.* 1999). Hinds *et al.* (2001) offer separate guidance for young people, parents and professionals who become involved in end-of-life decisions, indicating that dialogue needs to begin at diagnosis, and continues when a child's disease progresses, through to the initiation of end-of-life discussions. This indicates that there are many factors that are considered when such decisions are made. In many situations, however, parents want and seek both cancer-directed therapies and optimal symptom management and supportive care; it is not a choice of one over another (Bluebond-Langner *et al.* 2007).

Futility of treatment

Almost all of the professionals gave examples of where tensions arose in a clinical team, where more treatment was offered to a family when it was known that the treatment would not influence the final outcome, where there was a slimmest of hopes of cure and where quality of life could be affected significantly. The phrase, 'just because we can should we' was mentioned on a number of occasions. There were situations recounted of a third bone-marrow transplant being offered, when professionals might well predict either severe side effects of therapy requiring intensive care or in the worst case, a child/young person dying in transplant. Once again professionals sought to support families in their final decision and recognised that for some families it was the right decision for them to keep going with more therapy, but others were troubled that the information regarding outcome was either not explicit and less than honest or that it was received and perceived differently than the way the information was intended. Some professionals perceived a difference between those with a haematology and oncology diagnosis, where it was felt that the line was less clear and there was a greater temptation to offer more therapy, because one might imagine there is more to offer.

A number of examples were shared of where disagreements, most often not shared within a team,

created tension and these had an affect on working relationships. It may well be in these situations that the goal of therapy was not understood by all. Families might understand the goal and have had time to weigh up the cost benefit of further therapy. More junior nursing staff might not have access to this information, and might therefore make assumptions about the nature of the decisions being made, the nature of informed consent and the role of medical staff in offering more therapy. There may be some concerns that the obligation to do minimal or no harm to the patient is not being upheld (the ethical principles of *nonmaleficence*). Open communication in the team is clearly important, as is the need to document both the content and the nature of these interactions for all staff to understand family's perspectives so that they can continue to be supportive in their role, irrespective of their personal opinions.

Allocation of resources

Professionals mentioned access to some drugs, which were either unlicensed or expensive, leading to what is termed a *post-code lottery* for prescribing where medicines were available to some children in some parts in the United Kingdom but not other parts. Thus, there were examples of families seeking private funding to pay for these medicines, which when offered, and then withheld, led some families to go to extraordinary lengths to acquire them. There were also examples of trial drugs being withheld at the end of a trial, despite the fact that there had been a clear benefit to a child. In addition to access to medicines, some professionals were concerned about access to timely therapy, where limited resources due to poor staffing in some parts of the country led to bed closures and delays to children's treatment. There were clearly day-to-day concerns to ensure all patients were treated fairly and equally (the ethical principle of *justice*).

Conclusion

The children's and young people's cancer nurses are in a position to advocate for patient rights and to identify and help resolve ethical conflicts. They are ideally placed to do this, within the content of the multi-professional team, as they work closely with families day to day in more often intimate encounters. Threading through the accounts of professionals were two factors that for me influenced and impacted on ethical issues: open communication, and the nurses' ability and position in the team to truly be an advocate for the patient.

Open communication with CYP although believed to be a good thing, can still not be taken for granted. The word cancer still evokes strong feelings and there remain, despite the best efforts of some professionals and organisations, two dominant themes in society that CYP do not get cancer and that if they do they will die. So it is not surprising that some families will go to enormous lengths and cause themselves more anxiety and stress by protecting their children from knowing they have cancer. The implications of not knowing, as highlighted by many professionals, is that CYP are prevented from being involved in decisions that affect them, and they may be absent from treatment-related discussions. In the short term, difficulties arise for professionals in knowing how best to prepare children for the journey they are to embark upon. In the long term, lack of knowledge of what has happened to them may prevent them from making wise health choices in the future.

Experience as a child/young person's cancer nurse was clearly a prerequisite for being instrumental in facilitating communication between the parents and the child, and parents and the healthcare team. They have the skills to be able to step back from situations, draw on previous similar situations as well as their in-depth knowledge of children's cancer care to look critically at cases and enter ongoing debates. They were certainly able to articulate their own values, and able to put these on one side in order to draw on ethical principles in situations of conflict. But there were times recounted where nurses did not always feel that their views were valued and some perceived a medical dominance in such discourse that prevented them advocating for their patients. Strategies, such as multi-professional forums where clinical cases can be discussed and where there are open and frank discussions about clinical decisions, particularly difficult ones, were in place in many of their institutions. Clinical ethics meetings were commonplace, where professionals were able to draw on the expertise of a range of disciplines. Forte (2002) offers to nurses a structure to help resolve ethical conflicts, and teaching such a strategy early on in a nurse education would be welcomed:

1. Identify the issue and constructively summarise the facts of the case or conflict;
2. Identify the ethical principles involved;
3. Address the conflict with the persons involved, through a family conference or a meeting between colleagues;
4. If conflict is not resolved locally, consult the clinical ethics committee within the hospital.

The nature of care in children's and young people's cancer care will continue to evolve; future challenges of technology and limited resources, although not known in detail, can be anticipated. The clinical speciality will evolve and nurses will continue to specialise to meet these ongoing demands. Ethical conflicts will remain constant as we are challenged to deliver individualised care in an increasingly complex environment. Accommodating clinician expertise, parental decisional authority and child assent/consent would seem to be the key elements in any model of decision-making in children's and young people's cancer care (Whitney *et al.* 2006). We all have a responsibility to ensure that our own organisations seek ways to both document and maybe improve how we use ethical principles in our decision-making. The families in our care deserve nothing less.

Acknowledgements

Thank you to those colleagues who gave up their valuable time and offered wise reflections on the ethical issues they face in children's and young people's cancer care: Nigel Ballantine, Pharmacist, Birmingham Children's Hospital, Birmingham; Jamie Cargill, CNS Children with Leukaemia, Bristol; Amber Conley, Practice Nurse Educator, Great Ormond Street Hospital for Children NHS Trust, London; Dr Martin William English, Paediatric Oncologist, Birmingham Children's Hospital, Birmingham; Monica Hopkins, Advanced Nurse Practitioner, Alder Hey Children's NHS Foundation Trust, Liverpool; Dave Hobin, Paediatric Oncologist, Birmingham Children's Hospital, Birmingham; Rachel Hollis, Lead Cancer Nurse, St James'

Hospital, Leeds; Sue Morgan, Teenage Cancer Trust Consultant Nurse, St James' Hospital, Leeds; Sue Neilson, Children's Community Oncology Nurse, Birmingham Children's Hospital, Birmingham; Barry Pizer, Paediatric Oncologist, Alder Hey Children's Hospital, Liverpool; Louise Soanes, Teenage Cancer Trust Consultant Nurse, Royal Marsden Hospital, London; and Joanna Stone, CNS Neuro-Oncology, Royal Marsden Hospital, London.

References

Abbe, M., Simon, C., Angiolillo, A., Ruccione, K. & Kodish, E.D. (2006) A survey of language barriers from the perspective of pediatric oncologists, interpreters, and parents. *Pediatric Blood and Cancer*, **47**, 819–824.

Ablett, S. (2002) *Quest for Cure: UK Children's Cancer Study Group – The First 25 Years*. Trident Communications Ltd., London.

Alderson, P. (1993) *Children's Consent to Surgery*. Open University Press, Buckingham.

Angiolillo, A.L., Simon, C., Kodish, E., Lange, B., Noll, R.B., Ruccione, K. & Matloub, Y. (2004) Staged informed consent for a randomised clinical trial in childhood leukemia: Impact on the consent process. *Paediatric Blood and Cancer*, **42**, 433–437.

Barnes, E. (2005) Caring and curing: Paediatric cancer services since 1960. *European Journal of Cancer Care*, **14**, 373–380.

Beale, E.A., Baile, W.F. & Aaron, J. (2005) Silence is not golden: Communicating with children dying from cancer. *Journal of Clinical Oncology*, **23**, 3629–3631.

Bishop, J. (2000) Partnership in care. In: *The Child with Cancer: Family Centred Care in Practice* (ed. H. Langton). Bailliers Tindall, Edinburgh.

Bluebond-Langner, M. (1978) *The Private Worlds of Dying Children*. University Press, Princeton, New Jersey.

Bluebond-Langner, M., Belasco, J.B., Goldman, A. & Belasco, C. (2007) Understanding parents' approaches to care and treatment of children with cancer when standard therapy has failed. *Journal of Clinical Oncology*, **25**, 2414–2419.

Cornock, M. (2010) Hannah Jones, consent and the child in action: A legal commentary. *Paediatric Nursing*, **22**, 14–20.

Dawson, A. & Spencer, S.A. (2005) Informing children and parents about research. *Archives of Disease in Childhood*, **90**, 233–235.

DoH (2010) *National Cancer Survivorship Initiative Vision*. Department of Health, London.

Dixon-Woods, M., Young, B. & Heney, D. (2005) *Rethinking Experiences of Childhood Cancer: A Multidisciplinary Approach to Chronic Childhood Illness*. Open University Press, England.

Eder, M.L., Yamokoski, A.D., Wittmann, P.W. & Kodish, E.D. (2007) Improving informed consent: Suggestions from parents of children with leukemia. *Pediatrics*, **119**, 849–859.

Edwards, J. (2001) A model of palliative care for the adolescent with cancer. *International Journal of Palliative Nursing*, **7**, 485–488.

Eiser, C. & Havermans, T. (1992) Children's understanding of cancer. *Psycho-Oncology*, **1**, 169–181.

Ellis, R. & Leventhal, B. (1992). Information needs and decision making preferences of children with cancer. *Psycho-Oncology*, **2**, 277–284.

Field, M.J. & Behrman, R.E. (2004) Defining, interpreting, and applying concepts of risk and benefit in clinical research involving children. In: *Ethical Conduct of Clinical Research Involving Children*, pp. 113–145. The National Academies Press, Washington DC.

Forte, K. (2002) Ethical issues. In: *Nursing Care of Children and Adolescents with Cancer* (eds C. Rasco-Baggott, K. Patterson-Kelly, D. Fochtman & G.V. Foley), 3rd edn. W.B. Saunders Company, Philadelphia, Pennsylvania.

Friebert, S. & Kodish, E. (2003) The right to decide. *Journal of Clinical Oncology*, **21** (May 1 supplement), 70s–73s.

Gibson, F. (2005) Evidence in action: Fostering growth of research-based practice in children's cancer nursing. *European Journal of Oncology Nursing*, **9**, 8–20.

Gibson, F. (2009) Multiprofessional collaboration in children's cancer care: Believed to be a good thing but how do we know when it works well. Editorial. *European Journal of Cancer Care*, **18**, 327–329.

Gibson, F., Richardson, A., Hey, S., Horstman, M. & O'Leary, C. (2005) *Listening to Children and Young People with Cancer*. Unpublished report submitted to Macmillan Cancer Relief. Available from Gibsof@gosh.nhs.uk

Gibson, F. & Soanes, L. (2001) Long-term follow-up following childhood cancer: Maximising the contribution of nursing. *European Journal of Cancer*, **37** (15): 1859–1868.

Goldman, A. (1998) *Care of the Dying Child*. Oxford University Press, Oxford.

Grinyer, A. (2009) *Life after Cancer in Adolescence and Young Adulthood: The Experience of Survivorship*. Routledge, London.

Hinds, P. (2008) Truth telling, not telling, and listening. *Cancer Nursing*, **31**, 415–416.

Hinds, P.S., Oakes, L., Furman, W., Quargnenti, A., Olson, M.S., Foppiano, P. & Srivastava, D.K. (2001) End-of-life decision making by adolescents, parents, and healthcare providers in pediatric oncology. *Cancer Nursing*, **24**, 122–136.

Hinds, P.S., Drew, D., Oakes, L.L., Fouladi, M., Spunt, S.L., Church, C. & Furman, W.L. (2005) End-of-life care preferences of pediatric patients with cancer. *Journal of Clinical Oncology*, **23**, 9146–9154.

Horstman, M. & Bradding, A. (2002) Helping children speak up in the health service. *European Journal of Oncology Nursing*, **6**, 75–84.

Jefford, M. & Moore, R. (2008) Improvement of informed consent and the quality of consent documents. *Lancet Oncology*, **9**, 485–493.

Kelly, D. & Gibson, F. (2008) Developing an integrated approach to the care of adolescents and young adults with cancer. In: *Cancer Care for Adolescents and Young Adults* (eds D. Kelly & F. Gibson), pp. 229–247. Blackwell Publishing, Oxford.

Last, B. & van Veldhuizen, A. (1996) Information about diagnosis and prognosis related to anxiety and depression in children with cancer aged 8–16 years. *European Journal of Cancer*, **32A**, 290–294.

Mayall, B. (2002) *Towards a Sociology for Childhood: Thinking from Children's Lives*. Open University Press, Maidenhead.

Masera, G., Chesler, M.A., Jankovic, M., Ablin, A.R., Ben Arush, M.W., Breatnach, F., Eden, T., McDowell, H.P., Epelman, C., Bellani, F.F., Green, D.M., Kosmidis, H.V., Nesbit, M.E., Wandzura, C., Wilbur, J.R. & Spinetta, J.J. (1997) SIOP working committee on psychosocial issues in pediatric oncology: Guidelines for communication of the diagnosis. *Medical and Pediatric Oncology*, **28**, 382–385.

Masera, G., Spinetta, J.J., Jankovic, M., Ablin, A.R., D'Angio, G.J., Van Dongen-Melman, J., Eden, T., Martins, A.G., Mulhern, R.K., Oppenheim, D., Topf, R. & Chesler, M.A. (1999) Guidelines for assistance to terminally ill children with cancer: A report of the SIOP working committee on psychosocial issues in pediatric oncology. *Medical and Pediatric Oncology*, **32**, 44–48.

Ranmal, R., Prictor, M. & Scott, J.T. (2009) Interventions for improving communication with children and adolescents about their cancer (Review). *Cochrane Database of Systematic Reviews 2008*, Issue 4.

Ruccione, K. (2009) The legacy of pediatric oncology nursing in advancing survivorship research and clinical care. *Journal of Pediatric Oncology Nursing*, **26**, 255. doi 10.1177/1043454209343179.

Skeen, J.E. & Webster, M.L. (2004) Speaking to children about serious matters. In: *Psychosocial Aspects of Pediatric Oncology* (eds S. Kreitler & M.W. Ben Arush), pp. 281–312. John Wiley & Sons, England.

Sobo, E.J. (2004) Good communication in pediatric cancer care: a culturally-informed research agenda. *Journal of Pediatric Oncology Nursing*, **21**, 150–154.

Spinetta, J.J., Jankovic, M., Masera, G., Ablin, A., Barr, R.D., Ben Arush, M.W., D'Angio, G.J., Van Dongen-Melman, J., Eden, T., Epelman, C., Martins, A.G., Greenberg, M.L., Kosmidis, H.V., Oppenheim, D. & Zeltzer, P.M. (2009) Optimal care for the child with cancer: A summary statement from the SIOP working committee on psychosocial issues in paediatric oncology. *Pediatric Blood and Cancer*, **52**, 904–907.

Stiller, C.A. (1994) Population based survival rates for childhood cancer in Britain. 1980–91 *British Medical Journal*, **309**, 1612–1616.

Twycross, A., Gibson, F. & Coad, J. (2008) Guidance on seeking agreement to participate in research from young children. *Paediatric Nursing*, **20**, 14–18.

Whitney, S.N., Ethier, A.M., Fruge, E., Berg, S., McCullou'gh, L.B. & Hockenberry, M. (2006) Decision making in pediatric oncology: Who should take the lead? The decisional priority in pediatric oncology model. *Journal of Clinical Oncology*, **24**, 160–165.

Woodgate, R.L. & Yanofsky, R.A. (2010) Parents' experiences in decision making with childhood cancer clinical trials. *Cancer Nursing*, **33**, 11–18.

Yap, T.Y., Yamokoski, A., Noll, R., Drotar, D., Zyzanski, S. & Kodish, E. (2009) A physician-directed intervention: teaching and measuring better informed consent. *Academic Medicine*, **84**, 1036–1042.

Zwaanswijk, M., Tates, K., van Dulmen, S., Hoogerbrugge, P., *et al.* (2007) Young patients', parents' and survivors' communication preferences in pediatric oncology: Results of online focus groups. *BMC Pediatrics*, **7**, 35.

Suggested further readings

Alderson, P. & Morrow, V. (1995) *Ethics, Social Research and Consulting with Children and Young People*. Barnardo's, Essex.

Eiser, C. (2004) *The Quality of Life: Children with Cancer*. Lawrence Erlbaum Associates, Publishers, London.

Kreitler, S. & Ben Arush, M.W. (eds) *Psychosocial Aspects of Pediatric Oncology*. John Wiley & Sons, England.

15

Withholding and Withdrawal of Treatment: Ethical, Legal and Philosophical Aspects of Paediatric Intensive Care Nursing

Karen Harrison-White

'Children may become hopelessly entrapped in intensive care units where the machinery is more sophisticated than the code of law and ethics governing its use'.

(Stinson & Stinson 1981:5)

Introduction

Advances in both technology and medicine have increased our ability to prolong life beyond the point at which survival, or survival with a reasonable quality of life, would have previously been achievable or imaginable (Le Fanu 1999). This new capability is accompanied by immense clinical, moral, legal, sociocultural and economic responsibilities and dilemmas – dilemmas that confront the ambitions of medicine and the values of those who provide care (Moore *et al.* 2008). Approximately 80% of deaths in paediatric intensive care units (PICUs) occur following a decision to limit or withdraw life-sustaining treatment (Goh *et al.* 2001), which in English law must be made with strict reference to the best interests of the child (Inwald 2008).

As outlined by the Royal College of Paediatrics and Child Health (RCPCH 2004), ethically withholding and withdrawing life-sustaining treat-

ment are arguably equivalent but emotionally they often feel very different. If the decision from the beginning is to offer only palliative care, in the best interests of the child, then this decision requires that resuscitative care is inappropriate. However, if the decision to withdraw is taken after treatment and intention to sustain life has been commenced, then the decision will lead to a change in care with active withdrawal of life-sustaining treatment with a subsequent emphasis on palliative care (RCPCH 2004). Some health-care professionals and parents find the second route psychologically and emotionally more distressing, but on the other hand in this situation it may be comforting for the parents to believe that maximum treatment was offered.

It is always necessary in acute scenarios to give life-sustaining treatment until enough clinical information is available and consultation has occurred with the parents and a suitably senior multidisciplinary health-care team. The question of whether there are moral differences between withholding and withdrawing treatments or between acts and omissions is one on which health-care professionals continue to disagree. There is still philosophical and legal life left in debating the moral and conceptual differences and implications of these issues (Hope 2000). Burns *et al.* (2001) demonstrated that a considerably higher proportion of doctors (78%) compared with nurses (57%) agreed or strongly agreed that the act of withholding and withdrawing are ethically the same. During the course of this chapter, consideration will be given to the ethical, legal and philosophical aspects of nursing a Paediatric Intensive Care (PIC) patient once the decision has been made to withhold or withdraw treatment. Pivotally, the unique role that the nurse can play in these scenarios will be debated.

Royal College of Paediatrics and Child Health (2004) framework

The RCPCH (1997, 2004) produced an excellent framework for clinical practice which consisted of a compassionate and sensitive approach towards withholding or withdrawing life-sustaining treatment from children. This framework was not intended to be applied in a prescriptive, rigid way but rather it attempts to guide individualistic management, whilst fundamentally holding the best interests and rights of the child central to the decision-making process, framed within the law.

Within the framework, the RCPCH (2004) states that they believe three fundamental principles apply to withholding and withdrawing treatment: duty of care and the partnership of care, the legal duty and respect for children's rights. These will be revisited later in this chapter in relation to the unique role of the nurse.

In order to contextualise this chapter, it is important to consider the circumstances in which it would be deemed appropriate to withhold or withdraw treatment from a child; circumstances in which treatments would only sustain *life* and neither restore health nor confer any other benefit and therefore are no longer deemed to be in the child's best interests. According to the RCPCH (2004), there are five situations where it might be ethically and legally defensible to withhold or to withdraw life-sustaining medical treatment and these have been briefly outlined below.

When *brain stem death* is confirmed, the patient is legally defined as dead. The patient's organs may still function due to extraordinary medical assistance, for example, ventilation: such assistance can suitably be withdrawn.

Permanent vegetative state (PVS) may ensue following cerebral insults, for example, trauma or hypoxia. It should persist for 4 weeks or longer or become permanent before it could be predicted that recovery of consciousness will never occur and the child will be completely reliant forever on others for care. Diagnosis will depend on the fulfilment of certain clinical criteria and requires detailed assessment. In such circumstances, it may be deemed appropriate to withdraw treatment whilst ensuring that the patient receives optimal nursing care.

In the *no-chance situation*, treatment potentially delays death but improves neither life's quality nor potential. In these circumstances, it would be deemed futile and burdensome and not in the child's best interests to prolong life; hence, there is no legal obligation for the health-care team to continue care. Importantly, if such futile care is given it may be deemed 'inhuman and degrading treatment' under Article 3 of the European Convention on Human Rights.

In the *no-purpose situation*, the child may survive following the treatment but it would not be deemed to be in the child's best interests. For example, the child may have such an irreversible impairment that it would be unreasonable to expect them to continue. Indeed, prolonging treatment might worsen the child's condition with the likelihood of further deterioration.

The *unbearable situation* occurs when the child and/or family articulates that further treatment is more than can be tolerated; they may wish to have current treatment withdrawn or to refuse further treatment irrespective of medical opinion that it could be of potential benefit.

It is important to consider which patients these circumstances can be related to. Within neonatal practice, recent statistics demonstrate that discussions with parents with regards to withholding or withdrawing treatment may have occurred in up to 70% of deaths in neonatal intensive care units in the United Kingdom (UK) (McHaffie 2001). An example of a neonatal scenario where treatment may not be commenced or may be discontinued is the non-resuscitation of a baby at birth suffering with a congenital abnormality that is incompatible with survival, for example, anencephaly or severe prematurity, where the infant is likely to have a poor neurological outcome.

Between 43% and 72% of deaths in PICUs in the UK and other countries where it has been studied can be attributed to withdrawal of treatment (McCallum *et al.* 2000). Outside of the intensive care setting, similar decisions are applied in the management of children with chronic conditions but little data is available (Liben & Goldman 1998). It is estimated that at least 12 in 10000 children are living with a life-threatening condition in this country (RCPCH 2003). Many of these children receive palliative care at home, where decisions with regards to withhold invasive and intensive interventions are frequently made (Goldman *et al.* 1990). An example of when it would be deemed appropriate to withhold treatment in childhood would be in the case of a seriously neurologically impaired child suffering from a terminal illness where it would be deemed inappropriate to offer ventilation or resuscitation measures.

During the course of this chapter, reference will be made to the following two scenarios to enable the thread of the main issues in relation to withholding and withdrawing treatment to be linked to practice.

Scenario A

Scenario A involves a 13-year-old boy (Toby) with Duchenne Muscular Dystrophy (DMD) who spent prolonged periods of time in hospital requiring increased levels of non-invasive respiratory support. In collaboration with Toby and his family, it was deemed in his best interests to withhold the formation of a tracheostomy and to institute invasive ventilation. Toby articulated that his life would be intolerable if he could not communicate with the outside world. Physically, Toby was unable to move unaided and to then remove his power of speech, due to the tracheostomy, would have constituted an *unbearable situation*. Approximately a year after this decision, Toby died from acute respiratory failure.

Scenario B

In scenario B, an 18-month-old toddler (Grace) suffered a traumatic brain injury following a fall from an airport trolley. The toddler was not brain stem dead but had sustained a severe head injury, and after reviewing all of the clinical data the likely neurological outcome was extremely poor, constituting a *no-purpose* situation. The decision was made to withdraw ventilatory support and the child died.

All members of the health-care team together with the parents have the common goal of restoring health and sustaining the life of a child (endorsed by the Children Act 1989 and United Nation's Convention on the Rights of the Child 1989). As already discussed, advances in technology make it possible to offer treatment even when the scenario is hopeless. Such treatments may prolong life but offer no foreseeable benefit for this child and pivotally may inflict further suffering. As highlighted by the RCPCH (2004), all treatments offered to children now and in the future must be in the child's best interests.

As outlined by the RCPCH (2004), there is no one ethical framework that can be applied to embrace all the nuances of withdrawing and withholding treatment in children, but the RCPCH referred to the following overarching ethical theories and principles when writing their 2004 document. *There is a duty of care and the partnership of care* in which the health-care team has a primary duty to sustain life and restore health. Even if the child cannot be restored to health, there is an absolute duty to minimise pain and suffering as far as is possible. In satisfying these objectives, the health-care team will enter into a partnership of care, the terms of which are to serve the best interests of the child. The duty of care also embodies the notion that the ascertainable wishes of the child will be respected. Children should be listened to and informed as much as possible to enable them to participate at an age appropriate and capacity level with any decisions that are made.

There is also a *legal duty* in which health-care professionals fulfil their legal duty bound by the law. As highlighted by the RCPCH (2004), the law surrounding the withholding and withdrawal of treatment from children is complex and at times confusing, but it is clear that any treatment or practice given with the primary intention of causing death is unlawful. The Children Act (1989) does not refer directly to the practices of withholding or withdrawing treatment; however, it does state inter alia that:

- The child's welfare is the overriding consideration;
- Attention should be paid to the ascertainable wishes of the child;
- Children of sufficient understanding and maturity may be able to refuse medical, psychiatric or other assessments.

As outlined by the RCPCH (2004), a number of judgements related to withdrawing and withholding treatment have established that:

- There is no obligation to give futile or burdensome treatments and that such acts could constitute battery.
- When children are dying, treatment goals may be altered.
- When the vegetative state is deemed, permanent feeding and other medical treatments can be discontinued, although it is good practice to seek legal advice in such cases.
- Treatment may be withdrawn if it is deemed not to be in the patient's best interests.

Finally, *respect for children's rights* must be upheld. The United Nations Convention on the Rights of the Child (1989) ratified by the British Government outlines fundamental principles on how children should be treated. The RCPCH (2004) deemed that the following articles were the most pertinent:

- Article 3 states that action-affecting children should have *their best interests* held in central position.
- Article 24 confirms that children have a right to the highest possible standards of health-care provision.
- Article 13 confirms the right of the child to freedom of expression and to seek, receive and communicate information.
- Article 12 confirms that a child who is capable of forming views has the right to impart those views and for their views to be considered in accordance with age and maturity.

Test cases have proven that the courts have accepted that it is legally permissible to withdraw treatment if it would inflict an intolerable existence on the child. As outlined by the RCPCH (2004), although it is fundamentally important to operate within the law it is as important to define best practice in relation to the particular interests of the child and the family rather than just presenting and achieving the minimum legal requirement. We must of course be cognisant of what is legally required, but what is ethically appropriate may set our practice above the legal minimum requirement. If there is dissent between the health-care team and the child and parents as to what is in the child's best interests, it is best practice to consult the courts. It is unusual to have to resort to the courts as full, open and timely discussions with the child and parents usually allow for all perspectives to be considered and any disagreements to be resolved (Cartlidge 2007).

Ethical, legal and professional considerations

As outlined by Purcell (1997) for clinicians confronted with the emotive issue of withdrawing and withholding treatment in a child, it is so important to harness ethical theories, ethical principles, professional codes of conduct and the law to overlay some objectivity to the decision-making process. The legal underpinnings have already been considered; we should now turn our attention to ethical theories, principles and professional codes.

The ethical theory of *utilitarianism* or consequentialism promotes the concept of the 'greatest happiness for the greatest good' and actions are judged to be *right* or *wrong* by the nature of their consequences (Beauchamp & Childress 2001). Leading proponents of this theory were J.S. Mill (1806–1873) and J. Bentham (1748–1832). With reference to both scenario A and B, it could be argued that on balance the greater good was achieved for Toby and Grace by the act of withholding treatment for Toby and withdrawing for Grace. For Toby, his autonomy and his family's wishes were respected and he died dignifiedly. For Grace, the consequences of continuing treatment may have condemned Grace and her family to a life of severe and intolerable disability. Of course, from a disability perspective there are proponents who would offer contradictory arguments; such arguments will be explored later.

The ethical theory of deontology, or non-consequentialism, focuses on duties and laws that should be followed regardless of the consequences. As outlined by Purcell (1997), the outcome of a particular action does not make it *right* or *wrong* but the moral intentions of that action are what count. If the intentions are good, then the consequences that are directly based on those intentions are judged to be good. A famous exponent of deontology was Immanuel Kant (1724–1804). Deontologists assert that an act that affords *good* in one situation should be applied in other like situations. With reference to Toby's scenario, the moral intention was to respect his wishes and his autonomy. From a health-care professionals' perspective, the appropriateness of Toby's wishes were obvious to all those around him. In Graces' scenario, the moral intention was not to offer treatments that would not confer any benefit and could be construed to be of *no purpose* (RCPCH 2004).

The ethical and legal correctness of an action is judged in the UK by whether the clinician was acting in accordance with a practice that is accepted by an appropriate peer group, as encompassed in the *Bolam* test (Bolam versus Frien Barnet Hospital Management Committee 1957). With reference to the *Bolam* test, when making such decisions as those outlined above, it has to be questioned whether clinicians in different PICUs in the UK would have made similar decisions. If there is uncertainty amongst the health-care professionals as to the correct course of action or irresolvable disagreements with the parents, then clinicians should turn to the courts for guidance. In a recent example reported in the Daily Telegraph (2009), a baby, known by the initials OT, died following his parents' defeat in an attempt to overturn a ruling giving hospital staff the power to withdraw life-sustaining treatment. Baby OT had a rare metabolic disorder, had suffered brain damage and was in respiratory failure. A spokesman for the British Medical Association stated in the article that: 'Cases like this are very distressing and we have every empathy with the parents, but when the parents and the clinical team don't agree on the treatment for the child in question, the only way forward is to go to the courts and for the courts to decide on what is in the best interests of the child, which is paramount' (Telegraph 22nd March 2009).

It could be argued that rather than considering the utilitarian and Kantian theories, there should be a focus on virtue ethics, which highlights the importance of the agent who performs an action or makes a choice (Beachamp & Childress 2001). From this perspective, we should act in ways that reveal the virtues, even if that means doing what may be conceived as bad or bringing about undesirable consequences. It is really interesting to examine Toby and Graces' case from this perspective. In both scenarios, the health-care team were working collaboratively with the children/families to address what was deemed to be in the child's best interests and this is where the *virtue* side of both cases comes into play. The issue is no longer about saving a child's life but rather acting strictly within their best interests, even though the consequence for both children was ultimately death.

As highlighted by Purcell (1997), ethical principles can make theories more accessible and applicable in ethical debates. Within the context of medical health-care ethics, the notions of beneficence, non-maleficence, respect for autonomy and justice have been widely accepted as the four cornerstone principles that need to be considered when making ethical judgements (Gillon 1992; Beauchamp & Childress 2001). Beneficence refers to a moral obligation to act for the benefit of others. The principle of non-maleficence refers to the obligation not to cause harm and has often been considered to be the fundamental moral principle underpinning medical ethics (Beauchamp & Childress 2001). Beneficence and non-maleficence are preserved in the Nursing and Midwifery Council (NMC 2008) Professional Code of Conduct for medical staff and can be traced back to the fourth century BC Hippocratic Oath. Autonomy refers to the capacity of the individual 'to think, decide, and act on the basis of such thought and decision freely and independently and without … let or hindrance' (Gillon 1992:60). Justice refers to the principle of equity and fairness and is often discussed in relation to the fair distribution of health-care resources.

It is useful to work these ethical principles into real scenarios: let us examine and apply them in relation to Toby's scenario. In terms of *beneficence* from Toby's perspective, he could not conceive any benefit from having a tracheostomy and invasive ventilation, even though these treatment modalities could have prolonged his life. He perceived there to be no benefit in having an existence without being able to speak, when this was the last motor activity that he had intact. From the perception of *non-maleficence*, Toby and his family deemed the formation of a tracheostomy and invasive ventilation to constitute *harm*. This is where these ethical principles are so interesting: for one person a treatment option could offer benefit and for another harm, and this is why it is so pivotal that cases are considered individualistically. Examining the perspective of *autonomy*, Toby's autonomy was respected. In relation to children under 16 years of age, the Children Act (1989) requires that there is regard to the 'ascertainable wishes and feelings of the child concerned considered in the light of their age and understanding' (section 1(3)(a) cited in Dimond 2008). In Toby's case, although he was only 13, he truly understood the reality of his situation and the perceived ramifications of the treatment options. It could, however, be argued that it is difficult to anticipate the full reality of a treatment until it is experienced: in Toby's case a tracheostomy and invasive ventilation. From the perspective of *justice*, Toby had access to advanced treatment modalities but he decided with his family and the health-care team that it was inappropriate and most importantly not in his best interests to utilise them. Conversely, in not utilising these treatment options, other children would benefit from the availability of scarce high dependency and intensive care facilities thus enhancing their access to such services.

These principles commonly conflict in practice; even in Toby's case, the decision to respect his autonomy and to offer only beneficial nursing treatments did arguably hasten death thereby not protecting fully the principle of *non-maleficence*. Of course, clinically it is all about balancing these competing principles to act in the best interests of the child. Interestingly when studying doctors' and nurses' use of ethical theories in practice, Robertson (1996) found that when principles were in conflict nurses valued patient autonomy more highly and physicians valued beneficence. Our Professional Code of Conduct (NMC 2008) also steers us in the right direction when considering withdrawing and withholding treatment, although it is not directly referred to.

The role of the nurse when treatment is withheld or withdrawn

The remainder of this chapter will turn to consider the unique contribution that PIC nurses can potentially make when care is withheld or withdrawn in paediatrics. In PIC environments, nurses generally care for children on a one-to-one basis, often working long shift patterns. In working so closely with the child and family, nurses have the privileged opportunity to forge close relationships and may be in a position to understand and contextualise the unique family perspective. With reference to the instances when care can be legally and ethically withheld or withdrawn, this understanding can be particularly valuable when judgements are being made about *futility* and *quality or life* issues.

Futile care prolongs suffering and fails to improve the quality of life for a child (Akpinar *et al.* 2009). The term futility is notoriously difficult to quantify or qualify (Hoyt 1995; ten Have & Janssens 2002; Gedge *et al.* 2007) leading to immense complexities when applied to decision-making. However, decisions with regards to withholding and withdrawing care are increasingly based on the concept of *futility* (Lofmark & Nilstun 2002; Melia 2004). PIC nurses can potentially contribute to discussions with the parents and the wider health-care team as they get to know and understand the child and family with particular reference to *futility* and *quality-of-life* issues.

Many infants and children who have their care withheld or withdrawn do not have underlying disabilities but have suffered from an illness or accident and decisions around *futility* and *quality of life* are base upon future predictions of outcome. However, when considering whether to withhold or withdraw treatment in a child with an underlying disability, it is important to really understand the nature of the underlying disability to prevent incorrect judgements being made about the child's quality of life. As highlighted by Werth (2005), when end-of-life decisions are being made about an individual incapable of making autonomous decisions, either due to the disability, age or due to the intensive care treatments, it will be the value judgements of others that will determine if a person lives or dies. This fact highlights the importance of nursing and medical staff taking the time to really understand the nature of a person's disability to contextualise their being. Generally, concern has been raised about the lack of education that health-care professionals have with regards to providing services to people with disabilities in the current health-care system (Gill 2000). As highlighted by Werth (2005), the behaviour of health-care professionals towards people with disabilities can be affected by quality-of-life judgements when making end-of-life decisions. Saigal (2009) stated that despite wide interest in this subject area, there is no universal agreement on the definition of what constitutes *quality of life* especially in children. Gill (2000:530) reviewed the literature and stated that

> … health professionals significantly underestimate the quality of life of persons with disabilities compared with the actual assessments made by people with disabilities themselves. In fact, the gap between health professionals and people with disabilities in evaluating life with disability is consistent and stunning.

Arguments relating to *futility* and *quality-of-life* issues allow the health-care team to make decisions that may ultimately lead to death, whereas patients' advocates argue that such decisions should reside with the patients or their advocates and those who know them best (Helft *et al*. 2000). Reassuringly, research by Burns *et al*. (2001) demonstrated that physicians and nurses believe that quality-of-life determinants should only be judged from the perspective of the child and family rather than associated with particular chronic disorders. It is pivotally important that these considerations are fully understood and debated within the health-care team and family in order that a *best interest* judgement can be made. As outlined by Tibballs (2007), *best interests* is based on an evaluation of *quality of life*, *futility* and comparison of *burdens versus benefits* with and without treatment. The most common ethical and legal justification for withholding and withdrawing treatment rests on the *best interests* of the infant or child. It has to be remembered that often decisions are being made about a previously well infant or child, who has suffered an acute illness or accident, and the family and health-care team may not understand the ramifications of allowing

the child to live or it may be difficult to predict the full extent of the disability.

Best interest decisions can be difficult to make and are based on the subjective views of the decision-maker; it can potentially encourage a weakened approach to decision-making processes (Kennedy 1992). As highlighted by Inwald (2008), it is so important that the decision-maker has an in-depth knowledge of the child and family. The nurse may be able to support the child and parents in articulating and advocating for their perspectives and contributing to a fuller dialogue for the health-care team to consider. After discussions are formally held with the family and health-care team, it is often the nurse who is then asked questions by family members at the bedside, thus adding another layer of acquired knowledge from a nursing perspective. The nurse can usually quickly decipher how much the family has understood of the discussions and the unique family perspective following the consultation.

It has to be considered how much value is placed on nursing knowledge of the child and family when decisions are made in relation to withdrawing and withholding treatment. Despite recommendations to include nurses, families and other health-care professionals in decisions relating to withdrawing and withholding treatment (RCPCH 2004), it is evident that care-giving colleagues and patients and families are not always fully involved in this process (Ferrand *et al*. 2003; Sprung *et al*. 2003). The legal jurisdiction for decisions about withdrawing or withholding treatment rests with the consultant doctor in-charge (BMA 2001) and perhaps it is therefore understandable and somewhat inevitable that some consultants will fail to fully confer with colleagues. The burden of responsibility for some consultants must seem immense when making such decisions, and as highlighted by Slomka (1992) when power rests with a dominant group there is no requisite for negotiation.

From a nursing perspective, the failure to consult is a complex issue and perhaps can be related to the perceptions of the importance of nursing knowledge by those outside of the profession. According to Carper (1978) and more recently Edwards (1998) and Wainwright (1999), nursing knowledge and patterns of knowing rest on the art of nursing and aesthetics. It is so important that nursing knowledge and understanding are not seen as second rate when compared to scientific technological medical knowledge (Pattison 2006). Falk-Rafael (1996) suggests that if nurses want to gain power, they need to distance themselves from the caring qualities of nursing and assimilate medical norms. As highlighted by Pattison (2006) following on from Falk-Rafael's (1996, 1998) arguments, there is an assumption that caring does not require a knowledge base and that this paradigm only serves to perpetuate the low status of power assigned to caring nurses.

The changing nature of nursing may shift this power balance as more nurses are elevated to managerial roles or undertake advanced clinical roles (DoH 2006, 2008a). However, as highlighted by Pattison (2006), it is evident that whilst medical power may be weakening it currently still remains dominant in critical care environments. Some elements of knowledge are shared; however, medical knowledge still seems to be superior to nursing (Coombs & Ersser 2004). Jones (2008) argues that nurses have been the *invisible* leaders in health service provision, whilst the public perceive that they provide care and others manage and lead. Lord Darzi's final report, *A High Quality Workforce* (DoH 2008b), strongly acknowledges the need to develop and support nursing in their leadership roles at every level within the NHS (Jones 2008). As outlined by Clark (2008), in this challenging health-care system nurses must be prepared to rise to the challenge of embodying leadership in their roles.

Although the medical professions have received guidance on how to manage withholding and withdrawing treatment, neither the Royal College of Nursing nor the NMC have produced guidance on the nursing roles in withdrawing or withholding treatment scenarios (Pattison 2006). As highlighted by Rashotte *et al*. (1997), critical care nurses frequently express strong feelings of responsibility and accountability in relation to this scenario but such expressions can occur without the requisite professional or organisational underpinning power required allowing a genuine voice in decision-making to occur (Sorlie *et al*. 2001; Nathaniel 2006). In not having guidelines from the professional body, a powerful message is given that nurses do not play an important professional role within this situation. It also potentially blocks nurses from engaging in learning about the guidelines, ethics

and law in relation to this subject area, thus undermining the contribution that they can make when discussing aspects of withholding and withdrawing treatment in PIC settings. Research conducted by Street *et al*. (2000) demonstrated that nurses did not rate their contributions to be highly important in the decision-making process with regards to withholding and withdrawing treatment, and in only 3 of the 22 cases nurses included themselves as having made the final decision. Street (2000) suggests that perhaps it is more advantageous to play the role of advocate if you do not perceive yourself to be the *final decision-maker*. Interestingly, the nursing input was highly valued by the medical staff who perceived that they played a much greater role in the *final* decision-making process. Street (2000) also found that there was a significant difference in the weight given by nursing staff to parents' wishes and their beliefs regarding the perceived suffering and future quality of life compared to doctors. Doctors understandably perceived that the most important factor in making withholding and withdrawing decisions focused on prognostic factors related to the disease process rather than personal beliefs in relation to suffering and quality of life (Street 2000).

To really support the family and health-care team, it is so important that nurses have a working knowledge of the ethical, legal and practical issues related to withholding and withdrawing treatment (Street 2000; Crawford & Way 2009). In research conducted by Street (2000), 8 of the 22 nursing respondents were aware of the RCPCH (1997) guidelines but only 2 had actually read them! As highlighted by Meyer (2002), whether prepared or not, PIC staff members can find themselves abruptly entwined with distressed families during end-of-life scenarios and those families will probably hold the staff and their knowledge in high regard. Interestingly, doctors' awareness of the RCPCH (1997) guidelines was high, 17 out of 18 respondents knew that they existed, but only 12 had actually read them and 4 found them helpful (Street 2000).

It could be questioned as to how much the child, family and health-care team can benefit from an experienced and well-informed nurse during times of withholding and withdrawing treatment. PIC nurses can really support both the family and the medical staff during discussions about withholding and withdrawing treatment as they have been shown to be highly skilled within this domain, arising from their experience (Way 2003). Forbes *et al.*'s (2008) research demonstrated that particularly more junior medical staff found it difficult to have such discussions with parents. When critical decisions are being made with regards to withholding and withdrawing treatment, 58% of junior medical staff and 38.5% of senior medical staff reported receiving no specific training in relation to communicating with parents. Baverstock & Finlay (2008) identified that new consultants found responsibility and decision-making at the end of life to be one of the biggest changes from being a registrar.

An experienced, knowledgeable PIC nurse who knows the child and family can really support the medical team in talking with the family and eliciting what is in the best interests of the child. Sadly though, all too often the PIC bedside nurse and a senior member of the medical team will talk with the family but little if any discussion occurs between the health-care professionals prior to the meeting with the family, thus reducing the opportunity for the nurse to offer support or guidance. In fact, the nurse may enter into a consultation without knowing the direction that the discussion will take from a medical perspective. Of course, the bedside nurse may be very junior and not in a position to support the medical staff but they should still be exposed to discussion prior to the meeting with the family to ensure that they are prepared. Critically though, as outlined by Doherty (2008), four out of five nurses lack basic pre-registration training in end-of-life care, reported by the National Audit Office (NAO). The NAO recommended that the NMC should aim to improve this situation when reviewing nursing programmes. In the research by Burns *et al.* (2001), it was demonstrated that doctors and nurses agreed that doctors usually instigate discussion to limit life-sustaining treatment and that the families infrequently are the first to commence these discussions. Nurses were significantly more likely than doctors to report that they also often initiate such discussions highlighting the need for specialist training in this area.

Not surprisingly, Randolph *et al.* (1997) noted significant variability amongst PICU doctors and nurses with regards to attitudes relating to restrict-

ing life-sustaining treatment and concluded that parents could receive different approaches based on who was caring for their child. Interestingly, Gill (2005) argued that the differences in professional perspectives could be traced to the fundamental differences between professional roles. PICU doctors focus on monitoring the different treatments given to a patient whilst nurses concentrate on the holistic care of the patient. As a consequence, doctors will have a propensity to prolong treatment before an end-of-life decision is made. Critically though in a study by Studdert *et al.* (2003), doctors reported disputes amongst doctors whilst nurses reported disputes with doctors regarding leadership and availability but the doctors perceived these interactions as not constituting a significant conflict. Puntillo & McAdam (2006) undertook a systematic review with the aim of evaluating practical interventions for improving communication and collaboration between nurses and doctors when dealing with end-of-life issues. They found that an increase in shared decision-making can result from a better understanding and respect for the perspectives and burdens of those felt by the different professions. Puntillo & McAdam (2006) predicted that with effective communication and collaborative practice, the quality of end-of-life care will improve markedly. From a parental perspective, communication with the child and family with regards to treatment plans and shared decision-making are pivotal to the delivery of high quality care at the end of life (Meert *et al.* 2009); this can only occur if the health-care teams work together effectively.

If nurses are not consulted or their opinion considered, they may suffer *moral distress*. Moral distress (MD) is a relatively new concept in health-care ethics and is said to be a person's reaction when he/she knows the correct course of action but does not take it (Austin *et al.* 2009). This phenomenon can occur when a sense of moral responsibility is not acted on owing to internal personal constraints or due to external barriers (Nathaniel 2006). As highlighted by Nathaniel (2006), professionals report distress when their moral values are at odds with the realities of the workplace. Davies *et al.* (1996) demonstrated that nurses experienced moral distress when they were not listened to in decision-making processes; they felt frustration, anger and sadness. Oberle & Hughes (2001) conducted a qualitative study examining nurses' and doctors' experience of ethical issues that occurred in end-of-life decisions. Their study demonstrated that the core issue for both professions was witnessing suffering. Uncertainty about the most appropriate action was a source of moral distress with competing values, hierarchy, communication and scarce resources emerging as themes. The nursing staff in particular identified that they suffered moral distress when they were unable to impact on decision-making. Some nurses have cited prolonged treatment beyond any hope of survival as *torture*. A nurse relayed her experience of caring for a child with overwhelming congenital problems: 'you just hated to come in and see your name beside his name … it was hard. … He was so sick and they were just keeping him going, keeping him going and going and going. He was just dying in front of our eyes, but the doctors wouldn't give up. …' (McGibbon 2004 cited in Austin 2009:61).

Meyer *et al.* (2002) demonstrated in their research that parents rated nurses as very involved in their child's care at the time of death; indeed nurses were considered to be more involved at the end of life than friends or close family members. This highlights the need for nurses' contribution to this process to be valued and supported and in turn also reiterates the requirement for nurses to be informed with regards to withdrawing and withholding treatment. Although it is important for the profile of PIC nurses that they are informed and able to participate in decision-making processes with regards to withholding and withdrawing treatment, the most important factor is that the child and parents are supported in making a decision that is in the best interests of the child. Parental involvement in decision-making in relation to withdrawal and withholding treatment is high in PIC (Lynn 2008; Moore *et al.* 2008) and there is widespread agreement that parents should be involved in decision-making (Singh *et al.* 2004; Pinnock & Crosthwaite 2005). The role of the nurse should be to support the parents in making the correct decision based on the nurses' unique knowledge of the child and the family, underpinned by ethical, legal and professional knowledge. As highlighted by Longden & Mayer (2007), as health-care professionals we have a responsibility to proactively empower parents to make the correct decisions; this view has

been endorsed by the Paediatric Intensive Care Society (2002). Meyer *et al.* (2006) identified from their research a simple guidance to improve paediatric end-of-life care that included the need for honest and complete information, access to staff, communication and care coordination, support by staff, emotional expression, protection of the parent–child relationship and respect of faith. Meyer *et al.* (2002) also demonstrated that 70% of parents felt that they were informed about their child's prognosis; however, staff reluctance and anxieties to prognosticate in potential end-of-life scenarios, unwillingness to impart bad news or to diminish futility can limit the parents' ability to make informed end-of-life decisions (Van der Heide *et al.* 1998). Interestingly, Burns (2001) demonstrated that nurses were less satisfied with the quality of communication in relation to withholding and withdrawing treatment than doctors.

Loss of control has been identified as a very difficult issue that people face in a medical crisis (Williams & Koocher 1999). Of course, parents in particular struggle with the sense of loss of control because their traditional role is threatened (Meert *et al.* 2009). Meyer *et al.* (2002) demonstrated that nearly one quarter of parents reported that if able they would have made different decisions in relation to their child's care, although they were not able to determine whether the parents would have fundamentally changed their end-of-life decision-making. Parents who have loss of control experiences and regrets may be at an increased risk of complicated bereavement. It has to be questioned whether nurses could reduce the level of parental loss of control feelings, by working more closely with the child and family. End-of-life decisions are usually staged over a number of days. Stark *et al.* (2008) demonstrated that in half of all the cases researched, more than one discussion with the families occurred before a final decision was reached which is consistent with previous reports (Garros *et al.* 2003). Stark *et al.* (2008) showed that it was obvious that there was a gradual shift in focus from discussion with regards to limitation of treatment, to treatment withdrawal. It is here that nurses can support parents along this continuum because they are with the child and family 24 h a day. Nurses could also potentially guide the health-care team to the correct timings and content of meetings. However, Gill (2005) noted an inverse relationship between decision-making influence and the amount of time spent directly with a patient. Forbes *et al.* (2008) in a recent audit of 50 inpatient deaths demonstrated that discussions concerning withdrawing of life-sustaining medical treatment had a propensity to occur late in the course of the illness indicating that opportunities for discussion could have occurred earlier.

Recommendations

- The unique role that nurses play at the end of life should be recognised and utilised more fully.
- The NMC in the UK should give guidance to nurses with regards to their responsibilities when care is withheld or withdrawn.
- Nurses need to have a working knowledge of the ethical, legal and practical issues related to withholding and withdrawing treatment.
- The use of interprofessional education should be considered to support nurses and doctors working more effectively together in end-of-life scenarios.
- Nurses need to be supported in the strategies that they can invoke to take a more active role in decision-making processes.

Conclusion

When examining the roles of both doctors and nurses in relation to withholding and withdrawing treatment, it is obvious that both professions offer unique contributions within this scenario. The nursing contribution, however, could be stronger and more valued to ensure that the best interests of the child are protected and the experience of the child and parents is optimised during this crisis. Perhaps, the key to unlock this situation is better pre- and post-registration interprofessional training where doctors and nurses learn together how to effectively manage withholding and withdrawing treatment. By learning together, the professions might begin to understand and respect each other's distinctive contributions and perspectives (Barr 2005).

Reflective scenario

A father, whose 1-year-old son (baby RB) was born with congenital myasthenic syndrome (CMS), is going to the high court in an attempt to stop a hospital from withdrawing the ventilatory support that is keeping the child alive. CMS affects the ability to breathe independently and severely reduces movement. The doctors who are treating baby RB claim that his quality of life is so poor that it is not in his best interests to sustain his life. They are allegedly being supported in their action by the baby's mother, who is separated from his father. Pivotally, if the hospital succeeds in its application, it will be the first time a British court has gone against the wishes of a parent and ruled that ventilation can be withheld or withdrawn from a child who does not have brain damage. Lawyers for the father claim that the child's brain is not affected by the condition, arguing that it has meaningful responses to stimuli and he is able to recognise his parents.

Three questions

1. Utilising the RCPCH (2004) guidelines, on what basis is the hospital claiming that ventilatory support should be withdrawn on baby RB?
2. Why has this case been referred to the high court?
3. Why is this case so complex?
4. If you were nursing baby RB, what information would you want to know to support/refute your opinion that ventilation should be withdrawn?

References

Akpinar, A., Senses, M.O. & Er, R.A. (2009) Attitudes to end-of life decisions in paediatric intensive care. *Nursing Ethics*, **16** (1), 83–92.

Austin, W., Kelecevic, J., Goble, E. & Mekechuk, J. (2009) An overview of moral distress and the paediatric intensive care team. *Nursing Ethics*, **16** (1), 57–68.

Baverstock, A. & Finlay, F. (2008) What can we learn from the experiences of consultants around the time of a child's death? *Child: Child Health and Development*, **34** (6), 732–739.

Beauchamp, T.L. & Childress J.F. (2001) *Principles of Biomedical Ethics*, 5th edn. Oxford University Press, Oxford.

Bolam versus Friern Barnet Hospital Management Committee (1957) 2 AII ER 118.

BMA (2001) *Withdrawing and Withholding Life – Prolonging Medical Treatment: Guidelines for Decision – Making*, 2nd edn. British Medical Association, London.

Burns, J.P., Mitchell, C., Griffith, J.L. & Truog, R.D. (2001) End-of-life care in the pediatric intensive care unit: Attitudes and practices of pediatric critical care physicians and nurses. *Critical Care Medicine*, **29** (3), 658–664.

Carper, B.A. (1978) Fundamental patterns of knowing in nursing. *Advances in Nursing Science*, **1**, 13–23.

Cartlidge, P. (2007) (ed.) *Ethical, Legal and Social Aspects of Child Healthcare*. Elsevier, Oxford.

Clark, L. (2008) Clinical leadership: Values, beliefs and vision. *Nursing Management*, **15** (7), 30–35.

HMSO (1989) *Children Act, 1989*. Her Majesty's Stationary Office, London.

Coombs, M. & Ersser, S.J. (2004) Medical hegemony in decision-making – a barrier to interdisciplinary working in intensive care? *Journal of Advanced Nursing*, **46**, 245–252.

Crawford, D. & Way, C. (2009) Just because we can, should we? A discussion of treatment withdrawal. *Paediatric Nursing*, **21** (1), 22–25.

Daily Telegraph Reporter (2009) Courts are right to make decisions on Baby OT treatment withdrawal cases, said British Medical Association. Daily Telegraph, London. 22 March 2009. http://www.telegraph.co.uk/news/newstopics/politics/lawandorder/5032507/Courts-are-right-to-make-decisions-on-Baby-OT-treatment-withdrawal-cases-said-British-Medical-Association.html (accessed 15/10/09)

Davies, B., Cook, K. & O'Loane, M. (1996) Caring for dying children: nurses' experiences. *Pediatric Nursing*, **22**, 500–507.

DoH (2006) *Modernising Nursing Careers – Setting the Direction*. Department of Health, London.

DoH (2008a) *Towards a Framework for Post – Registration Nursing Careers: A National Consultation*. Department of Health, London.

DoH (2008b) *A High Quality Workforce: NHS Next Stage Review*. Department of Health, London.

Dimond, B. (2008) *Legal Aspects of Nursing*, 5th edn. Pearson Education Ltd., Essex.

Doherty, L. (2008) Survey shows 'woeful' lack of basic training in end-of-life care. *Nursing Standard*, **23** (13), 6.

Edwards, S.D. (1998) The art of nursing. *Nursing Ethics*, **5**, 393–400.

Council of Europe (2003) *European Convention on Human Rights 2003*. Council of Europe, Strasbourg.

Falk Rafael, A.R. (1998) Power and caring: A dialectic in nursing. *Advances in Nursing Science*, **21**, 29–42.

Ferrand, E., Lemaire, F., Regnier, B., Kuteifan, K., Badet, M., Asfar, P., Jaber, S., Chagnon, J., Renault, A., Robert, R., Pochard, F., Herve, C., Brun-Bruisson, C. & Duvaldestin, P. (2003) Discrepancies between perceptions by physicians and nursing staff of intensive care unit end-of-life decisions. *American Journal of Respiratory and Critical Care Medicine*, **167**, 1310–1315.

Forbes, T., Goeman, E., Stark, Z., Hynson, J. & Forrester, M. (2008) Discussing withdrawing and withholding of life-sustaining medical treatment in a tertiary paediatric hospital: A survey of clinical attitudes and practices. *Journal of Paediatrics and Child Health*, **44**, 392–398.

Garros, D., Rosychuk, R.J. & Cox, P.N. (2003) Circumstances surrounding end of life in a pediatric intensive care unit. *Pediatrics*, **112**, 371.

Gedge, E., Giacomini, M. & Cook, D. (2007) Withholding and withdrawing life support in critical care settings: Ethical issues concerning consent. *Journal of Medical Ethics*, **33**, 215–218.

Gill, C.J. (2000) Health professionals, disability and assisted suicide: An examination of relevant empirical evidence and reply to Batavia (2000). *Psychology, Public Policy and Law*, **6**, 526–545.

Gill, M.B. (2005) PICU Prometheus: Ethical issues in the treatment of very sick children in paediatric intensive care. *Mortality*, **10**, 262–275.

Gillon, R. (1992) *Philosophical Medical Ethic*. John Wiley & Sons, Chichester.

Goldman, A., Beardsmore, A. & Hunt J. (1990) Palliative care for children with cancer – home hospital or hospice? *Archives of Disease in Child*, **65**, 641–643.

Goh, A.Y. & Mok, Q. (2001) Identifying futility in a paediatric critical care setting: A prospective observational study. *Archives of Disease in Childhood*, **84**, 265–268.

Have, ten H. & Janssens, D. (2002) Futility, limits and palliative care. In: *The Ethics of Palliative Care: European Perspectives* (eds H. ten Have & D. Clark, D.). Open University Press, Buckinghamshire.

Helft, P.R., Siegler, M. & Lantos, J. (2000) The rise and fall of the futility movement. *The New England Journal of Medicine*, **343**, 293–296.

Heide, van der A., Maas, van der P.J. & Wal, van der G. (1998) The role of parents in end-of-life decisions in neonatology: Physicians' views and practices. *Pediatrics*, **101**, 413–418.

Hope, T. (2000) Acts and omissions revisited. *Journal of Medical Ethics*, **26** (4), 227.

Hoyt, J.W. (1995) Medical futility. *Critical Care Medicine*, **23**, 621–622.

HMSO (1998) *Human Rights Act*. Crown Copyright, HMSO, London.

Inwald D. (2008) The best interests test at the end of life on PIC: A plea for a family centred approach. *Archives of Disease in Childhood*, **93**, 248–250.

Jones, L. (2008) Leadership in the 'new' NHS. *Nursing Management*, **15** (6), 32–35.

Kennedy, I. (1992) *Treat Me Right: Essay in Medical Law and Ethics*. Oxford University Press, Oxford.

Le Fanu, J. (1999) *The Rise and Fall of Modern Medicine*. Abacus, London.

Liben, S. & Goldman, A. (1998) Homecare for children with life threatening illness. *Journal of Palliative Care*, **14**, 33–38.

Lofmark, R. & Nilstun, T. (2002) Conditions and consequences of medical futility – from a literature review to a clinical model. *Journal of Medical Ethics*, **28**, 115–119.

Longden, J.V. & Mayer, A.P.T. (2007) Family involvement in end-of-life care in a paediatric intensive care unit. *Nursing in Critical Care*, **12** (4), 181–187.

Lynn, G. (2008) End of life decision-making in paediatrics. *Journal of Paediatrics and Child Health*, **44** (7–8), 389–391.

McCallum, D.E., Byrne, P. & Bruera, E. (2000) How children die in hospital. *Journal of Pain Symptom Management*, **20**, 417–423.

Meert, K.L., Briller, S.H., Myers Schim, S., Thurston, C. & Kabel, A. (2009) Examining the needs of bereaved parents in the paediatric intensive care unit: A qualitative study. *Death Studies*, **33**, 712–740.

Meyer, E.C., Burns, J.P., Griffith, J.L. & Truog, R.D. (2002) Parental perspectives on end-of-life care in the pediatric intensive care unit. *Critical Care Medicine*, **30** (1), 226–231.

Meyer, E.C., Ritholz, M.D., Burns, J. & Truog, R.D. (2006) Improving the quality for end-of-life care in the pediatric intensive care unit: Parents' priorities and recommendations. *Pediatrics*, **117** (3), 649–657.

McHaffie, H.S. (2001). *Crucial Decisions at the Beginning of Life*. Radcliff Medical Press, Abingdon.

Melia, K. (2004) *Health Care Ethics: Lessons from Intensive Care*. Sage Publication, London.

Moore, P., Ketteridge, I., Gillis, J., Jacobe, S. & Isaacs, D. (2008) Withdrawal and limitation of life-sustaining treatments in a paediatric intensive care unit and review of the literature. *Journal of Paediatrics and Child Health*, **44**, 404–408.

Nathaniel, A. (2006) Moral reckoning in nursing. *West Journal Nursing Research*, **28**, 419–38.

NMC (2008) *The Code: Standards of Conduct, Performance and Ethics for Nurses and Midwives*. Nursing and Midwifery Council, London.

Oberle, K. & Hughes, D. (2001) Doctors' and nurses' perceptions of ethical problems in end-of-life decisions. *Journal of Advanced Nursing*, **33**, 707–715.

Pattison, N. (2006) A critical discourse analysis of provision of end-of-life care in key UK critical care documents. *Nursing in Critical Care*, **11** (4), 198–208.

PICS (2002) *Standards for Bereavement Care*. Paediatric Intensive Care Society, Sheffield.

Pinnock, R. & Crosthwaite, J. (2005) When parents refuse consent to treatment for young children. *Journal of Paediatrics and Child Health*, **41**, 369–373.

Puntillo, K.A. & McAdam, J. (2006) Communication between physicians and nurses as a target for improving end-of-life care in the intensive care unit: Challenges and opportunities for moving forward. *Critical Care Medicine*, **34** (11 Suppl), S332–S340.

Purcell, C. (1997) Withdrawing treatment from a critically-ill child. *Intensive and Critical Care Nursing*, **13**, 103–107.

Rashotte, J., Fothergill-Bourbonnais, F. & Chamberlain, M. (1997) Pediatric intensive care nurses and their grief experiences: A phenomenological study. *Heart Lung*, **26**, 372–386.

Randolph, A.G., Zollo, M.B., Wigton, R.S. & Yeh, T.S. (1997) Factors explaining variability among caregivers in the intent to restrict life-support interventions in a paediatric intensive care unit. *Critical Care Medicine*, **25**, 435–439.

Robertson, D. (1996) Ethical theory, ethnography and differences between doctors and nurses in approaches to patient care. *Journal of Medical Ethics*, **22**, 292–299.

RCPCH (1997) *Withholding or Withdrawing Life Saving Treatment in Children: A Framework for Practice*. Royal College of Paediatrics and Child Health, London.

RCPCH (2003) *A Guide to the Development of Children's Palliative Care Services. Report of a Joint Working Party of the Association for Children with Life-threatening or Terminal Conditions and their Families and the Royal College of Paediatrics and Child Health*. Royal College of Paediatrics and Child Health, London.

RCPCH (2004) *Withholding or Withdrawing Life Sustaining Treatment in Children*. Royal College of Paediatrics and Child Health, London.

Saigal, S. (2009) Measurement of quality of life of survivors of neonatal intensive care: Critique and implications. *Seminars in Perinatology*, **32** (1), 59–66.

Singh, J., Lantos, J. & Meadow, W. (2004) End-of-life after birth: Death and dying in a neonatal intensive care unit. *Pediatrics*, **114**, 1620–1626.

Slomka, J. (1992) The negotiation of death: Clinical decision making at the end of life. *Social Science and Medicine*, **35**, 251–259.

Sorlie, V., Forde, R., Lindseth, A. & Norberg, A. (2001) Male physicians' narratives about being in ethically difficult care situations in paediatrics. *Social Science Medicine*, **53**, 657–667.

Sprung, C.L., Cohen, S.L., Sjokvist, P., Baras, M., Bulow, H., Hovilehto, S., Ledoux, D., Lippert, A., Maia, P., Phelan, D., Schobersberger, W., Wennberg, E. & Woodcock, T. (2003) End of life practices in European intensive care units: The ethics study. *Journal of the American Medical Association*, **290**, 790–797.

Stark, Z., Hynson, J. & Forrester, M. (2008) Discussing withholding and withdrawing of life-sustaining medical treatment in paediatric inpatients: Audit of current practice. *Journal of Paediatrics and Child Health*, **44**, 399–403.

Stinson, R. & Stinson, P. (1981) On the death of a baby. *Journal of Medical Ethics*, **7** (1), 5–18.

Street, K., Ashcroft, R., Henderson, J. & Campbell, A.V. (2000) The decision making process regarding the withdrawal or withholding of potential life-saving treatments in a children's hospital. *Journal of Medical Ethics*, **26**, 346–352.

Studdert, D.M., Burns, J.P., Mello, M.M., Puopolo, A.L., Truog, R.D. & Brennon, T.A. (2003) Nature of conflict in the care of pediatric intensive care patients with prolonged stay. *Pediatrics*, **112**, 553–558.

Tibballs, J. (2007) Legal basis for ethical withholding and withdrawing life-sustaining medical treatment from infants and children. *Journal of Paediatrics and Child Health*, **43**, 230–236.

UN (1989) *United Nations Convention on the Rights of the Child (UNCRC)*. United Nations, New York.

Way, C. (2003) In their own words: Paediatric intensive care nurses' experiences of withdrawal of treatment. *Paediatric Intensive Care Nursing*, **4** (1), 17–31.

Wainwright, P. (1999) The art of nursing. *International Journal of Nursing Studies*, **36**, 379–385.

Werth, J.L. (2005) Concerns about decisions related to withholding and withdrawing life-sustaining treatment and futility for persons with disabilities. *Journal of Disability Policy Studies*, **16** (1), 31–37.

Williams, J. & Koocher, G.P. (1999) Medical crisis counseling on a pediatric intensive care unit: Case examples and clinical utility. *Journal of Clinical Psychology in Medical Settings*, **6** (3), 249–258.

Suggested further reading

RCPCH (2004) *Withholding or Withdrawing Life Sustaining Treatment in Children*. Royal College of Paediatrics and Child Health, London.

16 Palliative Care of Children: Some Ethical Dilemmas

Vicki Rowse and Martin Smith

There are two components of children's palliative care: their life and their death. Both raise ethical and social issues which are challenging for professionals and which will be examined from the perspectives of continuing life and end of life.

Continuing care and life: an introduction

One of the challenges for the twenty-first century is the legacy of rapid technological and medical advance during the twentieth century, as well as devices enabling closer monitoring and more complex surgery – there are new medicines, new techniques and, as a result, higher expectations. In addition, modern communication allows us to *speak* to the other side of the world, to explore billions of ideas and papers and to research a myriad of information relating to our health and well-being from the comfort of our homes. Now *miracles* in survival are reported all around the world in minutes and, as a consequence, our expectations of what is possible are raised higher and higher by the media. Practitioners in paediatric palliative care are beginning to ask the question 'We can treat but should we?'

The Royal College of Paediatrics and Child Health (RCPCH 2004) outlines five situations where it may be ethical and/or legal to withhold treatment (see Appendix 1 and Chapter 17). The first two may have some impact in children's acute palliative care, but the last three are increasingly becoming high profile also. They are: (1) the *brain dead* child, (2) the child in permanent vegetative state, (3) the child in the no-chance situation, (4) the child in the no-purpose situation and (5) the child in the unbearable situation.

The World Health Organisation (WHO 1998) defines paediatric palliative care as 'the active total care of the child's body, mind and spirit and also involves giving support to the family. It begins when illness is diagnosed, and continues regardless of whether or not a child receives treatment directed at the disease'. They go on to say that 'health providers must evaluate and alleviate a child's physical, psychological, and social distress' and, importantly, recognise the multi-faceted lives that children have: 'Effective palliative care requires a broad multidisciplinary approach that includes the family and makes use of available community resources; it can be successfully implemented even if resources are limited. It can be provided in tertiary care facilities, in community health centres and even in children's homes' (WHO 1998).

Ethical and Philosophical Aspects of Nursing Children, First Edition. Edited by Gosia M. Brykczyńska and Joan Simons.
© 2011 Blackwell Publishing Ltd. Published 2011 by Blackwell Publishing Ltd.

This is a far-reaching statement, covering all aspects of a child and the family's health, social, spiritual and environmental needs which points us in the direction of thinking about the whole child, not just the part that is dealt with by medical practitioners. If we use the WHO definition of palliative care to examine the nature of ethical issues encountered when working with this group of children and young people, we will soon realise that palliative care is far from a straightforward area of holistic health-care provision for children.

It begins when illness is diagnosed, and continues regardless of whether or not a child receives treatment directed at the disease.

For some families, diagnosis comes quickly. This could be before birth or soon after, or following an acute life-threatening episode. For others, there is uncertainty for years, either seeing their child deteriorate or feeling that something is wrong, but no one can identify the cause. Frequently, this lack of diagnosis is problematic for parents coming to terms with their child's condition, and trying to organise care and treatment. Great uncertainty is created as doctors cannot say what the disease process or prognosis will be, inhibiting families' ability to plan and in many cases access effective financial or practical support. The children can be hospitalised frequently either due to acute episodes of illness, for investigations or for palliative surgery. Some parents cope well with not knowing, but others live in fear that their child will die and there is considerable stress as a result.

For those with a quick diagnosis, there is a steep learning curve of medication, investigations and interventions in order to care for their child. There is no preparation for this other than in the hospital, and parents are often sent home not knowing what the future holds.

Today it is expected that a child born extremely prematurely will survive. While acknowledged that this is a life-threatening situation, modern equipment, techniques and drugs have enabled us to treat these tiny babies, and, many do survive. Via the media, we hear of the *miracle babies* who survive being born at 23 weeks and less than a pound in weight. It is extremely difficult for parents catapulted into this situation, making decisions under very stressful and unknown conditions; they are led by the advice of the medical and nursing teams caring for their baby. However, we do not yet know much about long-term effects, and are parents really able to make an informed decision about the long-term well-being of their child? The EPICure Study (2009), started in 1995, is following 219 children born before 26 weeks' gestation to assess the outcomes of extreme prematurity. So far, just under half have serious disabilities that are likely to impact on their daily life. The most common serious disability was learning difficulties followed by cerebral palsy and impaired vision or hearing. To account for technological advances since 1995, a second study, EPICure 2, was started in 2006, and first results are awaited later in 2009 (Johnson *et al.* 2009).

An example from practice is of twins born at 24 weeks, both with significant difficulties in the first weeks of life, when one was resuscitated a number of times. Both babies survived, one with some visual difficulties and a degree of developmental delay, the other profoundly disabled with a vastly reduced quality of life compared to their sibling. This child died following a lifetime of hospital admissions for chest infections, surgery, investigations and treatments. Their mother once expressed a view that if she had known what the future held, she would have requested that her child was not resuscitated repeatedly as she felt there was little quality of life.

The active total care of the child's body, mind and spirit

Disabled children and those with palliative care needs have the same rights as all other children, but how do they fulfil the five outcomes of *Every Child Matters* (2004) which are: (1) to be healthy, (2) stay safe, (3) enjoy and achieve, (4) make a positive contribution and (5) achieve economic well-being.

In recent years, there has been a steady increase in the seeking of legal opinion on whether to continue the treatment of severely ill or disabled children. This marks a change in the attitude of parents towards medical professionals; they are now more willing to challenge and seek advice to support their views. The debate is always around the child's quality of life and best interests. One of the first cases was that of David Glass in 2004 brought to the courts by doctors who believed he was in pain and at the end of his life; but his parents challenged this assessment, on the basis that the doctors were seeing David at a particularly low time in his life, and did not know him as a person outside of the hospital. After considerable legal battles, the parents won their case (Glass v The United Kingdom ECHR 113, 9.3.2004). David is now in his twenties. Subsequently, Charlotte Wyatt was born at 26 weeks' gestation in 2003. Her parents fought for her to be resuscitated but initially lost their case ([2004] EWHC 2247 (fam) 1FLR 21). However, when Charlotte survived the winter and seemed to be thriving, the court reversed the earlier decision ([2005 EWHC 693 (fam) [2005] 2FLR480), and she is now treated as any other child in a life-threatening situation. However, she is a severely disabled child in foster care as her parents have since divorced. There are other cases that direct the decision-making processes, such as that of conjoined twins, Jodie and Mary, (Re: A (conjoined twins) [2000] 57 BMLR 1) as this ruling stated that parents' wishes are influential but not decisive. The most recent case is that of Baby OT whose short life was ended in March 2009 by a decision of The High Court judges despite his parents' wish that he be allowed to remain on life support (*Times Online* 2009). The parents' view was that he had some quality of life, while doctors felt that he was in intolerable pain and had no future due to a rare life-limiting metabolic condition (*BBC Online* 2009). These cases had different rulings, but all hinged on the *best interests* of the child rather than the wishes of the parents (Dyer 2004; Glover 2006).

Another area of difficulty for professionals is when a family have strong religious values, such as Jehovas' Witnesses who refuse blood transfusions even if this procedure would be life saving. When applied to a child, it is very difficult for doctors to balance best interests of the child's body with their spiritual needs as determined by the religion which their parents have chosen for them. Several cases have gone to court and judges have ruled that the children concerned were not able to understand the consequences of their decisions (Re: E (medical treatment: consent) 1993 FLR 386; Re: S (a minor) (medical treatment) 1994 FLR 1065). The RCPCH (2004) attempts to differentiate between the lives of disabled and non-disabled children with the premise that a situation seemingly unbearable to a non-disabled child and family may not be viewed in the same way by a disabled child and family.

They focus on the child's ability to interact meaningfully with those around them and their environment.

Providing support to the family

As professionals, we have a fine line to walk. Empowerment, expert patients, equity and family-centred care are the building blocks of our practice ethos, but to what extent are we actually supporting families? The reality of modern health care is that it is expensive and the needs of children and their families are increasing. There is government direction to improve joint working and shared budgets, but regulations and laws actually inhibit much of this effort. For example, the continuing health-care provision for children is currently under review. Children are assessed under the adult framework and, if judged to be eligible for fully funded health care, cannot legally access any social services' support unless there are safeguarding children's issues (see also Chapter 17).

Enabling informed consent is often difficult, as it is not possible to tell parents what the future holds; and the type and level of support required by each family varies enormously. Much of the support given to families is down to the dedication and goodwill of individual professionals working with them from all agencies. Increasingly, the Voluntary or Third Sector is also involved in advocating for services at a higher level, and is being used politically in place of statutory services. An example of this is the Association for Children's Palliative Care (ACT 2008) whose aims are to campaign, develop and disseminate best practice, and empower and support families (ACT web site 2009).

Understanding needs is also a problematic area because children with palliative care need to have a range of diagnoses and disease trajectories; there is no standard treatment or care pathway. Parents approach their child's condition and daily life in different ways dependent on a whole range of factors: their mental and physical health, relationships, family support, employment, finances, housing, etc. Supporting a family requires an open, trusting relationship; a clear understanding that their needs are recognised; honesty; and action. Frequently, families feel let down by professionals who say they will help, but either do not follow through or do not communicate often due to a feeling of help-lessness. Sometimes, the pendulum swings too far the other way, for example, the view that parents want home-based respite, so there is now a lack of short break respite in many areas (see Chapter 17). The reality is that families want a combination of care that is flexible enough to meet the needs of the whole family. Edwards (2008) debating the moral aspects of the Ashley Treatment (2009), where a severely disabled child received surgery and medication to prevent her growing and develop-ing adult physical characteristics, argues that if the family could 'rely on adequate support from sup-port agencies such as Social Services ... they would not need even to contemplate the interventions they opted for'. Although this is an American case, the situation in England is not dissimilar as shown by Charlotte Wyatt's case. Her father would like to care for her at home, but there was inadequate support for him as a single parent to enable this to happen (Brazier 2005). Edwards (2008) concludes that sup-port of disabled people in their own homes requires an adjustment of the social context.

At a more fundamental level, prenatal screening is another area where parents make choices. Those who choose not to have screening because they would not terminate a pregnancy have discussed what they would do in the event of their child being born with disabilities and have decided what course they want to take. Sometimes this is difficult for medical practitioners to manage, particularly if the family want to take the baby home to die rather than try any form of treatment. The parents of Faith and Hope Williams, born in November 2008, were advised to terminate the pregnancy but decided to give the babies a chance of life, partly on religious grounds. Sadly, both babies died, but having been supported in their decision may help the parent's grief process (Lewis 2008).

Health providers must evaluate and allevi-ate a child's physical, psychological and social distress.

Many children who receive palliative care are disabled, but not all, and illness is a personal thing. Not everyone will have the same response to the same disease or symptoms. So how does one judge the level of distress in all these areas, especially in an acute setting where staff only see a snapshot of the child compared to the family who live with them?

When a child is unable to communicate their wishes, either due to age, disability or perceived understanding, it is incumbent upon those around them to try and determine what they would wish. This is where the *best interests* test is employed, but we also have a responsibility to try and find out what the child might want by employing various communication strategies and advocating to assist them with communication. The person who knows them best and can understand their communica-tion may not be the best person, however, to inter-pret their views (Rowse 2007). How many young people actually tell their parents what they want or think if they know that it will upset them?

There are huge difficulties in communicating with children who have palliative care needs. It is known that sick children protect their parents with a form of collusion when they know that a decision might upset them, and it takes a very confident young person and open family to discuss diffi-cult treatment decisions. The case of a 13-year-old Hannah Jones (*Guardian* 2008) illustrates how diffi-cult it is for professionals to understand and accede to children's wishes. Hannah had leukaemia from the age of 5 and her treatment had caused cardiac complications to the extent that a heart transplant was the only option for continuing her life. Hannah chose not to have the transplant as she felt the risks of dying during or soon after were high and there was a possibility that her cancer would return with the immune suppression required to prevent organ rejection. She chose to take her chance, but almost ended up in court as professionals in the hospital and social services initially felt that her parents were preventing her from having treatment. She employed a great deal of courage in convincing the child protection team that she knew exactly what she was doing, and that she knew what was best for her. Hannah's mother's echoed views of many par-ents of severely ill or disabled children, that until you have been in the situation you cannot under-stand what it is like, only surmise. Subsequently, Hannah underwent a successful heart transplant.

But who can make that judgement when the child itself cannot let us know, and when is it a controversial move? How do parents live with the criticism? The Ashley Treatment has provoked considerable debate, both for and against, but the key considerations are as follows: (1) Is the quality of life not worse than before? (2) Is the treatment being undertaken for the right reasons? (3) At what point is it a step too far (Edwards 2008)? Ashley's parents have been very open about their decision, using a weblog to publicly answer their critics, and they were clearly supported by the Medical Ethics Committee in making their decision – all factors that help the parents manage the mental and emotional aspects of such a decision.

Treatment decisions that are easier to make are such as the use of BIPAP ventilation, a treatment that enables a young person to receive overnight non-invasive ventilation. This improves quality of life and is increasingly used by young men with Duchenne muscular dystrophy. However, it also extends their life and leads to new complications which may or may not be resolvable, and may or may not impact on the quality of their daily life. Similar issues arise for individuals with cystic fibrosis, where advances in care and treatment have extended their expected lifespan from less than 10 years to 37 years today (Contact-a-family 2008); but this has also given rise to a new set of problems and challenges for those affected with the disease and for their physicians, such as progressive liver disease, osteoporosis and fertility and pregnancy issues (Littlewood 2004).

A broad multidisciplinary approach that includes the family

Again this is an admirable objective, but in practice it appears that a *palliative* diagnosis also gives rise to the view that any related issues are likewise health issues, with social services' practitioners being very clear that the health service should fund respite or home-based care, as it is required due to the child's health needs. Meanwhile, National Health Service (NHS) practitioners are unable to provide support during social or family crisis, such as when there are difficulties with finances, travel, housing or relationships. The dichotomy is that on the one hand children are seen as integral to their family with significant interdependencies, but on the other hand as individuals when an assessment of care needs is being processed, which often does not fully include the whole family. To deliver effective palliative care in practice, it should be *impossible* to separate a child's health, education and social needs.

An increasing problem for young people with anticipated shortened lives is the transition to adult care. Survival to adulthood was rare in the past, and as a result adult services had very little expertise or experience of the issues faced by these young people. In addition, they are relatively few in number so a model similar to Community Children's Nursing (CCN) is required to support them, but it is not available in adult care, which is either locality- or disease-focused. Many young people remain, therefore, under the care of paediatricians and children's wards, which inhibits their ability to function as young adults, particularly if they have communication difficulties. Allied to this is the inherent difficulty in making decisions for themselves and raising the profile of their needs so that services are developed to support them. This can result in the young person not being *allowed* to grow up by the facilities and the situation they find themselves in, and perhaps not having the chance or courage to discuss difficult issues with their parents due to dependency on them.

The question of how we can support parents and young people who are not ready to hear bad news, or deny that there is a problem, is a big one, and there are no easy answers. The children's hospice movement is going some way to addressing the issues with the development of facilities specifically for those aged 14–40 (the age range varies), where the young people can visit alone and have freedom to discuss issues pertinent to all youngsters such as alcohol, relationships, sex and drugs. If the young person is totally dependent on others for their care, this may be the only chance they get to say what they really think. The young person with disabilities relies so much on their parent or carer to organise everything for them, that they may have a very small social network, with very little privacy in their lives. Their activities may be entirely led by and within the family environment – so there is little experience of adolescent freedom for the youngster or young adult.

It can be provided in tertiary care facilities, in community health centres and even in children's homes.

This seems an odd statement given that children are now at home more than anywhere else. But it is rare to ask the parent of a disabled child if they can actually cope with them. Modern society expects individuals to cope and is not terribly sympathetic when they do not. Trends affect what is available, and there is often a complete swing from one perspective to another. For example, in the nineteenth century, children with disabilities who managed to survive were an accepted part of the community. But by the early twentieth century, many disabled children were institutionalised in residential homes or schools. Since the Children Act of 1989 promoted the family environment as being the best place for children, the availability of residential care has been vastly reduced, and it is now expected that the parent of a disabled baby or child will take them home and care for them or give them up for fostering and adoption, which is a meagre choice. There is little discussion as to whether they will be able to manage what is required of them, and certainly in the early stages there is little social or financial support. Children under 5 do not get respite care very easily, and social services are so pressured by work that the thresholds are very high for referrals of children with disabilities; moreover, the referral criteria themselves are unclear even to the social workers. The Children Act of 1989 says that all disabled children are children in need, but not all children are accepted by social services onto their casebooks.

Children with unstable health are often excluded from school because they are unwell or unstable so that they are frequently sent home or to hospital. Housing is frequently inadequate for their needs and equipment unavailable in more than one place, limiting the children's social activities. Family Link schemes are promoted as being the best respite option for younger children, but carers are few and far between and are often poorly equipped and poorly paid for the role they undertake (Family Link Program). In short, the rhetoric of integrating children to the community is only partially addressed, with parents potentially carrying a heavy burden of care, with an uncertain future.

End-of-life care: an introduction

It is a well-known fact that the number of children and young people dying compared to adults is relatively small, but what may not be so widely known is that these numbers are also in decline. Statistics from the Department of Health

highlight that 3,568 0–19-year-olds died in 2004 compared to 3,914 in 2001. This death rate in the 20–30 age range is higher with 4,500 deaths in 2001, but is also now on the decrease with 4,166 deaths occurring in 2004 (DoH 2006). The reasons behind this decline could be multiple, but improvement in medical support and ongoing research into drug therapy and treatment must be contributory factors. However pleasing this numerical decrease may be, it is of scant benefit to families and professionals when faced with providing end-of-life care for an individual child or young person, and the diverse challenges that are raised. In fact, the very ability to prolong life can in reality make an already difficult situation and decision far harder, and these issues more profound.

Kurz (2001) asserts that every person, regardless of age, has the right to die with dignity. However, Jacobs (2005) found that ethical issues surrounding the terminal phase of a child's life can emerge with a great intensity and be a difficult path to traverse. This could be due to the small numbers of children dying compared to adults, but is more likely to be due to western cultural beliefs and anticipation of life expectancy, and the emotions that a child's death and dying bring. In addition to these ethical difficulties, it must be remembered that the actual point that a child or young person moves from a palliative care phase to an end-of-life phase can often be difficult for the professional and family to identify and acknowledge. However, this transition is an important component of palliative care as Liben et al. (2008) identify, and is where the focus of care moves from an active approach to a comfort-based one. But at what stage do we as clinicians withdraw active treatment?

The tightrope of choice

RCPCH (2004; see Appendix 1) details five situations where it may be considered both ethical and legal to withdraw or withhold life-sustaining medical treatment. Although it is useful and necessary to have these situations identified in writing, it is extremely difficult in practice when we are confronted with these circumstances. It must be remembered, however, that the decision to withhold life-sustaining treatment does not mean that all care is ending, but that a different form of treatment is to be provided, namely, support treatment at the end of life (see also Chapter 15).

As professionals, we are aware that working with people in such a highly emotive situation is incredibly challenging and demanding. Nevertheless, despite an array of pitfalls including the ethical issues that will be discussed, we must not only be empathetic, but must also maintain our professionalism. One way in which potential issues or conflicts can be reduced in children or young people with a chronic palliative care need is by utilising an *end-of-life care* plan. These are especially useful as they ensure that the child/young person and families' needs are recognised, acted upon and disseminated to the professionals involved. End-of-life care plans are fairly recent concepts as indicated by ACT (2004) and although useful, it must be remembered that they are neither set in stone nor infallible. We must not forget that parents, care givers and the child/young person themselves may change their mind at short notice about where and how their child or they themselves wish to be cared for and what treatment they want provided, as was the case with young Hannah Jones (De Bruxelles 2008).

Acute decisions

Unfortunately, one area in which the end-of-life care plan's shortcomings are highlighted is in acute situations such as emergency departments and paediatric intensive care units (PICUs) (see Chapter 15). Unforeseen events to a well, healthy child, such as severe trauma, can demand that end-of-life and treatment decisions be made quickly and under pressure with all the associated ethical dilemmas and challenges that arise in these situations. Lack of awareness by acute staff of community services can impact negatively on the available options for children and families. However, is it that simple? Is it just a question of raising the awareness of professionals, children and their families about the choices and options and then the individual needs that are met? Children sometimes die as the result of an acute episode, perhaps in PICU or NNU. It is now recognised in adult terminal care that many would like to be at home but do not know how to ask, and it could be questioned how often do parents and/or children say they want to be at home,

or are given the chance to explore this option. Reverse retrieval from intensive care units can and does happen, but is far from straightforward to organise; it requires commitment and dedication from professionals involved, and courage and trust on the part of parents. Difficulties with end-of-life care plans can also arise when a child's family are clear of what they want for their child should a life-threatening episode occur, but others involved such as school staff and respite carers do not feel comfortable with *doing nothing* or are scared of the prospect of the child dying on them. These care plans require support for everyone whom the decision impacts upon, not just those involved in its formulation.

An area in which it would seem there are less ethical challenges for health professionals is that of the environment in which the end-of-life care is provided. After all, as professionals, should we not just allow the parents to choose where they want to be with their child for the final days and then facilitate this without regard? An initial professional response could be that the family want their child to have their final care at home/hospital/hospice and we will enable this to happen, regardless. But is this meeting the best needs of the child/young person and their family? Providing care in any of the aforementioned environments has both positive and negative implications and challenges for all involved. It must be remembered that the family are going through one of, if not the, most important and traumatic periods of their lives and to allow them to do so without professional support and advice is both unethical and, potentially, negligent. Case study 16.1 is an example of how professionals who know the family and have a good relationship with them can explore and discuss options for providing end-of-life care. In this scenario, inclusion of the child in the discussions had been considered with the family but parental wishes were that he was not told as they deemed him to be too young.

Case study 16.1

A meeting has been arranged with the family of a 6-year-old boy who is moving from active treatment to end-of-life care. The parents are fully aware of the aim of the meeting and are given a choice of where it is to be held, which they chose to be in the hospital. Attending this meeting were the boy's parents along with their paediatric consultant and their community oncology nurse specialist who have both worked with them since diagnosis and have a good working, professional relationship with them. The aim of this discussion is to give the parents the information to make an informed choice about where they want the future care for their child to be provided. All options are explored prior to the decision being made for the child to have their care at home provided by the children's community nurses' team with both the local hospital and children's hospice aware and able to offer support if required.

Children's involvement

The issue of whether or not to inform the child or young person of their impending death, regardless of where the situation arises, is the one area that seems to be a common problem when providing terminal care and is particularly challenging as highlighted by Vince & Petros (2006) and Liben *et al.* (2008). It appears to be a common wish of the parents of the child/young person that they do not want them to be told of their imminent death. The reason behind this seems to be that of the family wanting to *protect* and *shelter* the child/young person. Vince & Petros (2006), however, argue that if a child is capable of understanding their situation, then medical teams have an ethical duty to inform them and involve them in the process of their own death. This argument is supported by Kurz (2001), who acknowledges that the child should be kept fully informed whenever possible and involved in the decision-making process as much as possible. However, there are a multitude of factors that have an impact on the decision-making process in this huge ethical minefield. These conversations require knowledge of what is appropriate to say, based on the cognitive ability of children at different ages, and confidence on the part of the professional and parent that they have the tools to manage such a conversation (Slaughter 2005). Many parents will feel ill equipped to deal with questions from

the child, which usually occur at unexpected times, often once the professionals have left, and the child has had time to think (Slaughter 2005). Unfortunately, across the country, there is patchy psychological support for children and families at end of life, being a relatively new and under-resourced area of children's care.

The UN Convention on the Rights of the Child (UNCRC 1989) stipulates that 'Parties shall assure to the child who is capable of forming his or her own views the right to express those views freely in all matters affecting the child, the views of the child being given due weight in accordance with the age and maturity of the child'. Surely, therefore, it is a simple process of informing the child or young person of their impending death and awaiting their views on this subject.

In spite of this, it is the term 'capable of forming their views' that can cause further confusion and conflict at an already difficult period. What is the identifiable age at which a child becomes cognitively able to express their views and opinions on their care during the terminal phase of their life? Unfortunately, it is a recognised fact that some children and young people with a life-limiting illness may not live long enough to develop autonomy, or may have a disability which affects this process. The most common way of assessing the ability of a child or young person is by using the Fraser Guidelines, (Gillick v West Norfolk and Wisbeach AHA (1984:1 ER 373), (1985:3 All ER 423) (1986 AC 112)). These rulings stated that a child deemed competent could consent to treatment, but Lord Donaldson in 1991 (RE: R (A Minor) (Wardship: consent to treatment) 3 WLR 592) stated that a Gillick competent child meant one who was intelligent and should be listened to, but who could be overruled by parents or doctors.

Although the Fraser guidelines were not specifically developed with paediatric palliative care/terminal care in mind, further difficulties and ethical challenges have not surprisingly arisen since that ruling and have (sadly) led to legal proceedings and much publicised media attention. These ethical minefields have included situations such as that described earlier of Hannah Jones. It is likely that such cases will continue to increase as the boundaries of medical technology seem, at present, to be limitless, therefore ensuring that the ethical debate and issues will continue. Indeed, it could be argued, as Crawford & Way (2009) highlight, that medical technology has evolved faster than medical ethics and legislation.

In our case study, it was agreed that the professionals involved would not tell the child of their impending death unless they asked outright, or a conversation was had with them in which they raised the subject, which satisfied all parties' feelings and viewpoints. However, it was not just the ethical dilemma of whether or not to tell them about their impending death that came out of the meeting with their family. Care dilemmas were also raised as they decided that they wanted all care, whenever possible, to be provided at home, medication to be oral and that specific professionals were to be involved in their care.

Community-based care

Providing end-of-life care in the community can be very difficult with multiple challenges, and a number of conditions need to be in place for it to work, as highlighted by Stajduhar & Cohen (2009), cited by Hudson & Payne (2009), to ensure that effective support is provided for those dying at home. These include the desire of both the family and the child to be at home, adequate support from health-care professionals, the financial means for a carer (preferably two carers) to be at home to deliver care and the ability to provide symptom management. In addition, it should be acknowledged that other requirements might include balancing the needs of the individual child and family with the needs of the greater community nursing caseload. A further factor is that the staff involved need to be adequately trained, skilled and supported, as well as provided with the required resources to fulfil their role, and this is not always that straightforward to arrange.

While the family may wish to have the support of one to two professionals who know them well, it is not always sustainable in the community setting for several reasons. For example, a CCN service that is normally delivered from Monday to Friday between 9 a.m. and 5 p.m. will increase provision to 24/7 when a family chooses to have their child at home to die. This means the staff work an overnight on call system and visit at weekends,

immediately adding the stress of overtime to the heightened emotions of caring for a dying child and their family. If, as in several local examples, end-of-life care unexpectedly continues for several months, one or two members of staff would burn out in a relatively short time. So there is an equilibrium to be maintained in balancing the wishes of the family and the needs of the staff so that effective care can be maintained for all children under the care of the staff.

Other difficulties that arise, regardless of the environment, are based upon questions which may or may not be answerable. For example, how long will the child live, what symptoms/other symptoms will appear and what will happen next and when? How can we, as professionals negotiate care and support with the family if we are unsure of what will happen ourselves? There have been situations when professionals being open with families go through with them the symptoms and effects of drugs, the likely end-of-life sequence of events and probable effects on the child; but when these have not happened as outlined, families have been thrown into emotional confusion, and their coping mechanisms have been eroded, along with their trust in the professional caring for their child (Davis & De Valming 2006:497–509).

Bereavement care

Ethical issues do not just end when the child has died and require further exploration and consideration. Parents, siblings, the wider family and, in some cases, other parties such as education/respite workers and social workers will also need bereavement support. Questions such as who is best able to provide that support frequently arise. Should it be the nurse or medical professional who may have a long-term relationship with the family and other agencies but with minimal or no-trained counselling skills? Alternatively, should a referral be made to a service that does have the training, skills and resources but does not know the family? If indeed such a local service were available, who would they be able to support? Where would this support be provided and would it be for a defined length of time? Practitioners should advocate that this process of bereavement support needs to be not only led by the family, but also aided by professionals who know their own limits, can recognise the abnormal and direct them appropriately. However, this can also raise difficulties as the family, and immediate professionals, may well have strong emotional bonds with each other which could make it harder to make an informed, impartial and rational choice. If it is the nurse or medical professional that provides bereavement support, boundaries and support mechanisms must be put in place for that individual. After all, are we less ethically and morally responsible for our colleagues' well-being than that of our clients?

Burnout is a real issue for staff providing support for children with palliative/end-of-life care, and we are all vulnerable to the effects of this. Features highlighted by Hynson (2006:14–27) include fatigue, depression, anxiety, irritability and insomnia. Within the author's CCN practice environment, the necessity of support for professionals during and after caring for a child with palliative or end-of-life care needs is well recognised and actively provided for, both formally and informally, to help reduce the risk of burnout amongst staff. This takes place in the forms highlighted by Price *et al.* (2005) such as formal and informal clinical supervision, peer support and effective team working, as well as good managerial back up and understanding of the challenges for the individual staff member. Hospice staff are potentially more vulnerable to burn out due to the essence of their work being about supporting families through short lives and a continual exposure to sad events as highlighted by Hynson (2006:14–27) and Papadatou (2006:521–532).

Conclusion: getting it right?

So how do we find out what we should do? Parental feedback on the service experience which they have received is an exceptionally valuable tool in all areas of health care. So why should end-of-life care be any different? According to Burnell & O'Keefe (2004), concerns raised surrounding this issue include the lack of ability to gain informed consent prior to participation. This is due to the fact that during the consent phase, there is no way to predict how difficult the parents and family will find it to answer the research or audit questions. The common theme of health-care professionals wanting to *shelter* the family from as much pain as possible also plays a role in this respect (Brykczynska 1998) (see also Chapter 19).

The problem with ethical issues are that although some aspects are apparent to all, there are some *grey* areas in which one individual may see issues as clear cut with obvious answers and another person may view them as complex and contentious. The purpose of this chapter was not to give the reader all the answers but to give examples from practice and allow for further exploration and discussion. However, one current theme throughout all aspects of palliative care for children, young people, their families and the professionals involved are that difficult challenges and decisions have to be faced. Only through good, effective, honest communication, support and working together can these challenges be faced and managed in the best interests of the children, who are at the centre of everything we do.

Reflective scenario

Imagine you are a community children's nurse caring for 7-year-old James and his family; you have known them since James' diagnosis 5 years ago, with a degenerative metabolic condition. James has an expected life span of 10 years or so, he is now wheelchair dependent, gastrostomy fed and has difficulties communicating with those who do not know him well. He lives at home with his Mum and Dad, Sheila and Mark, and two siblings, Oliver who is 10 and Molly who is 5. He has a supportive network of family and carers, including his learning support assistant Mandy and respite carer Pauline who have known James for 2 years. Shelia and Mark are very clear that, when the time comes, they want James to die at home, but they also want him to enjoy life to the full and have all treatment possible until he gives up.

James has developed a severe and life-threatening chest infection for the second time in 6 months. The doctors caring for him feel it may be time to let him die, but his parents want full treatment including ventilation as he survived the last chest infection and they feel that he will cope with this one too.

Think about your role in supporting the family through this difficult time.

What needs to be discussed?
Who should be involved in the discussions?
What needs to be put in place?
What information do the family need?
What will be needed if he recovers?
What will be needed if he is not going to recover?
What is required for the wider group of people involved? Consider LSA, respite carers, siblings, doctors, ward staff and yourself.
Who should/could be involved at each stage?

References

ACT (2004) *A Framework for the Development of Integrated Multi-agency Care Pathways for Children with Life Threatening and Life-limiting Conditions.* The Association for Children's Palliative Care, Bristol. http://www.act.org.uk/ (accessed 28 March 2009).

ACT (2008) The Association for Children's Palliative Care Website, Bristol. http://www.act.org.uk/ (accessed 9 September 2008).

BBC Online (2009) Baby in right-to-life battle dies, 21 March 2009. http://news.bbc.co.uk/1/hi/uk/7956845.stm (accessed 9 November 2009).

Brazier, M. (2005) An intractable dispute: When parents and professionals disagree. *Medical Law Review,* **13** (3), 412–418.

Brykczynska, G. (1998) Can nursing research be a caring process? In: *Nursing Research – Setting New Agendas* (ed. P. Smith), pp. 108–138. Edward Arnold, London.

Burnell, R.H. & O'Keefe, M. (2004) Asking parents unaskable questions. *The Lancet,* **364** (9436), 737–738.

Contact a family website (2008) *Cystic Fibrosis Background.* Contact a family, New York. http://www.cafamily.org.uk/Direct/c93.html (accessed 9 September 2008).

Crawford, D. & Way, C. (2009) Just because we can, should we? A discussion of treatment withdrawal. *Paediatric Nursing,* **21** (1), 22–25.

Davies, D. & De Valming, D. (2006) Symptom control at the end-of-life. In: *Oxford Textbook of Palliative Care for Children* (eds A. Goldman, R. Hain & S. Liben). Oxford University Press, Oxford.

De Bruxelles, S. (2008) Dying girl Hannah Jones wins fight to turn down transplant. *The Times,* 11 November 2008.

DoH (2006) *Palliative Care Statistics for Children and Young Adults.* The Stationery Office, London.

Dyer, C. (2004) Baby should be allowed to die, UK court rules. *BMJ,* **329**, 875.

Edwards, S.D. (2008) The Ashley treatment: A step too far, or not far enough? *Journal of Medical Ethics,* **34**, 341–343, doi:10.1136/jme.2007.020243

EPIcure Study (12 March 2009). http://www.epicure.ac.uk/about-us/news/first-report-published-from-the-11-year-assessments (accessed 27 March 2009).

Glover, J. (2006) Should the child live? Doctors, families and conflict. *Clinical Ethics,* **1**, 52–59.

Hudson, P. & Payne, S. (eds) (2009) *Family Carers in Palliative Care.* Oxford University Press, Oxford.

Hynson, J.L. (2006) The child's journey: Transition from health to ill-health. In: *Oxford Textbook of Palliative Care for Children* (eds A. Goldman, R. Hain & S. Liben). Oxford University Press, Oxford.

Jacobs, H.H. (2005) Ethics in pediatric end-of-life care: A nursing perspective. *Journal of Pediatric Nursing,* **20** (5), 360–368.

Johnson, S., Fawke, J., Hennessy, E., *et al.* (2009) Neurodevelopmental disability through 11 years of age in children born before 26 weeks gestation. *Pediatrics,* **124** (2), 249–257.

Kurz, R. (2001) Decision making in extreme situations involving children: Withholding or withdrawal of life supporting treatment in paediatric care. Statement of the ethics working group of the Confederation of the European Specialists of Paediatrics (CESP). *European Journal of Paediatrics,* **160**, 214–216.

Lewis, P. (2008) Conjoined twin Faith dies on Christmas Day. *The Guardian,* Saturday 27 December 2008.

Liben, S., Papadatou, D. & Wolfe, J. (2008) Paediatric palliative care: Challenges and emerging ideas. *The Lancet,* **371** (9615), 852–865.

Littlewood, J. (2004) Looking back over 40 years and what the future holds. *27th European Cystic Fibrosis Conference,* Birmingham. http://www.cftrust.org.uk/aboutcf/whatiscf/cfhistory/Levy_Lecture_04_-_JL.pdf (accessed 9 September 2008).

Papadatou, D. (2006) Healthcare provider's responses to the death of a child. In: *Oxford Textbook of Palliative Care for Children* (eds A. Goldman, R. Hain & S. Liben). Oxford University Press, Oxford.

Percival, J. & Lewis, P. (2008) Teenager who won right to die: 'I have had too much trauma.' *The Guardian,* www.guardian.co.uk/2008/nov/11/child-protection-health-hannah-jones, 11 November 2008.

Price, J., McNeilly, P. & McFarlane, M. (2005) Paediatric palliative care in the UK: Past, present and future. *International Journal of Palliative Nursing*, **11** (3), 124–126.

Rowse, V. (2007) Consent in severely disabled children: Informed or an infringement of their human rights? *Journal of Child Health Care*, **11** (1), 70–78.

RCPCH (2004) *Withholding or Withdrawing Life Sustaining Treatment in Children: A Framework for Practice*, 2nd edn. Royal College of Paediatrics and Child Health, London.

Slaughter, V. (2005) Young children's understanding of death. *Australian Psychologist*, **40** (3), 179–186.

Stajduhar, K. & Cohen, C. (2009) Family caregiving in the home. In: *Family Carers in Palliative Care* (eds P. Hudson & S. Payne), pp. 149–168. Oxford University Press, Oxford.

The Ashley Treatment (2009). http://ashleytreatment.spaces.live.com/ (accessed 28 March 2009).

Times Online (2009) Parents given hours to appeal for Baby OT's right to life. http://business.timesonline.co.uk/tol/business/law/article5944097.ece.

UNCRC (1989) *General Assembly of the United Nations Convention on the Rights of the Child*. United Nations Convention on the Rights of the Child, The Stationery Office, London.

Vince, T. & Petros, A. (2006) Should children's autonomy be respected by telling them of their imminent death? *Journal of Medical Ethics*, **32**, 21–23.

WHO (1998) *WHO definition of Palliative Care*. World Health Organisation, Geneva. http://www.who.int/cancer/palliative/definition/en/ (accessed February 2009).

Suggested further readings

Ewing, B. (2008) Children's Wishes: Holistic revelations in Art. *Journal of Holistic Nursing* **26** (2), 147–154.

Goldman, A., Hain, R. & Liben, S. (eds) (2006) *Oxford Textbook of Palliative Care for Children*. Oxford University Press, Oxford.

Stuber, M. (2004) Spirituality in children confronting death. *Child and Adolescent Psychiatric Clinics of North America* **13** (1), 127–136.

Part IV

Philosophical Considerations in Professional Practice

If you have ever been to hospital what did the nurses do to help you?

Came in and spoke to me often which made me not so worried.   (Girl 10yrs)

I have never been to hospital, but I suspect they would soothe you if bad news occurred. (Boy 8yrs)

The nurse brought me ice cream, she talked to me to keep me calm and she gave me medicine.

She talked to me and not Mum and told me what had happened.   (Girl 11yrs)

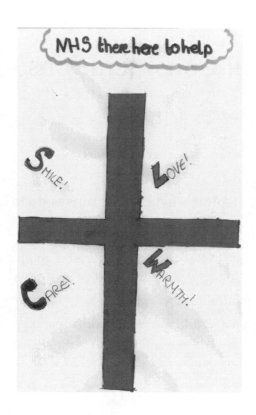

17 Researching Children and Young People: Exploring the Ethical Territory

Bernie Carter

'I believe that clinical research is now far safer than routine clinical care in today's children's hospitals'.

(Lantos 2004:147)

Introduction

This chapter nestles fairly innocuously in the middle of this textbook, its presence seemingly not an exception, nothing obviously strange about its inclusion. However, the fact that it is here at all reflects a fairly fundamental shift in the past 10–20 years within two arenas: research and ethics. Previously, many of the seminal research textbooks failed to address children, and many ethics texts which addressed children failed to consider research. The fact that children were largely invisible within seminal generic research textbooks reflected their social invisibility; even today, children are often just addressed in generic research textbooks in terms of their being members of a *vulnerable group*.

Arguments for and against children's involvement in research

Whilst many, myself included, would argue that framing children simply in terms of their vulnera-

bility oversimplifies their capacities, competence and agency (Carter 2009), there is historical context that explains why the protection offered to children within the regulations has value. Prior to the regulation of medical research, there was little to prevent medical experimentation. The Lübeck vaccine disaster in which 77 infants died and 208 infants became ill with tuberculosis (Bonah 2002) was a turning point in medical research leading to the 'first published discussion on medical research using human subjects, approximately two decades before the Nuremberg Trial and the Code of Nuremberg' (Jacobson *et al.* 2009:3291). Disasters like Lübeck or the potential for such catastrophes remain at the heart of protectionist attitudes to human subjects', and particularly children's, involvement in experimental research. Indeed, these fears have reignited recently in the USA as a result of the *Kennedy Krieger lead paint study* which resulted in a landmark case held in a US Court of Appeals. The court records state that:

> Apparently, it was anticipated that the children, who were the human subjects in the program, would, or at least might, accumulate lead in their blood from the dust, thus helping the researchers to determine the extent to which the various partial abatement methods worked.

Ethical and Philosophical Aspects of Nursing Children, First Edition. Edited by Gosia M. Brykczyńska and Joan Simons.
© 2011 Blackwell Publishing Ltd. Published 2011 by Blackwell Publishing Ltd.

There was no complete and clear explanation in the consent agreements signed by the parents of the children that the research to be conducted was designed, at least in significant part, to measure the success of the abatement procedures by measuring the extent to which the children's blood was being contaminated. *It can be argued that the researchers intended that the children be the canaries in the mines but never clearly told the parents* (emphasis added). (*Ericka Grimes v Kennedy Krieger Institute Inc. No 128; 24-C-99-000925 and 24-C-95066067/CL 193461*

(Circuit Court for Baltimore City 2000:2–3))

Spriggs (2004:177) notes that the ruling from this study was that children should not be 'included in trials that do not have a therapeutic benefit and which include risk' and that this had caused alarm amongst some researchers and bioethicists who expressed deep concerns about the imposed blanket ban. Major problems can arise from an over-protectionist approach to researching children. Clinical practice was and is to a large degree guided by knowledge extrapolated from studies on adult patients (children being framed simply as mini-adults) (Punch 2002) or from proxy information about children derived from asking their parents. The ethical protection of children in terms of research has meant that they became concomitantly more vulnerable as recipients of care and interventions within practice. Notwithstanding the Kennedy Krieger lead paint study, there are many researchers and practitioners who would agree with Halila & Lötjönen (2003:36) who note that:

Children are well protected by international guidelines, sometimes even too well. This is one reason why treatments for children's diseases are too seldom based on evidence.

This in itself is an ethical issue.

Linked to the notion of protection was an underlying assumption that children were not capable of being included. Research was generally done *on* or *to* children without any real consideration of their wishes. When the perspective of the child was sought, parents acted as proxies for their children's experiences. Children's lack of capacity and capability in relation to consent meant that there was a risk that children would merely be used as 'a means to an end' (Lantos 2004:148). Children's presumed lack of capability as potential research subjects meant that they were categorised as being homogenously vulnerable. Yet, the notion of vulnerability is contested (Carter 2009). Coleman (2009:14) argues against a homogenous view of vulnerability and reasons the need for more nuanced categories of vulnerability, questioning 'what are vulnerable human subjects actually vulnerable *to*?' (emphasis in original). Coleman (2009) proposes considering vulnerability as phenomena which are consent-based, risk-based and justice-based. This challenge to the loose use of the concept of vulnerability, particularly in relation to children, means it is likely that researchers, reviewers, children and their parents will be in a position to make more informed decisions about risks, benefits and their involvement.

A move from *research on* to *research with* children

Researching about children's health and health care was, and still remains to a degree, perceived as being risky, difficult and challenging. Many of these challenges have been refuted as well as the claims that children lack adult maturity, that they are unreliable, predisposed to lying or making things up because they 'cannot distinguish between reality and fantasy' ` (see, e.g., Punch 2002; Kirk 2007). The dismissal of such a large constituent part of the population from research reflects the way in which society has *othered* and still does *other* children's perspectives, potential contributions, agency and contributions to research (Lahman 2008; Carter 2009).

However, in the past 20 or so years, there have been significant shifts in the discourse that surrounds children and young people within society, for example, in the UK, The Children Act (1989, 2004), The National Service Framework for Children, Young People and Maternity Services (DoH 2004) and Every Child Matters (HM Government 2004) which emphasise the need to improve the levels of children's participation. This has resulted in some shifts towards a more inclusive, child-centred set of policies which position children as active agents, able to report on their experiences, insightful into the practices of children and childhood. Whilst some of this discourse is undoubtedly rhetorical, it has opened up opportunities for children's nurses and other professionals and researchers to engage in research *with* rather than *on* children. Adopting this sort of stance has the potential to be more ethically sound as it means children may be less 'vulnerable to representations that others impose on them' (Barron 2000:33).

More recently again, the move has transferred attention from research that simply acknowledges children and recruits them as participants to a research agenda which is engaging – to a greater or lesser degree – with children as co-researchers. The move has been towards research *by* children about issues of importance to children. What is perhaps of ethical interest is that in our collective rush towards working alongside children as co-researchers we have not perhaps sufficiently considered the risks and benefits of children researching other children or of children being researched by children.

All of these moves have changed the map of research (regardless of whether the research being undertaken is on-with-by children) and there has had to be a concomitant response in terms of the ethical issues associated with undertaking research on-with-by children. What seems to have happened is that the arena of children's research ethics is seen as being particularly difficult, complex and unusual. This is perhaps surprising since many of the generic ethical issues that children's nurses are familiar with and have to consider, negotiate and resolve on a daily basis in practice are similar to those faced by researchers, albeit in a different context. However, researchers face particular challenges posed by a particular set of concerns and discourses related to the whole notion of children and research. These discourses create competing demands and tensions for researchers adding a degree of complexity that can sometimes feel overwhelming, crushing the would-be-researcher's quest, spirit and enthusiasm for *doing research*. Clearly, research does bring additional considerations, requiring children's nurses and researchers from other disciplines to navigate these challenges using a map that they may not be familiar with, using language different to that of everyday practice and placing constraints that can be both frustrating as well as bemusing. However, the map that guides research practice is not actually so very different to the more familiar maps that guide ethical clinical practice.

The difference between the ethics of practice and research

The thing that most clearly distinguishes research from clinical practice is that they have inherently different purposes, aims, methods and interventions. Figure 17.1 provides an overview of the differences. However, these boundaries can sometimes seem blurred as, for example, some clinical practice may be experimental or cutting edge but may not need to be categorised as research. In brief then, clinical practice can be said to refer to:

> ... interventions that are designed solely to enhance the well-being of an individual patient or client and that have a reasonable expectation of success.
>
> (NCPHS 1979)

Whereas a definition of research (regardless of whether the aim is to generate or test hypotheses) is defined in the Research Governance Framework as:

> ... the attempt to derive generalisable new knowledge by addressing clearly defined questions with systematic and rigorous methods.
>
> (DoH 2005:3)

Even though the aim of clinical practice is to engender benefit for the child and their family, it is clearly neither a risk-free nor ethically neutral endeavour. Previously, a distinction was drawn between so-called therapeutic and non-therapeutic research (and indeed, this remains a frequently used categorisation in the literature). However, this distinction is now seen as unhelpful, misleading and confusing, as a single research study may include elements that are potentially therapeutic (such as a medicine) as well as others which are non-therapeutic (such as an X-ray). Equally, so-called therapeutic research may carry more risks than non-therapeutic research. The Royal College of Paediatrics and Child Health (RCPCH), following on from the Declaration of Helsinki (WMA 2000, 2008) avoids the semantic tangles associated with the

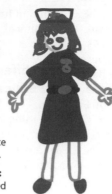

Clinical practice/treatment

Purpose:
intervention to diagnose, prevent, cure or palliate.

Aim:
to improve the individual's health status.

Methods:
practice-based use of tests which lead to clinically based advice, choice and intervention for an individual.

Rationale for treatment decision:
patient offered the best option based on pragmatic discovery.

Health-care research

Purpose:
a systematic investigation.

Aim:
to generate knowledge that could be of future benefit to other patients/people.

Methods:
research-based protocols and tools used to generate, analyse and synthesise data to (generally) generate aggregate findings.

Rationale for treatment decision:
treatment and/or intervention decision randomised and/or selected according to protocol.

Figure 17.1   Differences between clinical practice and health-care research (adapted from Alderson (2007:2280)).

terms therapeutic and non-therapeutic and highlights instead the:

> … principles that research involving children is important for the benefit of all children, and that a research procedure which cannot directly benefit the child is not necessarily unethical if the findings might benefit future generations of children. Research where there is no benefit to the individual child participant would have to be of minimal risk.
>
> (RCPCH & Hull 2000)

However, the fact that participation in a research study may bring no prospect of immediate or direct benefit to an individual child or group of children, although they may enhance future care and benefit children in the future (Kankkunen *et al.* 2002), clearly creates parameters that require a specific way of thinking about the ethical and other risks, concerns and issues.

Maps: the search for knowledge and knowing the (ethical) territory and setting your moral compass

Risk to children is a vital ethical concern within research and much attention has been paid to defining, determining and categorising risk. The RCPCH (2000:15) defines risk as 'a potential harm; the characteristics of risk include the probability of its occurrence, as well as its magnitude and dura-

tion' and further categorises it as being minimal, low or high risk (see Figure 17.2).

Whereas it might be relatively easy to determine risk associated with a study requiring additional blood tests or biopsies, what is less easy to do is to determine the ethics and risks associated with interview-based research and the degree of negative impact that such a study might have on individual children. Indeed, Brody *et al.* (2003:91–92) state that:

> Evaluations of potential risk associated with research protocols have almost exclusively emphasized physical risk, although others have acknowledged that risks associated with research participation may also include psychological, economic, and social elements.

Caldwell *et al.* (2004:805) further proposes that:

> When considering trial participation, parents and paediatricians are usually more concerned about the risks and benefits for the individual child than any societal benefit. … Currently there seems to be no coherent conceptual framework or criteria for judging whether the risks of research are reasonable in relation to what might be gained by the (child) research participant or society.

Clearly then, regardless of whether or not we spend much of our professional life undertaking research or if we are just about to start our first research project, we all need guidance to ensure that we are

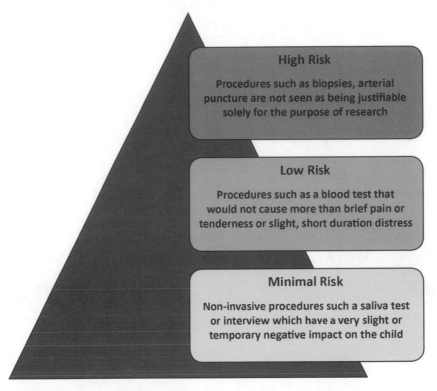

Figure 17.2   Degrees of risk (adapted from RCPCH (2000)).

ethical in the decisions we make, the risks we expose children to and the way that we practice as researchers. Research codes and governance frameworks are part of the structures that help provide guidance although they only provide part of the guidance we need. What is perhaps as important as being cognisant of the codes, rules, principles and legislation is to know the research territory and to be aware of the potential risks as well as the potential benefits. One way of thinking about how we can come to know this territory is through thinking about maps and how they have and continue to be used to guide other explorers and travellers to find their way through unfamiliar territory and landscapes in their search for knowledge and understanding.

Maps are representations of a land-or seascape. They can give you a good idea of the sort of features you are likely to come across, the types of preparation you should make and the sorts of dangers you might encounter. However, they do not actually show you the reality of the landscape. Quite often, maps are intrinsically beautiful presenting detailed information about the landscape they are representing. They can provide details, for example, on the lay of the land (whether it is flat, hilly or mountainous); where the rivers, roads, railways and canals are; where villages, towns and cities are positioned; as well as where dangers might exist such as quicksand, firing ranges and potholes. Having access to and knowledge of this type of information can be hugely important – it allows a traveller to have a sense of what they might come across and to prepare for their journey. But, however detailed, accurate, interactive and cleverly drawn a map is, it can only ever be a highly functional representation. However, in the same way that maps help guide a traveller exploring a new country, a research map can help to guide a researcher to plan, undertake and disseminate their research.

Research is often described as a journey (see Figure 17.3) with the researcher having to equip themselves for the journey by making appropriate preparations for the research project, undertaking the journey

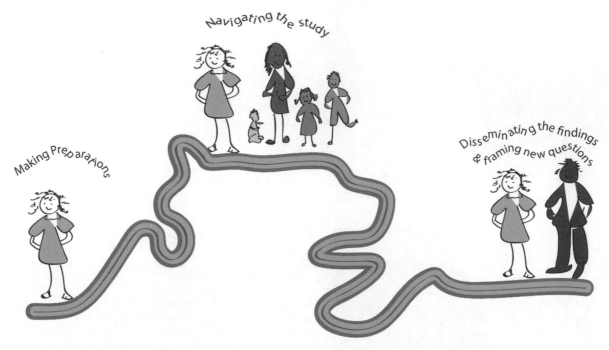

Figure 17.3   Key stages in the research journey.

itself by using a map to navigate their way through the challenges that the research presents and then finally disseminating their experiences of the journey and what they learned as a result and identifying the new research questions that arise. Thus, research is cyclical and some, but not necessarily all, of the ethical issues likely to confront the researcher and the participants can be prepared for.

In each of these phases, particular ethical challenges, concerns and issues need to be dealt with in order for the research to be as ethically sound as possible. In this chapter, the focus is on the first stage and if this stage is not undertaken well, the repercussions are felt through the rest of the study.

Making preparations

Ethical principles: guidelines and categories of research

One of the first ethical challenges a researcher has to consider is whether or not the research they are thinking about can be designed and implemented in a way that is ethical. Any research that involves human subjects has to be undertaken in a way that accords with 'three basic ethical principles, namely respect for persons, beneficence and justice' (The Council for International Organizations of Medical Sciences (CIOMS 2002)). If a research study cannot meet criteria around these three principles, then the research study is inherently unethical and cannot proceed. Other principles that underpin research include the principle of sufficient importance, scientific soundness, and utility (see King & Churchill 2000). The Bioethics Committee of the Canadian Paediatric Society (CPS-BC 2008:708) describes research in children as 'a moral duty based on several ethical principles', and they outline the principles as being:

- *Beneficence*: applying evidence-based care generated from research specific to children;
- *Non-maleficence*: avoiding harmful therapies extrapolated from adult patient data or experience;
- *Distributive justice*: allowing research benefits to be available to all populations;

- *Respect for informed consent*: supporting developing autonomy in children considering research participation; and
- *Respect for privacy and confidentiality*: providing confidentiality within the limits of legal requirements.

The guidance that governs and shapes ethical research is broadly the same regardless of the type of research that is being undertaken; research involving human subjects includes:

- Studies of a physiological, biochemical or pathological process, or of the response to a specific intervention – whether physical, chemical or psychological – in healthy subjects or patients;
- Controlled trials of diagnostic, preventive or therapeutic measures in larger groups of persons, designed to demonstrate a specific generalisable response to these measures against a background of individual biological variation;
- Studies designed to determine the consequences for individuals and communities of specific preventive or therapeutic measures; and
- Studies concerning human health-related behaviour in a variety of circumstances and environments (The Council for International Organizations of Medical Sciences (CIOMS 2002)).

These four broad categories of human subject research underpin the categorisation of children's health/health-care research. However, what marks research on-with-by children as something special is the fact that children are framed as a vulnerable group requiring particular protection. As proposed by the Medical Research Council (MRC 2004:5) children:

> ... require special protection because they are less likely than adults to be able to express their needs or defend their interests – they may not have the capacity to give consent.

Therefore, the first ethical question that a researcher is required to consider is whether the research question can be legitimately and effectively answered without exposing children to the risks and burdens that may arise from participation in a research study. Lantos (2004:149) argues that '[b]ecause we cannot minimise the risk of research to zero, our task is to both minimize risk and to somehow care for those people who are harmed as a result of their altruistic participation in research'. The default setting for all guidance is to protect children, and initially it may seem that adopting a strongly protective stance to children's potential involvement in research studies is desirable. The MRC (2004) in their guidance document, *MRC Ethics Guide: Medical research involving children*, clearly have this protective stance in mind in the advice they issue to researchers (see Box 17.1).

These are bedrock principles which underpin research involving children. They provide boundaries for researchers to work within, and they aim to protect children's interests and manage risks. They acknowledge children's capacity and competence to assent and dissent, they frame the way in which researchers should approach and engage with children and they accept that a child's family is an important part of their life and will to a greater or lesser degree be involved in decision making. What they perhaps overlook or do less well is to explicitly consider and promote children's rights. Hill (2005) suggests that the four rights embedded in the United Nations Convention on the Rights of the Child (UNCRC) are essential: welfare, protection, provision and choice and participation. Bell (2008:10) sees rights as fundamental to research practice with children as she clearly states:

> As children's rights exist in the moment when research interests and children's everyday lives intersect, continuing throughout the research process and beyond ... it is critical for research ethics guidelines to reflect human rights principles that also incorporate special considerations reflected within children's rights instruments such as the UNCRC.

The importance of acknowledging rights does need to be woven into guidelines which also protect. As new areas of medicine open up, for example, the biomedical enhancement of children, the strength of existing protections may not be sufficient to safeguard children's interests and protect them from risk and potential harm (Berg *et al.* 2009). However, in some – arguably many – situations, this protection can sometimes be over-interpreted. In the past, as Knox & Burkhart (2007:310) propose, this has meant that 'protecting children in research often got translated to excluding children from

---

Box 17.1   Principles proposed by MRC to guide research involving children.

- Research should only include children where the relevant knowledge cannot by obtained by research in adults.
- The purpose of the research is to obtain knowledge relevant to the health, well-being or health-care needs of children.
- Researchers can only involve competent children if they have obtained their informed consent beforehand.
- A child's refusal to participate or continue in research should always be respected.
- If a child becomes upset by a procedure, researchers must accept this as a valid refusal.
- Researchers should involve parents/guardians in the decision to participate wherever possible, and in all cases where the child is not yet competent.
- Researchers should attempt to avoid any pressures that might lead the child to volunteer for research or that might lead parents to volunteer their children, in the expectation of direct benefit (whether therapeutic or financial).
- Research involves partnership with the child and/or family, who should be kept informed and consent to separate stages of the project. Obtaining consent is a continuing process, rather than a one-off occurrence. Children and their families are likely to appreciate some recognition of their role in this partnership, such as a certificate of participation.
- Researchers must take account of the cumulative medical, emotional, social and psychological consequences of the child being involved in research. Children with certain conditions may be exposed to a sequence of research projects. It is advisable to consider the risks of a particular research procedure in the context of the child's overall involvement in projects by different researchers.

---

clinical trials'. This form of protectionism can actually marginalise children's interests. The first principle that research should 'only include children where the relevant knowledge cannot by obtained by research in adults' can sometimes be interpreted to prevent potentially important research from being undertaken. As with all ethical decisions, interpretation of principles is not always easy. As King & Churchill (2000:710) note:

> Principles can be used appropriately or clumsily, and good decisions depend a great deal on character and appreciation of context as well as on principled reasoning.

Some research studies or phases in research studies require particular ethical consideration, Phase 1 clinical trials, for example, where benefit may be particularly 'difficult to predict or determine' (Haylett 2009) and the ethics of enrolling children into such trials may be extremely contentious. Indeed, the ethical challenges and moral dilemmas faced by nurses caring for children entered into Phase 1 trials are now being explored, and Chang (2008) has identified the negative effect that this can have on the work life of nurses. In this and in other ethically challenging research

situations, the underpinning principles of respect for persons, beneficence and justice must be applied.

Risks and benefits need to be considered and all medical research is guided by the principle that the 'well-being of the individual research subject must take precedence over all other interests' (WMA 2008:A6, p. 1) and that 'medical research involving human subjects may only be conducted if the importance of the objective outweighs the inherent risks and burdens to the research subjects' (WMA 2008:B21, p. 3). What is not entirely clear from these seminal sets of guidance is exactly where children's nursing research fits. Clearly, some research undertaken by children's nurses is biomedical in nature although a significant amount of contemporary research is qualitative focusing on children's experiences and evaluating services. Currently, this sort of research would be generally deemed to be a minimal risk to children (see Figure 17.2) although there perhaps does need to be research undertaken to determine the qualitatively different risks incurred through the allegedly softer methods and methodologies. Mishna *et al.* (2004:449) note that:

> While some issues are similar to those in any research context, the nature of the researcher-

participant relationship, and the unstructured nature of qualitative research methods, add a dimension of risk.

Duncan *et al.* (2009:9) talk of their experiences in a qualitative study of the 'grey moments of research fieldwork when we find ourselves uncomfortable and without appropriate guidance or precedent'. In such studies, the risks to children and researchers are perhaps less obvious than those in clinical trials but they do exist. The complexity of issues and the fact that simple answers are unlikely to be forthcoming underpins Hopkins & Bell's (2008:5) stance where they suggest that:

> ... researchers must begin from an informed place to carefully assess the full extent of possible ethical issue while continuing to reflect upon their own positionality and constructs of the world.

Introducing issues of assent, consent and dissent

The shift to child-inclusive practices in research has meant that research has to be designed in such a way that two key concerns are dealt with. The first of these relates to how the potential child participants are informed about the study. The second concern relates to ensuring that children are able to decide whether to agree (assent or consent) to participate in the study. Whereas in the past, potential participants had to actively opt out of a study, potential participants now have to actively opt in to research.

In many ways, the ethical issues inherent in gaining children's assent and consent to research are similar to the ethical issues related to clinical practice-based assent and consent. What does perhaps separate research-oriented assent, consent documents and their supporting documentation (information sheets and letters of invitation) is the degree of scrutiny that they receive. Routinely, such documents are reviewed by Research Governance Committees and Ethics Committees and also sometimes by Children's (and Parents') Panels. The aim of this close level of scrutiny is to ensure that the documents are easy to understand, do not mislead and clearly indicate, amongst other things, what will happen to the child, what will be expected of them, what the risks and potential benefits might be

and, importantly, the fact that they do not have to take part. All of these measures aim to safeguard children's interests, providing a degree of ethical protection whilst promoting children's opportunities to participate in research. Increasingly, children are being involved in the process of developing assent (see, e.g., Ford *et al.* 2007) and consent documentation with the aim of trying to increase the level of assurance that the materials developed by children will be understood by children.

As previously indicated, there is now a fairly extensive literature, including numerous recommendations and guidelines, that addresses assent and consent, but as Bray (2007:451) rightly points out, many of these fail to consider qualitative approaches; perhaps of even more significance is that within this plethora of papers, 'there is little practical advice for researchers conducting research with children and young people to aid gaining assent'.

Children's understanding: research, proposals and information sheets

Contentiously perhaps, although the Holy Grail of information sheets and informed consent is for participants to fully understand the study, their participation, the risks and benefits, the outcomes and other factors, there is a view that understanding in-and-of-itself is not necessarily a problem (Eriksson & Helgesson 2005). Eriksson & Helgesson (2005:677) acknowledge that lack of understanding is a problem if it results from 'poor or inadequately communicated information, but not if it stems from the research participants deliberately choosing not to make the effort needed to acquire that understanding'. Whilst this proposal may initially seem to be contentious, we do well to consider that if people have the right to information then they equally should have the right to limit the amount of information they wish to be given. Many, possibly all, researchers have been faced with situations where they are following the research protocol to the letter and providing appropriate levels of information only to have the potential research participant express their willingness to participate before the explanation is complete. The judgement the researcher has to make is whether this does constitute informed consent. However, this issue aside, a considerable amount of work has been undertaken in the past 10 years to explore issues that relate to children's decision-making capacities and research.

The capacity to make decisions has most frequently been linked to the child's chronological age, with researchers searching for a delineator age which would readily allow the researcher to *know* that children below a particular age were unable to assent. However, more recent research which has acknowledged the multifactorial influences on decision making note that such capacities are 'highly context and situation dependent' (Brody *et al.* 2003:80). Disregarding context and solely using the blunt instrument of chronological age means that the sophistication and capability of some children is overridden. Ashcroft *et al.* (2003:17) drawing on Goodenough *et al.'s* (2003) excellent work, note that children's

> ... ability to understand and evaluate is context dependent and depends on their personal experience both of research and of social and family life, issues discussed at school in lessons, and so on; and third, that children's expertise in handling these issues might be quite variable, so that general rules cannot easily be made about children's decision-making capacity in the context of research.

Children with chronic illness are often viewed as a special case as many of them have a fairly sophisticated understanding of their own illness and disease causation (Ashcroft *et al.* 2003). Alderson (2007:2276) supports this when explaining that:

> Adversity may increase knowledge, skills and courage when children cope with disability or illness in ways that more fortunate people may not imagine.

Fernandez (2003:30) warns that researchers have a responsibility to respect children and we should not ignore 'those who might be understudied by virtue of their clinical characteristics (such as those with rare paediatric disorders)'. However, Wendler & Shah (2003) take a different stance and propose that the threshold for assent should be 14 years of age. Their thought-provoking paper resulted in a flurry of commentaries each providing detailed and passionate rationales as to why Wendler and Shah's proposition was flawed. Whilst there seems

to be a fairly lively consensus that 14 years is too high a limit, there is less consensus about a lower limit; typically, the age for assent is 7 years of age.

Interestingly and importantly, research has shown that children may struggle with some research-related concepts which lie outside their usual experience. Although Ashcroft *et al.* (2003) found that young children have the capacity to understand the purpose of research and are able to evaluate their potential involvement in it, other studies have identified limitations in children's understanding. The concept of research itself can be challenging for children and adults as seen in Spencer *et al.'s* (2004) work on an information sheet about research which participants found to be very useful. Concepts such as voluntariness and confidentiality may be incompletely understood by children (Ondrusek *et al.* 1998; Burke 2005) and understanding of rights may also need to be improved (Bruzzese & Fisher 2003). Ondrusek *et al.'s* (1998) study showed that 9-year-olds were capable of understanding the benefits and risks of research and John *et al.'s* (2008) work showed that the 6–8-year-olds had a partial understanding of the study (two-thirds of them understood they were going to have a blood test but did not know why). Wolthers (2006:296) found that from

> ... age of nine approximately 95% of the children felt they were able to read some or all of the written information, and in the six to eight year old group more than 85% felt that they were able to understand it when they were assisted by a parent. Furthermore, approximately half of the six year olds and more than two thirds in the seven to sixteen year old group felt they understood the verbal information completely; very few felt they did not understand it at all.

Much attention has been paid by researchers to creating sound information sheets (and other supporting documentation such as letters of invitation). Generally, information leaflets need to be developmentally appropriate, take cognisance of the target group of children and their particular resources, experiences, capacities, experiences and needs, and clearly state the purpose, risks and benefits of the study and what will happen to the children if they take part. Information sheets aimed at younger children tend to incorporate visual cues and images to help guide them; short sentences and plenty of

---

Box 17.2   Excerpt from an information sheet.

What would you need to do?

There are three bits in this project that you can take part in.

First of all, you could interview some of the other children on the activity days to find out what they think about the Diana Nurses.

In another bit of the project I would ask you to take some photographs of your life and the way that the Diana Nurses help you. I would also like you to make a scrapbook using the photos you have taken and putting in some stories, or drawings or other things.

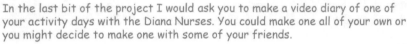

To make sure everyone can join in this bit I would give you a little camera and I would get the pictures developed and give you a scrapbook.

I would need to borrow the photos and the scrapbook for a little while but I would give it back when I had finished with it.

In the last bit of the project I would ask you to make a video diary of one of your activity days with the Diana Nurses. You could make one all of your own or you might decide to make one with some of your friends.

I will help you if you need help.

---

white space on the page can help ensure that a child does not feel overwhelmed by the prospect of reading the sheet (see Box 17.2).

The readability of information sheets can at times cause problems as they are often written at an inappropriate level for the target audience. Creating clarity in information sheets requires a particular skill set from the researcher and an appreciation of the children they are planning to inform. Words and concepts that researchers use as shorthand such as protocol, proposal, research, anonymity, confidentiality, risk and benefit need to be translated into language that is clear, unambiguous, accessible and which does not patronise the children who may potentially participate. When this is done well, then as Burke notes,

> ... even complicated procedures, involving multiple steps, can be explained to all of the age groups from whom assent would be requested.

Bruzzese and Fisher's study showed that being taught about the *Research Participants' Bill of Rights* increased children's (and adults') comprehension of some of these difficult concepts. Bray tackles this issue, and in her study she developed an activity (words and pictures) board to support reciprocal discussion between herself and the children considering her study. She reports that this activity facilitated their understanding about the study and their potential involvement, and enhanced their ability to make an informed choice about whether to assent.

However, despite very stringent efforts to communicate effectively things can go awry (see Box 17.3).

What is clear is that however good an information sheet is, it can only provide part of the information process. Dialogue, not 'simply chatting' (Beach & Proops 2009:182), is a crucial element that supports the process of helping children understand the research study and making an informed decision about whether to participate. Ungar *et al.* (2006:S32) warns that:

> ... informational documents may be useful, they should be viewed only as a supplement for a discussion between the investigator and the child who is a potential research participant.

Following on from the process of informing the child/parent(s), there is a complex (mostly invisible) process that the researcher and potential participant

Box 17.3   A lesson from the research field: the case of an anemone coming for tea.

In one of my studies, a child who had assented to be part of the study and who was clearly enjoying the research suddenly asked me when the *anenome* was arriving. Somewhat bemused I started to try and unravel what she meant and she was adamant that I had told her mother about an anemone. It took quite a lot of detective work to track the misunderstanding back to her having overheard me talking to her mother about anonymity in the study. She had decided that meeting an anemone would be quite exciting and was a tad disappointed when I explained that the *anenome* was the thing I'd explained to her at the beginning of the study. This misunderstanding did not affect the quality of her assent or the relationship we had established but it did provide me with a warning that all my dialogue within the family home should be accessible regardless of whom it was primarily directed at.

are unlikely to be fully consciously aware of. This process involves the potential participant interpreting the information, assessing the risks and benefits, responding to intuition and considering other factors such as altruism and motivation. It often involves sharing ideas and thoughts with other people.

Whereas an adult participant may make a decision about participating in a research study on their own, children's participation involves a much more complex process. It always involves at least a dyad (parent–child) and often involves a triad (parents–child). The degree to which children feel able to make decisions of this nature may reflect the ways in which more routine decisions are made within the family. A more democratic approach to family life may better prepare a child for this sort of decision than an autocratic approach to decision making. Ashcroft *et al.* (2003) report that children tend to underestimate the degree of authority they have to make decisions, and Brody *et al.* (2003) support this view when they highlight the ethical importance of appreciating the limits that adolescents may perceive in terms of their opportunity to genuinely exercise their individual right to personal autonomy. Parental influence can be profound on children's decisions and perceptions of their freedom to choose whether to participate or not. Joffe (2003:10) proposes a fairly simple model of decision making (see Figure 17.4a) (which, he accepts, creates a *shadow of the truth*) with the child's influence and decision-making responsibility increasing over developmental time whilst the parents' influence and responsibility decreases.

Whilst the notion of a smooth acquisition of capacity over developmental time is attractive, it does not take into account contextual factors such as hospitalisation, challenges to health and any other experiences that may impact on the child and

their willingness to become a decision maker. The more ragged line (as shown in Figure 17.4b) may more accurately reflect the way in which children generally acquire the capacity to make decisions and their willingness to take them. It is important to note that children's willingness to take part in decision making and consent can be heavily influenced by context, how they are feeling and may shift; this is no different to adults. In Figure 17.4c, the steeper curve reflects the way in which an expert child (such as a child with a chronic illness who has substantial understanding of their medication and treatment regimes) may more quickly acquire a decision-making responsibility.

Reynolds & Nelson (2007) show how information is only one element in the decision-making process. Their data from diabetic adolescents and their parents showed how quickly and intuitively perceptions of risk magnitude were formed and how these decisions about research participation appeared to be based on affective responses to the information. These affective decisions seemed to be more prominent and fundamental to the final decision than the perceptions of probability based on the rational choice model. They propose that the subjectivity of decision making means that risk perception may be misaligned to the researchers' intended message. Clearly, this is an ethical issue that impinges on informed consent. Brody *et al.*'s (2003) work shows that although there are some areas of disagreement between adolescents and their parents, there is frequent agreement on decisions to participate as well as on matters such as their perceptions of risk, aversion, burden and benefit. Understanding risk and benefit is core to informed consent, yet risks extend beyond physical risk and include, amongst other factors, the risks

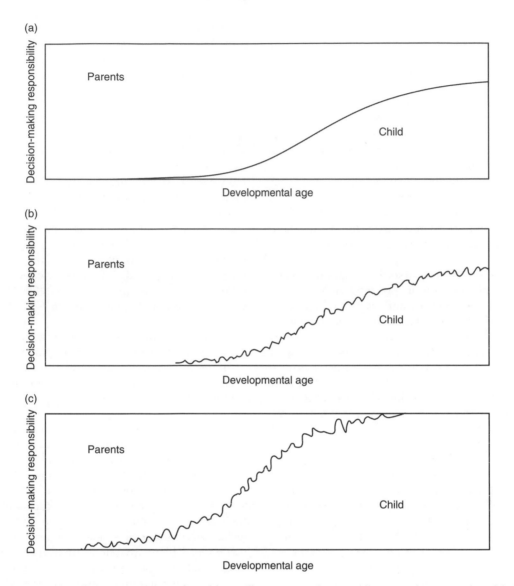

Figure 17.4 Decision-making responsibility (adapted from Joffe (2003)). (a) showing Joffe's original conceptual model, (b) showing a less smooth and more realistic profile of the acquisition of decision-making responsibility, and (c) showing how an expert child may more quickly acquire decision-making responsibility.

of 'intrusion, humiliation, embarrassment, misreport and misrepresentation' (Alderson 2007:2279).

Consent requires researchers to be reflexive and to 'assess their ethical obligations on an ongoing basis' (Mishna *et al.* 2004:462). This means that consent can never be seen as a single event; it needs to be dialogic, involving the children, their parents and the researcher(s) (Sammons 2009). Most important is the requirement that consent is always

honoured (Moeller 2003). Shilling & Young (2009:8) talk of consent being a 'social recognition of the role of parents' and that their decision 'might best be characterised as one that embodies an obligation of responsibility'.

Masty and Fisher's notion of the *goodness of fit* shows how a researcher can create what they call a *family-fitted* consent process by considering the following dimensions:

1. The child's current cognitive capacity to understand and his or her emotional readiness to make participation decisions about the issues posed by the specific research problems and design.
2. Contextual factors and characteristics that might affect parents' understanding of the nature of the child's disorder and the distinction between medical or mental-health treatment and intervention research.
3. The family's history of shared decision making for the child's health-related matters.
4. The child's autonomy strivings balanced with the parents' duty and responsibility to make decisions in their child's best interest.

Assent/consent forms, like information sheets, need careful preparation so that children can understand what they are agreeing to. Guidance is available to help both researchers and reviewers appreciate best practice in relation to the development of sound information sheets (see, e.g., http://www.nres.npsa.nhs.uk/applications/guidance/#PIS). They need to be kept clear and simple, reflecting the wording and style used in the information sheet. Generally, assent/consent forms provide a detailed breakdown of the individual elements that the child/parents is agreeing/consenting to. This means, in some research studies, that children/parents opt in to some elements of the study and opt out of other elements. A simple example of this could be that the child agrees to be interviewed but not to be audio-recorded. Although consent forms have the potential to become unwieldy if there are too many separate statements to agree/decline, Spriggs (2004:180), based on reflecting on the alarm created as a result of the Kennedy Krieger lead pain study, believes that:

> ... researchers and reviewers should be expected to contemplate and sign a statement that says: 'I would not hesitate to submit myself, or members of my own family, or anybody for whom I have any respect or affection, if in circumstances identical to those of the intended subjects'.

To pay or not to pay?

Payment of children to participate in research studies is a strongly contested area globally, the concern being that payments act as an undue inducement to participation. In the UK, the EU Directive 4d, directs that there must be no financial inducement (to either the child or their parent(s)) to enrol a child in a trial. A similar stance of 'no incentives or financial inducements are given except compensation' is found in the Clinical Trial Directive and similar wording exists in the Medicines for Human Use (Clinical Trial) Regulations (2004). Compensation which is allowable covers the family's time and expenses so that they are not out of pocket. However, these strictures for payment and participation in clinical trials apply only to children; adults can be paid. Although the prohibition does not cover research that falls outside the Clinical Trials Directive, questions about the nature and extent of payment remain troublesome. In an interesting paper which explores and raises the concerns associated with payment, Wendler et al. (2002:166) discuss the potential that payment has to:

> ... distort parents' decision-making; the opportunity for financial gain may lead parents to agree to research enrolment they otherwise would have opposed as contrary to their children's interests.

They further propose four types of payment: reimbursement, compensation, appreciation and incentive, each of which raises particular issues for the researchers and the children/families. The notion of payment being a destructive force and a slippery slope to inducing parents to inappropriately enrol their children in studies is presented by Fernhoff (2002) who provides a nice counterargument in this paper. The relative non-importance to parents of the materialistic and financial benefits of their child participating in a study compared to the opportunities for themselves and their child learning more about their child's disease was demonstrated in one study looking at possible new recruitment strategies for clinical trials (Rothmier et al. 2003). Weise et al. (2002) talk of the need to find a balance between a fair token gesture of appreciation and an inducement. They note that the American Academy of Pediatrics (AAP) recommend that any inducement could be reduced if the discussion of payment to a child happened after they have completed their involvement in the study. The ethics of this are not without challenge. In Iltis et al.'s (2006) detailed review of institutional policies in the USA, reasons for adopting a particular practice and the types of payment given were identified and the need to build consensus was highlighted.

Payment remains a difficult issue, and researchers in the UK undertaking non-clinical trial studies need to consider the ethical implications of whether they should offer payment,; and if so, what the payment should be. Research findings show that children often participate in studies based on an altruistic sense of wanting to help other children (Wolthers 2006), but this should not preclude them from receiving some form of payment.

Navigating the study

Most of the literature surrounding ethics and research on-with-by children focuses on the principles underpinning research – what is permissible and what needs to be borne in mind when designing and undertaking research. However, there is much less literature that reflects upon the real-life experiences of doing research and negotiating real-life ethical issues. Once a study has gained ethics and research-governance approval, the researcher faces the task of ensuring that they abide by the promises and statements they have made in the proposal. They are responsible for ensuring that letters of invitation are sent, the study is explained to each individual child and to their family and that informed assent and consent are achieved. The practical and pragmatic ethical management of a study with child participants is tricky and, as Duncan *et al.* (2009:1) note:

> Ethical dilemmas are unavoidable in the research setting. Sometimes we can pre-empt them, in which case protocols are likely to be in place and clear paths can be followed when they do arise. At other times they emerge spontaneously and force us to think about events we did not foresee.

As Daniel-McKeigue (2007) notes, the integrity of the research is an essential component in conducting ethical research. It is important to ensure that regardless of the pressures placed on the researcher to complete their study, they remain critically aware that 'children as research participants and as persons affected by research arrive with rights and retain their rights at all times' (Bell 2008:10). The researcher needs to be morally and ethically grounded at all times and in all aspects of their

study. They have the responsibility for navigating the everyday, minute by minute operation of the study drawing on their own expert knowledge and discussing with colleagues, as appropriate, any issues which arise. Diekema (2006:S11) notes that:

> ... the welfare of children participating in research depends on knowledgeable, caring, and responsible investigators who place the well-being of the research participant above all other aspects of the research project. Good research is ethical research.

The notion of ethical mindfulness (Guillemin *et al.* 2009) needs to underpin our research practice and our engagement with children and this sense of being ethically aware to concerns and issues will help us navigate the research territory in an effective and affective manner. Ethical practice requires a moral responsiveness which means that we are able to respond to the 'particularity and ambiguity' (Moeller 2003) of researching with individual children rather than making assumptions based on a more generic approach. Moeller (2003:W1) argues for a 'thoughtful interpretation of relevant regulations' being perhaps better able to 'serve the protection and empowerment of children involved in research'. The notion of the thoughtful researcher as an ethical researcher is important providing that their thoughtfulness is grounded in an appreciation of the many factors, including the need to ensure that children's rights are respected, protection is provided and knowledge is advanced.

Disseminating the findings

Since research is primarily focused on the generation of new knowledge, it is crucial that this knowledge is disseminated. Not to do so would be unethical practice, and there is now a strong imperative to ensure that research is disseminated widely, effectively and in a timely manner. Much of this dissemination occurs by professionals to other professionals through professional forms of communication including journal articles, conferences and networks. However, an issue of increasing ethical concern is the dissemination of research findings to participants. Part of the review responsibility of Ethics Committees is to consider and discuss how a study will be reported and disseminated and the ways in which participants and relevant community groups will be informed. Whilst this might be relatively simple in some studies, in others it may be particularly challenging due to the costs involved (Shalowitz & Miller 2008) and the sensitivity of reporting back after a period of time and the decisions that need to be taken in terms of whether it is aggregate or individual results that participants in clinical trials receive. Studies are beginning to address the issue of informing participants of the results of studies, and whilst it is a complex issue, the rights of participants to access to this knowledge are beginning to be influential. In the USA, Fernandez *et al.*'s (2003) study found few IRB-approved consent forms indicated the right for participants to receive a summary of the results and that further work is needed to explore researchers' views about the barriers they perceive hinder the return of results and the participants' views about what they need. The situation is further complicated when the participants are children, as questions arise as to whether results should be disseminated to them or their parents; this partly, of course, depends on many factors including the nature of the research itself.

Conclusion

Arguably then, Lantos' statement that opened the chapter about his belief that clinical research is safer than routine clinical care in today's children's hospitals may seem counter-intuitive, but it is likely to have a high degree of truth. The ethical issues and risks surrounding research mean that it is scrutinised far more closely than many routine aspects of clinical practice. Higher levels of reflexivity accompany research, and there is more -detailed monitoring, documenting and reporting of ethical concerns, incidents and issues than occurs in practice. Safeguards and systems are in place (although that does not mean that things cannot go wrong) to protect children, and the ethics of research involving children has been subjected to a much-heated and lively debate amongst researchers, academics and practitioners. Research is reviewed by experts and key stakeholders although much of it is still not designed and reviewed by children who are the target population. As we all develop confidence in the processes in place in relation to research involving children, we will be better positioned to share our anxieties and concerns and get the real experts – the children – to offer their perspectives on the research that will affect them and other children. Researching children's health will always be ethically challenging, but as Caldwell *et al.* (2004:809) state:

> Children might be left behind if government, researchers, and industry conclude that it's just too hard, too complicated, too risky, and too expensive. Children deserve better.

It is hard to argue against a plea that children deserve better. Ethically, better is the place we need to be.

Reflective scenario

You have created and piloted a range of information sheets, assent and consent forms to ensure that potential participants (age 6–18 years) will understand what will happen to them if they decide to participate in your study. You have got confidence in these documents but want to provide additional support to help ensure that they understand and are able to exercise their rights (e.g. their right to choose not to participate, anonymity and confidentiality). You also wish to ensure that they understand what a research project entails (e.g. what research is, the concept of risks and benefits and dissemination of findings).

1. What sort of activity or activities would you design to help the children and young people understand the key concepts of choice about participation, anonymity and confidentiality? Who might deliver this and how would you check their understanding?
2. How would you ensure that the children and young people who have given their assent or consent are able to exercise their right to withdraw from the study?
3. What sort of activity or activities would you develop to help children understand what a research project entails with a special focus on ensuring they understand the risks and benefits? Who might deliver this and how would you check their understanding?

References

Alderson, P. (2007) Competent children? Minors' consent to health care treatment and research. *Social Science & Medicine*, **65**, 2272–2283.

Ashcroft, R., Goodenough, T., Williamson, E. & Kent, J. (2003) Children's consent to research participation: Social context and personal experience invalidate fixed cutoff rules. *American Journal of Bioethics*, **3**, 16–18.

Barron, C.L. (2000) *Giving Youth a Voice: A Basis for Rethinking Adolescent Violence*. Fernwood, Halifax, Nova Scotia.

Beach, R. & Proops, R. (2009) Respecting autonomy in young people. *Postgraduate Medical Journal*, **85**, 181–185.

Bell, N. (2008) Ethics in child research: Rights, reason and responsibilities. *Children's Geographies*, **6**, 7–20.

Berg, J.W., Mehlman, M.J., Rubin, D.B. & Kodish, E. (2009) Making all the children above average: Ethical and regulatory concerns for pediatricians in pediatric enhancement research. *Clinical Pediatrics*, **48**, 472–480.

Bonah, C. (2002) 'Experimental Rage': The Development of Medical Ethics and the Genesis of Scientific Facts. Ludwik Fleck: An answer to the crisis of Modern Medicine in Interwar Germany? Society for the Social History of Medicine Millennium Prize Essay 2000. *Social History of Medicine*, **15**, 187–207.

Bray, L. (2007) Developing an activity to aid informed assent when interviewing children and young people. *Journal of Research in Nursing*, **12**, 447–457.

Brody, J.L., Scherer, D.G., Annett, R.D. & Pearson-Bish, M. (2003) Voluntary assent in biomedical research with adolescents: A comparison of parent and adolescent views. *Ethics & Behavior*, **13**, 79–95.

Bruzzese, J.M. & Fisher, C.B. (2003) Assessing and enhancing the research consent capacity of children and youth. *Applied Developmental Science*, **7**, 13–26.

Burke, P. (2005) Listening to young people with special needs: The influence of group activities. *Journal of Intellectual Disabilities*, **9**, 359–376.

Caldwell, P.H.Y., Murphy, S.B., Butow, P.N. & Craig, J.C. (2004) Clinical trials in children. *Lancet*, **364**, 803–811.

Canadian Paediatric Society (CPS) – Bioethics Committee (2008) Ethical Issues in health research in children. *Paediatrics and Child Health*, **13**, 707–712.

Carter, B. (2009) Tick box for child? The ethical positioning of children as vulnerable, researchers as barbarians and reviewers as overly cautious: A discussion paper. *International Journal of Nursing Studies*, **46** (6), 858–864.

Chang, A. (2008) An exploratory survey of nurses' perceptions of phase I clinical trials in pediatric oncology. *Journal of Pediatric Oncology Nursing*, **25**, 14–23.

Children Act (1989) http://www.legislation.gov.uk/ukpga/1989/41/contents

Children Act (2004) http://www.legislation.gov.uk/ukpga/2004/31/contents

Circuit Court for Baltimore City (2000) Circuit Court for Baltimore City, Case numbers: 24-C-99-000925 and 24-C-95066067/CL 193461 Ericka Grimes v Kennedy Krieger Institute Inc. and Myron Higgins, a minor, etc., et al. v Kennedy Krieger Institute, Inc., No. 129, September Term edn. pp. 1–103.

CIOMS (2002) *International Ethical Guidelines for Biomedical Research Involving Human Subjects*. The Council for International Organizations of Medical Sciences (CIOMS) in collaboration with the World Health Organization (WHO), Geneva.

Coleman, C.H. (2009) Vulnerability as a regulatory category in human subject research. *Journal of Law Medicine & Ethics*, **37**, 12–18.

Daniel-McKeigue, C.J. (2007) Cracking the ethics code: What are the ethical implications of designing a research study that relates to therapeutic interventions with children in individual play therapy? *The Arts in Psychotherapy*, **34**, 238–248.

DoH (2004) *The National Service Framework for Children, Young People and Maternity Services*. Department of Health, London.

DoH (2005) *Research Governance Framework for Health and Social Care*, pp. 1–55. Department of Health, London.

Diekema, D.S. (2006) Conducting ethical research in pediatrics: A brief historical overview and review of pediatric regulations. *The Journal of Pediatrics*, **149**, S3–S11.

Duncan, R.E., Drew, S.E., Hodgson, J. & Sawyer, S.M. (2009) Is my mum going to hear this? Methodological and ethical challenges in qualitative health research with young people. *Social Science & Medicine*, **69** (11), 1691–1699.

Eriksson, S. & Helgesson, G. (2005) Keep people informed or leave them alone? A suggested tool for identifying research participants who rightly want only limited information. *Journal of Medical Ethics*, **31**, 674–678.

Fernandez, C.V. (2003) Context in shaping the ability of a child to assent to research. *American Journal of Bioethics*, **3**, 29–30.

Fernandez, C.V., Kodish, E., Taweel, S., Shurin, S. & Weijer, C. (2003) Disclosure of the right of research participants to receive research results – An analysis of consent forms in the Children's Oncology Group. *Cancer*, **97**, 2904–2909.

Fernhoff, P.M. (2002) Paying for children to participate in research: A slippery slope or an enlightened stairway? *The Journal of Pediatrics*, **141**, 153–154.

Ford, K., Sankey, J. & Crisp, J. (2007) Development of children's assent documents using a child-centred approach. *Journal of Child Health Care*, **11**, 19–28.

Goodenough, T., Williamson, E., Kent, J. & Ashcroft, R. (2003) 'What did you think about that?' Researching children's perceptions of participation in a longitudinal genetic epidemiological study. *Children & Society*, **17**, 113–125.

Guillemin, M., McDougall, R. & Gillam, L. (2009) Developing "Ethical Mindfulness" in Continuing professional development in healthcare: Use of a personal narrative approach. *Cambridge Quarterly of Healthcare Ethics*, **18**, 197–208.

Halila, R. & Lötjönen, S. (2003) Why shouldn't children decide whether they are enrolled in nonbeneficial medical research? *American Journal of Bioethics*, **3**, 35–36.

Haylett, W.J. (2009) Ethical considerations in pediatric oncology phase I clinical trials according to the belmont report. *Journal of Pediatric Oncology Nursing*, **26**, 107–112.

Hill, M. (2005) Ethical considerations in researching children's experiences. In: *Researching Children's Experiences* (eds S. Greene & D. Hogan), pp. 61–86. Sage, London.

HM Government (2004) *Every Child Matters: Change for Children*. DfES/1081/2004 edn., pp. 1–32. DfES Publications, Nottingham.

Hopkins, P.E. & Bell, N. (2008) Interdisciplinary perspectives: Ethical issues and child research. *Children's Geographies*, **6**, 1–6.

Iltis, A.S., DeVader, S. & Matsuo, H. (2006) Payments to children and adolescents enrolled in research: A pilot study. *Pediatrics*, **118**, 1546–1552.

Jacobson, R.M., Ovsyannikova, I.G. & Poland, G.A. (2009) Testing vaccines in pediatric research subjects. *Vaccine*, **27**, 3291–3294.

Joffe, S. (2003) Rethink "Affirmative Agreement," but Abandon "Assent". *American Journal of Bioethics*, **3**, 9–11.

John, T., Hope, T., Savulescu, J., Stein, A. & Pollard, A.J. (2008) Children's consent and paediatric research: Is it appropriate for healthy children to be the decision-makers in clinical research? *Archives of Disease in Childhood*, **93**, 379–383.

Kankkunen, P., Vehvilainen-Julkunen, K. & Pietila, A.M. (2002) Ethical issues in paediatric nontherapeutic pain research. *Nursing Ethics*, **9**, 80–91.

King, N.M.P. & Churchill, L.R. (2000) Ethical principles guiding research on child and adolescent subjects. *Journal of Interpersonal Violence*, **15**, 710–724.

Kirk, S. (2007) Methodological and ethical issues in conducting qualitative research with children and young people: A literature review. *International Journal of Nursing Studies*, **44**, 1250–1260.

Knox, C.A. & Burkhart, P.V. (2007) Issues related to children participating in clinical research. *Journal of Pediatric Nursing*, **22**, 310–318.

Lahman, M.K.E. (2008) Always othered: Ethical research with children. *Journal of Early Childhood Research*, **6**, 281–300.

Lantos, J.D. (2004) Pediatric research: What is broken and what needs to be fixed? *The Journal of Pediatrics*, **144**, 147–149.

MRC (2004) *MRC Ethics Guide: Medical Research Involving Children*. Medical Research Council, London.

Mishna, F., Antle, B.J. & Regehr, C. (2004) Tapping the perspectives of children: Emerging ethical issues in qualitative research. *Qualitative Social Work*, **3**, 449–468.

Moeller, C.J. (2003) Moral responsiveness in pediatric research ethics. *American Journal of Bioethics*, **3**, 1–3.

NCPHS (1979) The Belmont Report. *Ethical Principles and Guidelines for the Protection of Human Subjects of Research*. National Commission for the Protection of Human Subjects of Biomedical and Behavioural Research, Washington, DC.

Ondrusek, N., Abramovitch, R., Pencharz, P. & Koren, G. (1998) Empirical examination of the ability of children to consent to clinical research. *Journal of Medical Ethics*, **24**, 158–165.

Punch, S. (2002) Research with children: The same or different from research with adults? *Childhood*, **9**, 321–341.

Reynolds, W.W. & Nelson, R.M. (2007) Risk perception and decision processes underlying informed consent to research participation. *Social Science & Medicine*, **65**, 2105–2115.

Rothmier, J.D., Lasley, M.V. & Shapiro, G.G. (2003) Factors influencing parental consent in pediatric clinical research. *Pediatrics*, **111**, 1037–1041.

RCPCH & Hull, D. (2000) Guidelines for the ethical conduct of medical research involving children. *Archives of Disease in Childhood*, **82**, 177–182.

Sammons, H. (2009) Ethical issues of clinical trials in children: A European perspective. *Archives of Disease in Childhood*, **94**, 474–477.

Shalowitz, D.I. & Miller, F.G. (2008) Communicating the results of clinical research to participants: Attitudes, practices, and future directions. *PLoS Med*, **5**, e91.

Shilling, V. & Young, B. (2009) How do parents experience being asked to enter a child in a randomised controlled trial? *BMC Medical Ethics*, **10**, 1–11.

Spencer, S.A., Dawson, A., Rigby, C., Leighton, N. & Wakefield, J. (2004) Informing patients about research: Evaluation of an information leaflet. *Quality in Primary Care*, **12**, 37–46.

Spriggs, M. (2004) Canaries in the mines: Children, risk, non-therapeutic research, and justice. *Journal of Medical Ethics*, **30**, 176–181.

Ungar, D., Joffe, S. & Kodish, E. (2006) Children are not small adults: Documentation of assent for research involving children. *The Journal of Pediatrics*, **149**, S31–S33.

Weise, K.L., Smith, M.L., Maschke, K.J. & Copeland, H.L. (2002) National practices regarding payment to research subjects for participating in pediatric research. *Pediatrics*, **110**, 577–582.

Wendler, D. & Shah, S. (2003) Should children decide whether they are enrolled in nonbeneficial research? *The American Journal of Bioethics: AJOB*, **3**, 1–7.

Wendler, D., Rackoff, J.E., Emanuel, E.J. & Grady, C. (2002) The ethics of paying for children's participation in research. *The Journal of Pediatrics*, **141**, 166–171.

Wolthers, O.D. (2006) A questionnaire on factors influencing children's assent and dissent to non-thera-peutic research. *Journal of Medical Ethics*, **32**, 292–297.

WMA (2000) Declaration of Helsinki. *Ethical Principles for Medical Research Involving Human Subjects*, pp. 1–5. World Medical Association, London.

WMA (2008) *Declaration of Helsinki. Ethical Principles for Medical Research Involving Human Subjects*, pp. 1–5. World Medical Association, London.

Suggested further readings

Christensen, P. & James, A. (2008) *Research with Children: Perspectives and Practices*, 2nd edn. Jessica Kingsley, London.

NREC (2009) Information Sheets & Consent Forms Guidance for Researchers & Reviewers. National Research Ethics Committee, Norway. http://www.nres.npsa.nhs.uk/applications/guidance/#PIS.

Tisdall, K., Davis, J. & Gallagher, M. (2008) *Researching with Children and Young People. Research Design, Methods and Analysis*. Sage Publications, London.

Web sites

Ethical issues in research with children: a reading list. http://www.nspcc.org.uk/Inform/research/reading_lists/ethical_issues_in_research_with_children_wda55732.html

NIHR Coordinated System for gaining NHS Permission (NIHR CSP) http://www.ukcrn.org.uk/index/clinical/csp.html

Medicines for Children Research Network http://www.mcrn.org.uk/

UNCEF – Child and youth participation resource guide http://www.unicef.org/adolescence/cypguide/index_ethics.html

18 Philosophical and Epistemological Aspects of Children's Spirituality

Rita Pfund

Introduction

Within the health-care setting, attention to detail would require that we nurture the spirituality of the child. Yet the spirituality of children and young people in health care tends to be explored almost exclusively in the context of critical illness, palliative care and death (Hall 2006; Hedayat 2006; Robinson *et al.* 2006; Price *et al.* 2007; Walters 2008; McSherry & Jolley 2009). But does this narrow remit cover the true essence of care which in child health encompasses the whole child – with a particular focus on the child's well-being biologically, emotionally, socially and spiritually? Exploring the topic via a literature search quickly establishes the many facets of spirituality with an abundance of child-focused literature, including an international journal dedicated specifically to children's spirituality (http://www.childrenspirituality.org/).

This chapter will explore the many facets of spirituality in childhood and during the young person's transition to adulthood. Before any conclusions can be drawn as to how the spiritual needs of children and young people can best be addressed within the health-care setting, the attitudes that health-care professionals hold on the subject in their personal lives needs to be examined; since these views impact on how spirituality is incorporated into the holistic care provided for children, young people and their families.

The concept of spirituality

The term *spirituality* within the public domain

What is the image commonly evoked by the word *spirituality*? Could it be argued that this image might be getting in the way of solving the problems surrounding the very concept itself, because for many it conjures up a vaguely religious concept – Christian, Eastern or *New Age*, or even the implication of something entirely abstract?

Readers might be forgiven for concluding that if one cannot touch, feel or measure it, it is of a spiritual nature. The *Penguin English Dictionary* (Garamonsway 1965:677) defines *spiritual* as 'of or like a spirit; having life, intelligence and will, but no body; concerned with the faculties of the soul, not materialistic; religious; given or inspired by God; holy; type of religious folk song'.

Ethical and Philosophical Aspects of Nursing Children, First Edition. Edited by Gosia M. Brykczyńska and Joan Simons.
© 2011 Blackwell Publishing Ltd. Published 2011 by Blackwell Publishing Ltd.

A basic Google search on the word *spirituality* (not at this point children's spirituality as the intention was to tease out the meaning adults associate with the concept) was revealing. Below is a sample of entries:

- 'Property or income owned by a church' (http://wordnetweb.princeton.edu/perl/webwn?s=spirituality).
- 'That which relates to or affects the human spirit or soul as opposed to material or physical things. Spirituality touches that part of you that is not dependant on material things or physical comforts' (http://www.livingwordsofwisdom.com/definition-of-spirituality.html).
- 'New age spirituality as the development of individual personal spiritual experiences. It is not any one specific philosophy, or set of religious beliefs. It is a journey through many paths and practices that leads to self-discovery' (http://www.livingwordsofwisdom.com/new-age-spirituality.html).
- And a final example from Wikipedia (http://en.wikipedia.org/wiki/Spirituality) which defines spirituality as 'matters of the spirit, a concept often (but not necessarily) tied to a spiritual world, a multidimensional reality of one or more deities. Spiritual matters regard humankind's ultimate nature and purpose, not as material biological organisms, but as spirits or energy with an eternal relationship beyond the bodily senses, time and the material world. The spiritual is contrasted with the physical and the temporary. A sense of connection is central to spirituality – connection to a reality beyond the physical world and oneself, which may include an emotional experience of awe and reverence. Spirituality may also include the development of the individual's inner life through practices such as meditation and prayer, including the search for God, the supernatural, a divine influence, or information about the afterlife. Spirituality is the personal, subjective aspect of formalised religion, mysticism, magic and of the occult.

The web site also helpfully advises the reader not to confuse the term with *spiritualism*.

Spirituality defined in relation to children and young people

> Think of our children as inheritors of our received wisdom and help them at all ages and stages to develop the abilities each has for skilfully testing it and making personally sensible meaning from it.
> Yust (2007:7)

Adding children into the picture, and moving on to professional data bases, the following will now examine the current state of knowledge around children's spirituality and how opposing aspects of religion and secularity overlap.

Bunge *et al.* (2008) examine the attention given to children in the Bible, and in doing so highlight two relevant issues:

- They found that it is much easier to study adult conceptions about children than the experiences of children themselves. It is difficult to know precisely how children were actually treated and raised and how they actually behaved. Moreover, the very questions we pose to children tend to shape their responses, and adult preconceptions about children additionally colour their interpretations of the children's answers.
- The increase in collaborative work and interest shown across disciplines, irrespective of religious background or profession – concerning the affairs of children – aids in the re-evaluation of ideas about children and the moral obligations of individuals, religious communities and nations towards the children themselves.

Bunge *et al.* refer to a web site – http://www.search-institute.org/spiritual-development which offers the most comprehensive, inclusive definition and explanation of children's spirituality (see Box 18.1) and illustrates clearly why the concept cannot just simply be deduced from an understanding of the spiritual world of an adult.

A further link on the same website informs of the results from a longitudinal study on children's spirituality. The site has also developed a preliminary working model of children's spirituality. Readers are encouraged to follow up the link to this three-dimensional model which is currently in its developmental stage, but promises to be very

---

Box 18.1　Spiritual development (Reprinted with permission from Search Institute®. Copyright © 2008 Search Institute, Minneapolis, MN; 800-888-7828; www.search-institute.org. All rights reserved.)

'Spiritual Development is, in part, a constant, ongoing, dynamic, and sometimes difficult interplay between three core development processes

- *Awareness or awakening* – being or becoming aware of or awakening to one's self, others, and the universe (which may be understood as including the sacred or divine) in ways that cultivate identity, meaning, and purpose
- *Interconnecting and belonging* – seeking, accepting, or experiencing significance in relationships to and interdependence with others, the world, or one's sense of the transcendent (often including an understanding of God or a higher power) and linking to narratives, beliefs, and traditions that give meaning to human experience across time.
- *A way of living* – authentically expressing one's identity, passions, values, and creativity through relationships, activities, and/or practices that shape bonds with oneself, family, community, humanity, the world, and/or that which one believes to be transcendent or sacred.

These human dimensions are embedded in and interact with other aspects of development; personal, familial, and community beliefs; values and practices; cultural and sociopolitical realities; traditions, myths, and interpretive frameworks; significant life events, experiences, and changes.

This framework suggests that spiritual development is a core developmental process that occurs for all persons, regardless of their religious or philosophical beliefs or worldview. Young people engage in these processes in many different ways with different emphases and levels of intensity (from highly engaged to passive). And many young people tap their own culture or religious tradition's belief systems, narratives, and community to give form to this process.' (http://www.search-institute.org/spiritual-development)

---

comprehensive and user-friendly (http://www.spiritualdevelopmentcenter.org/Display.asp?Page=DefinitionUpdate).

Linking children's spirituality to the life experience of children and theories of spirituality resulting from such work is not a new phenomenon. Bradford's (1995) work on children's spirituality was informed and shaped by his work with the Children's Society where he engaged with children and young people, not in a health-care context, but with socially and emotionally disadvantaged children and young people. The next section will explore why deducing a child's spiritual awareness from the experience of adults can be problematic.

Spirituality across the life cycle

St Thomas & Johnson (2007) explain that using a sensory approach children utilise non-verbal intelligence to navigate through their life experiences. The translation of their discoveries and insights do not pass through the filters of the verbal and analytical mind but instead remain as mythical truths which stand alone in need of further interpretation. Yust (2007) warns that we cannot disregard the tension between developmental theories and our understandings of spiritually infused pedagogies. Yust, like others, rejects the image of a child as a passive, yet-to-be-socialized not-yet-adult person!

Many theories on spirituality pertaining to children have been developed from the adult experience and perspective to be subsequently applied to a child's developmental stage. Gabarino & Bedard (1996) found that children's spirituality is invariably linked to developmental theories. Yet St Thomas & Johnson (2007) explain that most adults have discarded the roots of their own life myths, which were established long ago in the same child-like trial-and-error crucible. They also state that these myths evolved from their own personal translation and insights based on their own human relationships and cultural heritage. The authors suggest that in avoiding human vulnerability and pain,

Table 18.1   Stages of faith development by Fowler (1981).

Stage 0	*Nursed faith or foundation faith* (the struggle to trust and resist mistrust)	Age 0–4 years
Stage 1	*Chaotic faith or unordered faith* (imitating dependable adults in episodic ways)	Age 4–8 years
Stage 2	*Ordering faith* (learning the stories of one's group or community)	Age 7–11 years
Stage 3	*Conforming faith* (identifying with the views and opinions of others)	Age 12–18 years
Stage 4	*Choosing faith* (critically reflecting on what and how one believes)	Age 18–40 years
Stage 5	*Balanced faith or inclusive faith* (living with paradoxes and polarities)	Age 40+ years
Stage 6	*Selfless faith* (envisioning a sense of the unity of all things)	Later life

many adults have chosen to put away childhood memories, that have become too frightening, too painful, too vulnerable – to be able to feel again that innocent place of awe, wonder and powerlessness. This often causes a conflict for the adult who wishes to protect children by trying to hide the truth from them when faced with a child expressing spiritual distress, be this in relation to any adverse life event.

Barnes *et al.* (2000) explain that exploring children's faith development can illustrate how spirituality and religion may inform children's lives, play a part in children's moral formation, socialisation and induction into a sacred world view, as well as provide the child with inner resources. In addition, the authors acknowledge the aspects of spirituality and religion parents may bring to bear in relation to their children's emotional and physical health, as well as the religious or spiritual stance of the health-care provider.

Bradford (1995:60) bases his model of children's spirituality on the incremental stages of faith development found in the work of Fowler & Emery (1976). Readers might find themselves reminded here of the principles of moral development proposed by Kohlberg (http://psychology.about.com/od/developmentalpsychology/a/kohlberg.htm) and indeed Fowler himself was influenced by the pedagogical developments of this time, namely, the work of Kohlberg and Piaget (Fowler & Dell 2006). Faith development is seen to be independent of specific religious affiliation such as Christianity, Buddhism, Islam or Judaism, or even none (Table 18.1).

These have been refined through further research into a three-stage model by Fowler *et al.* (1991). Walker (2005) explains that these have been matched against children's developmental stages to enable practitioners to conceptually orientate their therapeutic process (Table 18.2).

Organic, intrapersonal, interpersonal, contextual and even supervenient factors can influence the course of spiritual development (Wagnener & Newton Malony 2006). However, children and young people with either physical or learning disabilities, or siblings of these children, including very young parents – such as adolescent parents finding themselves having to make decisions for very sick newborns – do not neatly fit into Fowler's faith and spirituality categories. Spiritual development could be delayed, but also it could be accelerated compared to the child's chronological age, for children and young people who have been confronted with adverse life events are often catapulted to a stage well beyond their years.

Sexson (2004:43) discusses a study undertaken by Fosarelli, asking 6000 children aged 6–18 'if you could get God to answer one question, what question would you ask God?' Whilst it was not possible to trace a publication of this particular study, Sexson in personal communication with Fosarelli reveals that children in the control group were more likely to questions such as 'why did the dinosaurs die?' Whilst children who had experienced major stresses would ask more specific questions, such as 'why did my dad die?' Sexon (2004) concludes that using this question in a spiritual assessment could be very useful.

Seeking spirituality in the reality of the lives of children and young people

Although the more recent framework of faith development cited above is available, for the purpose of this chapter the earlier framework spanning the full life cycle proposed by Fowler & Emery (1976) is utilised to explore examples around issues affecting children and young people, and how these can be linked back to spiritual components.

Table 18.2 Fowler's stages of children's faith development (Fowler *et al.* (1991), in Walker (2005:129).

Stage	Age	Characteristics
One	3–7	Children live in a world of fantasies, images, moods, stories, actions and examples. To move out of this, they need to develop rational thinking and a distinction between fantasy and reality.
Two	7–11	Mythic-literal stage. Story is of central importance; fairness and justice are central concerns. Children may become convinced of their exceptional goodness/badness.
Three	11–18	Synthetic-conventional faith. To reach this, children need good personal relationships and more awareness of the larger environment.

Nursed faith or foundation faith (0–4 years)

Hall (2006) demonstrated the views and values women have had of pregnancy and birth, and comments on the powerful, spiritual relationship they can experience with their unborn child. Within high risk pregnancies, Price *et al.* (2007) have found that spiritual expression was the key to maternal health and healing. Further examples in the literature mainly pertain to the experience of staff and parents caring for very sick neonates. Cadge & Catlin (2006) researched in an American hospital, health-care provider's constructs of meaning and investigated how health-care workers respond to the existential *why* question implicit in an infant's illness, suffering and sometimes death, which they observed daily. In their study, the authors found that more than 80% of the health-care workers surveyed drew strength from religious and spiritual teachings. Barnes *et al.*'s (2000) findings demonstrate how parents and health-care providers affect the spiritual development of a child. Meanwhile Waldron (2007) researching the emergence of language and symbol in the development of the young infant found that this could not be separated from the foundation faith which was being nurtured in the young child.

Chaotic faith or unordered faith (4–8 years)

The words *wonder* and *awe* and the concepts they represent are seldom found in academic texts, but they do appear to be intrinsic to how artists and writers capture the essence of childhood, such as Milne (1924) telling of the story about Christopher Robin and his friends' adventures. For many, the *Heile Welt* represents a place one can escape to in fiction, where nothing really bad happens and problems or conflict tends to be resolved successfully. St Thomas & Johnson (2007) explain how children of different cultures and different life experiences frequently navigate between inner and outer realities: the conflict of navigating through trauma along with the differences between cultures, languages and ethnicities places tremendous pressure on children to acculturate and integrate realities that very often do not easily fit together. However, according to St Thomas & Johnson (2007) the challenge still remains to create a connection that acknowledges the past and integrates the present differences in a way that supports hope for the future. The poem below seeks to explain to young children whose world is turned upside down by the arrival of a sick newborn baby brother, what is happening by giving simple explanations of the different physical environment, emotions felt and memories that can be taken into the future.

Our little baby brother
On Monday we went with dad to see our new
   baby brother.
We looked at him in the incubator. Tubes went
   into him.
There were lots of beeping and buzzing
   machines.
He was really really small
Really really tiny.
We stood on a chair and reached
   through a peephole into his incubator.
We held his hand and his fingers and toes.
They were really really small
Really really tiny.
We went to see him everyday – he was really
   very tiny.
Tubes went into him to help him breathe and
   eat.

And even the tubes were tiny.
Machines were buzzing and beeping. For our
    little baby brother
Who was really really small
Really really tiny.
We drew him pictures and talked to him.
And he started to breathe and to eat
Machines were buzzing and beeping
They told us how well he was doing, our clever
    baby brother
Who was really really small
Really really tiny.
We went to see our brother everyday,
and we all watched him get better and grow.
That is mum and dad and Isaac and me
and on Friday we'll take him home.
And when he's bigger we'll tell him the tale of
    the time when he was
Really really small
Really really tiny.

Source: Pfund (2007)

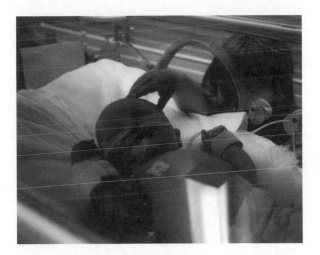

Mountain (2007) states that creative arts activities engage children in learning that is intimately related to spiritual development, involving self-understanding, understanding of relationships, wider environmental connectedness and connection with the divine. From her study and experience, she concludes that the current education system, driven by an economic-rationalist society, is not caring for the needs of the whole child. Yet, all aspects of the school curriculum should provide opportunities for spiritual experiences. Buchanan & Hyde (2008) explain how cognitive,

affective and spiritual dimension can be addressed within a curriculum, whilst Wills (2009) offers practical examples of a series of spirituality mornings run in a UK primary school (http://www.childrenspirituality.org/support/projects/spiritualitydays.asp).

On a typical *spirituality day*, the children (of any age group) will take part in activities which relate to personal and global issues. They will have a time for silence and reflection, will connect imagination to creativity through music, art, drama and creative writing, and will be given the opportunity to talk about how the experiences have affected their own personal lives. According to Mountain (2007), there is much research showing the interrelationship between the efficient working of the mind in understanding and learning and with the inner spiritual life and the life of the emotions.

Ordering faith (7–11 years)

Mountain (2007) states that as our society continues to develop in diversity and complexity, concern is being expressed by academics and professionals (Kegan 1994; Elkind 2001), that young people are not coping adequately and need help in developing understanding and meaning of the world around them. Mountain (2007) sees *The Hurried Child* image, *as* defined by Elkind (2001), as a reality in the school situation: according to her, the crowded curriculum means school time gives little space for quiet reflection on deeper personal and spiritual issues. Statistically, a staggering percentage of children experience adverse life events and loss of varying degrees and intensity, such as parental divorce. Many studies observe that even before parental divorce, children and adolescents suffer due to high levels of marital discord, ineffective and inconsistent parenting, diminished parental well-being and reduced parent–child affection (http://family.jrank.org/pages/413/Divorce.html).

Professionals need to be alert to the child who seeks the space for quiet reflection. The picture of the sheep having a tough time was presented to a maths teacher by a child becoming aware of the terminal nature of her long-term illness (Figure 18.1).

Pictures expressing the search for spiritual meaning are often drawn by children coming to terms

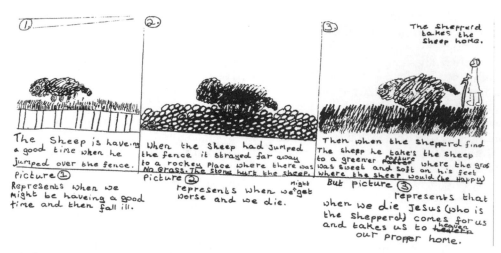

Figure 18.1 *Palliative Care Nursing of Children and Young People.* Oxford: Radcliffe Publishing; 2007. © Pfund. Reproduced with the permission of the copyright holder.

with terminal illness, either their own or that of other significant people in their lives. A very good selection has been published by Brown (2006), Brown & Warr (2008), Kinchin & Brown (2001) and Brown (1999). These pictures are typical for children experiencing adverse life events, but it is difficult to identify examples of art drawn by children who had no particular adverse life-trigger but are drawn for a professional, who then includes the drawing in a publication making it difficult to compare and contrast both types of drawings. This highlights the assertion made by Bunge *et al.* (2008) that much of what we know about children's spirituality is actually generated by adults and not by children themselves.

Children are exposed to the adult world problems of violence and environmental degradation which flood into our homes through the mass media, according to Mountain (2007). In addition to this, some children lead exceedingly busy lives. After-school activities distract children in various ways: the constant stimulation of video games and TV shows and the busy-ness stemming from extra lessons in music or sporting activities all lead to potential fragmentation of their core selves, whilst, as Mountain illustrates, demands and societal conflicts increasingly intrude upon their inner space.

In this atmosphere, the need for nurturing the thought processes that thrive in this inner space can easily be overlooked.

Human beings crave a sense of self, of security, a truth we can depend on, a world we can tame and understand – things we can believe in even if life becomes problematic. This is one of the differences between adult and child thinking acknowledged by St Thomas & Johnson (2007) and is superbly captured in the story of the little prince by St Exupery (1947). As Mountain (2007) asserts, spiritual development is given lip service in much of the educational literature and there is little attention given to designing and using methods to promote the spiritual dimension of the child.

Conforming faith (12–18 years)

Moncher & Josephson (2004) highlight changes in family structure over the last few decades affecting children of today, and that will influence the formation of the next generation of families. Consequently the authors describe an alarming increase of associated childhood emotional and behavioural problems, including problems such as criminal activity suicide, unplanned pregnancy and alcohol use. It is not surprising therefore that by far the most diverse literature could be identified for this age group. Subjects addressed pertained to resilience (Ahern *et al.* 2008), teenagers' perception of spirituality (Wintersgill 2008), exploring a measuring tool to assess spirituality,

(Harris *et al.* 2008), the role of spirituality in preventing early sexual activity (Doswell *et al.* 2003), religiousness and alcohol use in college students (Von Dras *et al.* 2007; Menagi *et al.* 2008), exploring health beliefs and health behaviours in college students (Wyatt *et al.* 2006; Nagel & Sgoutas-Emch 2007) and referrals for pastoral care comparing psychiatric versus surgical adolescent patients (Chapman & Grossoehme 2002). These samples highlight the scope of the evolving body of evidence within the subject of children's and young peoples' spirituality.

Choosing faith (18–40 years)

Young people in the transitional phase of spiritual development, but also many parents and healthcare providers will feature in these three final stages, thus forming part of the feedback loop to the first four stages of faith development found in the context of children's and young peoples' exposure to the health-care system. Gall (2006) conducted a study exploring this stage of faith development in relation to spirituality and coping with life stresses amongst adult survivors of child sexual abuse and found evidence of both negative and positive forms of spiritual coping. Individuals who experienced more severe forms of abuse relied more on negative forms of spiritual coping such as spiritual discontent (anger at God). In contrast, survivors who have integrated spirituality as a resource to be relied on in their daily lives may also use it in their coping with memories of abuse and as a method of creating meaning and integrating their history of abuse within a stronger sense of self. Gall concurs with Pargament & Brant (1998) that since negative spiritual coping is used less often than positive spiritual coping, it may serve as a signal of distress, or a *red flag* for psychological distress. It might be in this retrospective context that the stages of faith development are particularly revealing. Gall (2006) found a clear link in children who were abused at an earlier age and may have experienced a disruption in their development of a strong and secure sense of a benevolent God, and so, as adults, are less likely to turn to God and others for spiritual support.

Balanced faith or *inclusive faith* (40+) and *selfless faith* in later life

These stages of spiritual development become relevant from a service perspective in relation to professionals within health, education and social care. Topics examined here range from nurses' and carers spiritual well-being in the workplace (Fisher & Brumley 2008), nursing attitudes (Lundmark 2006), competencies (Van Leeuwen & Cusveller 2004; Baldaccino 2006), paediatrician characteristics associated with attention to spirituality and religion in clinical practice (Grossoehme *et al.* 2007), nurse education in general (Narayanasamy 2006; Hickey *et al.* 2008) and children's nursing (Kenny & Ashley 2005) in particular.

Addressing spirituality in child health care

According to Feudtner *et al.* (2003), spirituality is viewed as a vital aspect of the illness experience. Key concepts in nursing include concepts such as *dignity*, *respect* and *nurturing*, and Mason-Whitehead *et al.* (2008) find them interdependent, and often difficult to define. Interestingly, the concept of spirituality is omitted from their compilation of nursing concepts. In contrast, approaching the topic from a South African context, Tjale & Bruce (2007) in their concept analysis of holistic nursing care in paediatric nursing describe nursing activities as 'child and family focused, culturally sensitive, and congruent with family beliefs and values, planned to meet the physical, emotional, mental, spiritual, social and cultural dimensions of care' (p. 50).

In their 2003 study, Feudtner *et al.* set out to profile pastoral care providers' perception of the spiritual care needs of hospitalised children and their parents, barriers to better pastoral care, and to assess the quality of spiritual care in children's hospitals in the USA (Figure 18.2). No other studies from a paediatric context could be identified in the literature. Barriers to the provision pertained to

- Inadequate staffing of the pastoral care office;
- Inadequate training of health-care providers to detect patients' spiritual needs; and

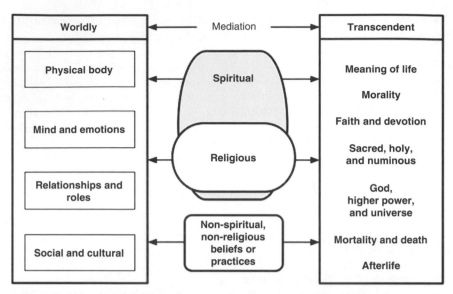

Figure 18.2   A model of spiritual, religious or other beliefs, activities and relationships mediating between domains of ordinary experience and transcendent concerns. Feudtner, 2003. Reproduced with the permission of the copyright holder.

- Being involved too late to be able to provide all the care that could have been provided.

These findings are confirmed by Weeding (2010) who affirms that spiritual support is clearly identified in the ACT Care Pathways (Elston 2004; ACT 2007, 2009), and has already been implemented locally (Wolff & Browne 2010). However, in Weeding's experience spiritual care is mainly requested in the form of religious support at the end of a child's life, and as such is heavily dependent for implementation on the interpretation of individual health-care professionals' caring modality for the child and its family.

Erickson (2008), presenting a case study of an adolescent who was left with severe disability following a car accident in which her mother and grandmother were killed, finds it helpful to look at spirituality as a journey. On this journey, each member of the health-care team plays a role in helping a child or an adolescent to find a sense of meaning, purpose and connectedness with others, and to recognise that there are questions that may never be answered or explained.

It is in these situations that the transfer of adult awareness of spirituality onto children and young people becomes most problematic. This can be seen in at least two major areas. The increasing numbers

of young people currently still remaining in paediatric care whilst transition arrangements to adult or adolescent services are being made can be a problematic issue. The lack of awareness of the spiritual needs of these youngsters can cause distress to the young patient, but also to professionals dealing with spiritual issues. Wilford (2008) describes his retort to a patronising approach by professionals giving him a grim prognosis:

> … when I was in hospital they said that I was critical, … that I was not very well … and there might be a chance that I might die they said in really simplistic terms like I was a child … and I said that we are all dying in a Tibetan sort of a sense Buddha and the Sylvia Plath sort of a way, and their faces sort of dropped, and they realised what they were dealing with then.

Likewise, interpreting as a spiritual experience an activity that a disabled child enjoys, and therefore is relaxed, overlooks the very real distress the same child might be experiencing but not have the verbal capacity to express. This can be a particular issue for children with degenerative illnesses, for whom we are unlikely to know whether their cognitive abilities are diminishing in line with their physical abilities and their capacity to express themselves (Pfund 2007). Distant memories and hallucinations might mean that this child is emotionally not in a safe environment and therapeutic play activities alone will not necessarily address these issues.

Weeding (2010), reflecting on how staff introduce the chaplaincy service to families with children who suffer from life-limiting and life-shortening conditions, concludes that the service should be introduced much earlier in the life path, as by far the greatest amount of time is spent addressing spiritual issues of the living who have no particular religious affiliation. The above examples also illustrate that the chaplain needs to be an integral member of the team delivering holistic care, as he or she needs to have an understanding of factors affecting a young patient's ability to express their needs and wants. The chaplain is also invaluable in guiding professionals in dealing with spiritual questions where perhaps they feel out of their depth, or where the issue raised by a young patient might be at odds with the professionals' own belief system.

Weeding's (2010) own experience is predominantly supporting parents of very ill, very young children. This might be representative for many hospital settings. Yet, addressing the spiritual needs of the entire family, according to Tanyi (2006), can assist in maintaining normalcy, cohesion and resilience in the midst of crises.

Health-care facilities often reflect a particular philosophy, and dedicated children's hospitals are more likely to have child-friendly and children-dedicated chapels. One such example is the much treasured Victorian chapel at the Hospital for Sick Children, Great Ormond Street, which has even special seating made for children as well as a chapel welcoming the whole family, parents, sick child, siblings and significant others (Figure 18.3).

Tanyi (2006) acknowledging the complex nature of spirituality considers *family* spirituality as a much broader concept, as it encompasses the individual's distinct spirituality, and that of the whole family unit, and is consistent with the multidimensional and ambiguous nature of spirituality. She describes family spirituality as the search for meaning and purpose in life, meaningful relationships, individual family member spirituality, family values, beliefs and practices which may or may not be religiously based, and the ability to appreciate transcendency.

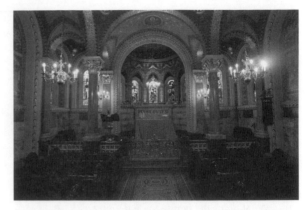

Figure 18.3   Victorian chapel at the Hospital for Sick Children, Great Ormond Street. Reproduced courtesy of Great Ormond Street Hospital.

Tanyi (2006) found that other disciplines such as social work and family therapy already have strategies to assess spirituality, but that no such formal guidelines exist within nursing. Some nursing models and theories of nursing do acknowledge the need to assess for spiritual distress and spiritual well-being, but these are not used much in practice in the UK. McEvoy (2003) warns that models have given rise to categorizations of culture, spirituality and religion. Whilst it is important for paediatric nurses to understand that whilst delineations can be made, there are also many intersecting factors that make separation of these issues difficult. He suggests that paediatric nurses should, perhaps, focus instead on understanding the individual child's or family's traditions, values and beliefs, and how these dimensions impact the health of the child. Sexson (2004:38) describes a mnemonic help to ask pertinent questions suggested by McEvoy (2003) as BELIEF, which stands for the following: a family's *belief* system, value system or *ethics*, how a family practices spirituality or religion *lifestyle*, a family's *involvement* in a community of believers, whether there is participation in religious orientated *education*, discussion of *future* events that might be affected by the family's spirituality, such as birth control, immunization, circumcision, abortion, transfusion of blood products and other events (Box 18.2).

However, in the context of child health it could be argued that incorporating carefully chosen

Box 18.2   Guidelines to spiritual assessment for families as suggested by Tanyi (2006:289) Reproduced with permission.

Meaning and purpose

Who or what does the family consider the most meaningful?
What gives the family meaning in their daily routines?
What gives the family peace, joy and satisfaction?

Strengths

What gives the family strength?
What helps the family to deal with crises?
What does the family do in order to rebuild their strength?

Relationships

What do family members like about their family?
Does the family have a relationship with God/Higher Power, universe or other? If yes, how do they describe it?
Is the family involved in community-based spiritual activities? If yes, which ones?

Beliefs

What are the family's beliefs? And what do these beliefs mean to their health?
Does the family practise rituals such as prayer, worship or meditation?

Individual family member spirituality

How do family members express/describe their spirituality?
And what does this mean to their health?
Are there conflicts between family members because of their spiritual views?

If yes, what is the impact, if any, on the individual and family's health?

Family's preference for spiritual care
How does the family describe/express their spiritual views?
Can the family give examples of how nurses can integrate their spiritual views when working with them?
Does the family consider anyone their spiritual leader?
And if necessary, can the spiritual leader be contacted to assist with providing care to the family?

Sources: Fitchett (1993), Maugans (1996), Hodge (2000), McEvoy (2000), Wilkinson (2000), Tanyi (2002).

These questions serve only as a guide to help nurses elicit spiritual information for each category. Nurses can, therefore, rephrase these questions according to the family's understanding and expressions of their spirituality.

questions such as in the example above is good practice and the sharing of information would be more acceptable to families rather than being asked similar questions by a multitude of different professionals. This is already required for the child *in need* through the CAF (Common Assessment Framework, http://www.dcsf.gov.uk/everychild-matters/strategy/deliveringservices1/caf/caf-framework/) This approach would be more time efficient, given that the main reason for neglecting spiritual care within the health-care system appears to be the need for prioritising work and the perceived lack of time to address this particular aspect of care.

A model of spirituality applied to holistic care of the child and family

Bradshaw (1994) states that spiritual care is inseparable from physical, social and psychological care, because it is indistinguishable from the wholeness of care. Yet in the current acute health-care climate, patients often experience a fragmented, technical, disease-oriented service. Henderson (2006) views this as a particular barrier to embracing holistic care for nursing staff especially those new to the health-care system. Within health care, different models of holistic care have been developed and utilised since the 1960s. Most nurses will be familiar with models based on *activities of living* such as Virginia Henderson's and the Roper, Logan and Tierney model which was based on it, or Orem's model emphasising the patient's participation in care or the *systems theory* as developed by King which regards patients as interconnected units forming a unique whole (Mason 1995). Having examined the various facets implicit in the concept of spirituality, the question is posed whether spirituality should be viewed as a separate aspect of the *activities of living*, or whether spirituality is a synergy of all the necessary living elements. If the latter were the case, it might make an otherwise abstract activity of living somewhat more tangible. For example, when meeting the need for *dignity* of clients of any age, this personal need overarches several other distinct activities of living, for example, privacy when toileting and bathing. Likewise, considering the need for patient dignity is also a nursing approach supporting the patient's spirit. If we were to substitute *emotional well-being* with the term *spirituality* – superimposing aspects of spirituality onto the activities of living – this move would pose little difficulty. Spirituality is a broader concept than simply emotional well-being and it encompasses not only aspects such as meeting faith requirements, but also exploring fears and worries. This then allows addressing factors that interfere with aspects of well-being such as sleep and personal comfort, maintaining contact with peers and so on.

An additional dimension is added by Miner-Williams (2005) who suggests that providing care in a spiritual manner is caring for the *person* in addition to caring for the patient – through the *manner* in which the nursing care is delivered. Such care has the potential to reach out and minister to the spirit of the patient, not only their body or psyche.

Feudtner *et al.* (2003) developed a broad model of spiritual care needs:

> … based on a dynamic and ecumenical interpretation of spirituality as those beliefs, activities, and relationships that mediate, influence, or modify the relationship between several domains of human experience and transcendent issues or concerns. (p. e67)

Like the prevailing philosophy around the activities of living, this model perceives spirituality as a mode of living – a process, an inquiry, a conversation – rather than a separate realm of life, isolated from other aspects of the person. Feudtner *et al.* (2003) conceptualise spiritual care needs as potentially encompassing a diverse array of human needs for which they give specific examples. Within the physical body, the experience of physical pain can lead to intense spiritual enquiry regarding the meaning of suffering – a predominantly spiritual endeavour. Likewise, there can be a connection to spirituality in the *relationships and roles* domain of human experiences, examples of which are hopes, fears, problematic relationships with family members or schoolmates, financial concerns, stigmatising cultural beliefs or one's understanding of illness and its treatment. The beauty of this model is that it has the flexibility and imagination to encompass all the elements that affect a child or young person in addition to any health concerns which might be the direct cause of the health concern itself or might be a consequence of the health concern.

This makes Feudtner *et al.*'s (2003) work perhaps the most enlightened tool we can currently apply when considering the spiritual needs of children and young people in the health-care environment.

Conclusion

This chapter has examined a wide range of issues pertaining to children's spirituality. But at the end of it can we agree, or do we even wish to agree, on one overarching definition of children's spirituality? Reminding ourselves of the components identified in the literature specifically pertinent to the spirituality of the child, there were three main domains within spirituality, namely, *a way of living, awareness or awakening* and *interconnecting and belonging* (http://www.search-institute.org/spiritual-development).

The difficulty with the ambition to find the *definitive* explanation of spirituality has to be the diversity and individuality which this huge area of humanness is addressing, and the risk of not addressing it at all, whilst there is uncertainty as to the meaning of spirituality itself. What makes up the *spiritual* nature of the child or young person has to be a synergy of the developmental stage, the *system* or the direct environment a child is growing up in, and the specific life events that a particular child experiences.

An aspect well known to child health professionals, but easily overlooked when applying principles which were established in the context of the care of adults and now transferred to children and young people, even when developmental stages are being considered, is the fact that children do not stagnate. Although a child at any given moment *is* at a particular developmental stage, the nature of being a child is such that development is continual; all the developmental issues affecting a child's spirituality continue also, often over many years, and the child will be re-evaluating and re-assessing his or her spiritual stance continually.

Feudtner *et al.* (2003) suggest that the concept of spirituality needs to be developed further so that the correct questions can be asked. In line with this, there needs to be an understanding of the illness experience longitudinally, during the course of prolonged hospital admissions or repeated admissions to clarify how the spiritual history of individual patients or families develops over time. Feudtner *et al.* (2003) also ask how spiritual care can improve patient outcomes, both spiritual in a sense of spiritual well-being,

and secular in terms of satisfaction with quality of life and the role doctors and nurses play to facilitate this. This underpins recent efforts that Barnes *et al.* (2000) describe as a new synthesis between medicine, religion and spirituality, extending notions of healing to include concern for the body, mind and spirit. Examples of how practical questions asked can address this issue can be found in the Barnes paper, and the Feudtner *et al.* (2003) paper.

There is an evolving body of knowledge, which currently is difficult to access. This is partly due to data bases that do not directly relate to child health can be difficult to tap into. Also, some work is in its developmental stage, such as the model put forward by the search institute (http://www.spiritualdevelopmentcenter.org/Display.asp?Page=DefinitionUpdate) and research not yet published by Fosarelli, but cited by Sexson (2004), which is likely to address the difficulty of getting a true reflection of a child's understanding of spirituality highlighted by Bunge *et al.* (2008) earlier.

Addressing the concerns of body, mind and spirit is likely to, in the longer term, assist in addressing the many issues expressed by young people as discussed earlier and which are discussed in other chapters in this book.

Spirituality can be considered only superficially by many nurses and health-care workers and dismissed as vague and an optional extra dimension to a child's personality, in a very pressured health-care environment. However, it might yet emerge as a subject area that is integral to children's and young peoples' care, as it has the potential to be inclusive of every aspect of life that challenges today's children and youth. It is encouraging to discover how topical aspects of spirituality are and that the concept is being addressed in education, social care, mental health and general child care. It is desirable to see child health-care workers engage much more in collaboration with other disciplines in promoting children's spiritual needs whilst interpreting the 'Every Child Matters' (http://www.dcsf.gov.uk/everychildmatters/) agenda. Nurses and health-care workers need to more fully embrace the spiritual needs of *all* children, not just the ones experiencing critical illness, palliative care and death.

Reflective scenario

Callum, now aged 15, has been diabetic since the age of 5. He is recovering from a life-threatening episode of keto-acidosis after a night out with his friends. He is aggressive and uncooperative. This is out of character for the young man. The diabetes services have known him for many years and have just started to discuss transition to adult services.

Over the years his parents had insisted on a very rigid regime of managing his diabetes, and consequently he had experienced few problems. Recently, his parents have split up, and Callum chose to live with his father. In an attempt to compensate for the disruption Callum has experienced, and also to help him become more independent, the management of his diabetes has been relaxed with Callum now managing his blood sugar monitoring, insulin injections and diet with parental support when he asks for it.

He is shocked to hear that the doctor has told his parents that when he was in a coma he only had a 30% chance of survival.

1. What information would you want to ascertain in a spiritual assessment of Callum and his family?
2. How would you incorporate the information gathered in the care planned for Callum?
3. Think of a child or young person you have cared for. With hindsight, which aspects of care could have been more holistic if spirituality in the context of Feudtner's (2003) work had been considered?

References

ACT (2007) *The Transition Care Pathway: A Framework for the Development of Integrated Multi-agency Care Pathways for Young People with Life-threatening and Life-limiting Conditions.* Association for Children's Palliative Care, Bristol.

ACT (2009) *Neonatal Pathway.* Association for Children's Palliative Care, Bristol.

Ahern, N.R., Ark, P. & Byers, J. (2008) Resilience and coping strategies in adolescents. *Paediatric Nursing,* **20** (10), 32–36, S1–S7.

Baldaccino, D.R. (2006) Nursing competencies for spiritual care. *Journal of Clinical Nursing,* **15**, 885–896.

Barnes, L., Plotnikoff, G., Fox, K. & Pendleton, S. (2000) Spirituality, religion, and pediatrics: Intersecting worlds of healing. *Pediatrics,* **104** (6), 899–908.

Bradshaw, A. (1994) *Lighting the Lamp.* Scutari Press, Harrow.

Bradford, J. (1995) *Caring for the Whole Child: A Holistic Approach to Spirituality,* p. 60. The Children's Society, London.

Brown, E. (1999) *Loss Change and Grief: An Education Perspective.* David Fulton Publishers, London.

Brown, E. & Warr, B. (2007) *Supporting the Child and the Family in Paediatric Palliative Care.* Jessica Kingsley, London.

Brown, E. (2006) Ritual and religion. In: *Oxford Textbook of Palliative Care for Children* (eds A. Goldman, R. Hain & S. Liben). Oxford University Press, New York.

Buchanan, M. & Hyde, B. (2008) Learning beyond the surface: Engaging the cognitive, affective and spiritual dimensions within the curriculum. *International Journal of Children's Spirituality,* **13** (4), 309–320.

Bunge, M.J., Fretheim, T.E. & Roberts, G.B. (2008) *The Child in the Bible.* Eerdmans Publishing Company, Grand Rapids, Michigan.

Cadge, W. & Catlin, E. (2006) Making sense of suffering and death: How health care providers construct meanings in a neonatal intensive care unit. *Journal of Religion and Health,* **45** (2), 248–263.

Chapman, T. & Grossoehme, D. (2002) Adolescent patient and nurse referrals for pastoral care: A comparison of psychiatric vs medical – surgical populations. *Journal of Child and Adolescent Psychiatric Nursing,* **15** (3), 118–123.

Doswell, W.M., Kouyate, M. & Taylor, J. (2003) The role of spirituality in preventing early sexual behaviour. *American Journal of Health Studies,* **18** (4), 195–202.

Elkind, D. (2001) The hurried child Reading (USA) Basic Books cited in Mountain, V. (2007) Educational contexts for the development of children's spirituality: Exploring the use of imagination. *International Journal of Children's Spirituality,* **12** (2), 191–205.

Elston, S. (2004) *Integrated Multi-agency Care Pathways for Children with Life-threatening and Life-limiting Conditions.* ACT, Bristol.

Erickson, D. (2008) Spirituality, loss and recovery in children with disabilities. *International Journal of Children's Spirituality,* **13** (3), 287–296.

Feudtner, C., Haney, J. & Dimmers, M. (2003) Spiritual care needs of hospitalized children and their families: A national survey of pastoral care providers' perceptions. *Pediatrics,* **111** (1), e67–72.

Fisher, J. & Brumley, D. (2008) Nurses' and carers' spiritual wellbeing in the workplace. *Australian Journal of Advanced Nursing*, **25** (4), 49–57.

Fitchett, G. (1993) Assessing. *Spiritual Needs: A Guide to Caregivers*. Augsburg Fortress, Minneapolis, quoted in Tanyi, R. (2006) Spirituality and family nursing. *Journal of Advanced Nursing*, **53** (3), 287–294.

Fowler, J.W. & Emery (1976) *Stages of Faith*. New York: Harper Row cited in Bradford J (1995) *Caring for the Whole Child: A Holistic Approach to Spirituality*. The Children's Society, London.

Fowler, J.W. & Dell, M.L. (2006) Stages of faith from infancy through adolescence: Reflections on three decades of faith development theory. In: *The Handbook of Spiritual Development in Childhood and Adolescence* (ed. E.C. Roehlkepartain), p. 35. Sage Publication, California.

Fowler, J., Nipkow, K.E. & Schweitzer, F. (eds) (1991) *Stages of Faith and Religious Development: Implications for Church, Education and Society*. Crossroads Press, New York cited in Walker S. (2005) *Culturally Competent Therapy*, pp. 129. Palgrave Macmillan, Basingstoke.

Garamonsway, G.N. (1965) *The Penguin English Dictionary*, p. 677. Penguin Books Ltd., Aylesbury.

Gall, T.L. (2006) Spirituality and coping with life stress among adult survivors of childhood sexual abuse. *Child Abuse and Neglect*, **30**, 829–844.

Garbarino, J. & Bedard, C. (1996) Spiritual challenges to children facing violent trauma. *Childhood*, **3** (4), 467–478.

Grossoehme, D.H., Ragsdale, J.R., McHenry, C.L., Thurston, C., DeWitt, T. & VandeCreek, L. (2007) Pediatrician characteristics associated with attention to spirituality and religion in clinical practice. *Pediatrics*, **119** (1), 117–123.

Hall, J. (2006) Spirituality at the beginning of life. *Journal of Clinical Nursing*, **15**, 804–810.

Harris, S.K., Sherritt, L.R., Holder, D.W., Kulig, J., Shrier, L.A. & Knight, J.R. (2008) Reliability and validity of the brief multidimensional measure of religiousness/spirituality among adolescents. *Journal of Religion and Health*, **47**, 438–457.

Hedayat, K. (2006) When the spirit leaves: Childhood death, grieving, and bereavement in Islam. *Journal of Palliative Medicine*, **9** (6), 1282–1291.

Henderson, V. (2006) The concept of nursing. *Journal of Advanced Nursing*, **53** (1), 21–34.

Hickey, D., Doyle, C., Quinn, S., O'Driscoll, P., Patience, D., Chittick, K. & Cliverd, A. (2008) 'Catching' the concept of spiritual care: Implementation of an education programme. *International Journal of Palliative Nursing*, **14** (8), 39–400.

Hodge, D.R. (2000) Spiritual ecomaps: A new diagrammatic tool for assessing marital and family spirituality.

Journal of Marital and Family Therapy, **26** (2), 217–228 quoted in Tanyi, R. (2006) Spirituality and family nursing. *Journal of Advanced Nursing*, **53** (3), 287–294.

Kegan, R. (1994) In over our heads: The mental demands of modern life Cambridge, MA Harvard cited in Mountain, V. (2007) Educational contexts for the development of children's spirituality: Exploring the use of imagination. *International Journal of Children's Spirituality*, **12** (2), 191–205.

Kenny, G. & Ashley, M. (2005) Children's student nurses' knowledge of spirituality and its implications for educational practice. *Journal of Child Health Care*, **9** (3), 174–185.

Kinchin, D. & Brown, E. (2001) *Supporting Children with Post Traumatic Stress Disorder*. David Fulton Publishers, London.

Lundmark, M. (2006) Attitudes to spiritual care among nursing staff in a Swedish oncology clinic. *Journal of Clinical Nursing*, **15**, 863–874.

Mason, G. (1995) Conceptual frameworks for planning care. In: *Child Health Care Nursing* (eds B. Carter & A. Dearmun). Blackwell Science, Oxford.

Mason-Whitehead, E., Mcintosh, A., Bryan, A. & Mason, T. (2008) *Key Concepts in Nursing*. Sage, London.

McEvoy M. (2000) An added dimension to the pediatric health maintenance visit: The spiritual history. *Journal of Pediatric Health Care*, **14** (5), 216–220 quoted in Tanyi, R. (2006) Spirituality and family nursing. *Journal of Advanced Nursing*, **53** (3), 287–294.

McEvoy, M. (2003) Culture and spirituality as an integrated concept in pediatric care *Am J Maternal/Child Nurs* **28** (1), 39–43 cited in Sexson, S. B. (2004) Religious and spiritual assessment of the child and adolescent *Child and Adolescent Psychiatric Clinics of North America*, **13** (1), 35–47.

McSherry, W. & Jolley, S. (2009) Meeting the spiritual needs of children and families. In: *Palliative Care for Children and Families* (eds J. Price & P. McNeilly) Palgrave, Houndmills.

Menagi, F.S., Harrell, Z.A. & June, L.N. (2008) Religiousness and college student alcohol use: Examining the role of social support. *Journal of Religion and Health*, **47**, 217–226.

Milne, A.A. (1924) *When We Were Very Young*. Methuen, London.

Miner-Williams, D. (2005) putting a puzzle together: Making spirituality meaningful for nursing using an evolving theoretical framework. *Journal of Clinical Nursing*, **15**, 811–821.

Moncher, F.J. & Josephson, A.M. (2004) Religious and spiritual aspects of family assessment. *Child and Adolescent Psychiatric Clinics of North America*, **13** (1), 49–70.

Maugans, T.A. (1996) The spiritual history. *Archives of Family Medicine* **5**, 11–16 quoted in Tanyi, R. (2006)

Spirituality and family nursing. *Journal of Advanced Nursing*, **53** (3), 287–294.

Mountain, V. (2007) *Educational Contexts for the Development of Children's Spirituality: Exploring the Use of Imagination International Journal of Children's Spirituality*, **12** (2), 191–205.

Nagel, E. & Sgoutas-Emch, S. (2007) The relationship between spirituality, health beliefs, and health behaviours in college students. *Journal of Religion and Health*, **46** (1), 141–154.

Narayanasamy, A. (2006) The impact of empirical studies of spirituality and culture on nurse education. *Journal of Clinical Nursing*, **15**, 840–851.

Pargament, K.I. & Brant, C.R. (1998) Religion and coping. In: *Handbook of Religion and Mental Health* (ed. H.G. Koenig). Academic Press, San Diego quoted by Gall, T.L. (2006) Spirituality and coping with life stress among adult survivors of childhood sexual abuse. *Child Abuse and Neglect*, **30**, 829–844, 840.

Pfund, R. (2005) Our little baby brother. *Critical Reflection RLO* (Reusable Learning Objective under development by the University of Nottingham).

Pfund, R. (2007) *Palliative Care Nursing of Children and Young People*. Radcliffe Publishing, Oxford.

Price, S., Lake, M., Breen, G., Carson, G., Quinn, C. & O'Connor, T. (2007) The spiritual experience of high risk pregnancy. *AWHONN The Association of Women's Health, Obstetrics and Neonatal Nurses*, **36** (1), 63–70.

Robinson, M.R., Thiel, M.M., Backus, M.M. & Meyer, E.C. (2006) Matters of spirituality at the end of life in the pediatric intensive care unit. *Pediatrics*, **118** (3), 719–729.

Sexson, S.B. (2004) Religious and spiritual assessment of the child and adolescent. *Child and Adolescent Psychiatric Clinics of North America*, **13** (1), 35–47.

St Exupery, A. (1947) *The Little Prince*. Picollo, London.

St Thomas, B. & Johnson, P. (2007) *Empowering Children through Art and Expression*. Jessica Kingsley, London.

Tanyi, R.A. (2002) Towards clarification of the meaning of spirituality: Nursing theory and concept development or analysis. *Journal of Advanced Nursing*, **39** (5), 500–509.

Tanyi, R. (2006) Spirituality and family nursing. *Journal of Advanced Nursing*, **53** (3), 287–294.

Tjale, A. & Bruce, J. (2007) A concept analysis of holistic nursing care in paediatric nursing. *Curationis*, **30** (4), 45–52.

Van Leeuwen, R. & Cusveller, B. (2004) Nursing competencies for spiritual care. *Journal of Advanced Nursing*, **48** (3), 234–246.

Von Dras, D.D., Smith, R.R. & Marx, D. (2007) Associations between aspects of spiritual well-being, alcohol use,

and related social-cognitions in female college students. *Journal of Religion and Health*, **46**, 500–515.

Waldron, S. (2007) The significance of the emergence of language and symbol in the development of the young infant. *Journal of Religion and Health*, **46** (1), 85–98.

Wagnener, L.M. & Newton Malony, H. (2006) Spiritual and religious pathology in childhood and adolescence. In: *The Handbook of Spiritual Development in Childhood and Adolescence* (ed. E.C. Roehlkepartain). Sage Publication, California.

Walker, S. (2005) *Culturally Competent Therapy*. Palgrave Macmillan, Basingstoke.

Walters, D. (2008) Grief and loss: Towards an existential phenomenology of child spirituality. *International Journal of Children's Spirituality*, **13** (3), 277–286.

Weeding, P. (2010) Transitions within acute care settings: The chaplain's perspective. In: *Perspectives on Palliative Care for Children and Young People – A Global Discourse* (eds R. P fund & S. Fowler-Kerry). Radcliffe Publishing, Oxford.

Wilkinson, J.M. (2000) *Nursing Diagnosis Handbook with NIC Interventions and NIC Outcomes*, 7th edn. Prentice Hall Health, Upper Saddle River, NJ. Quoted in Tanyi, R. (2006) Spirituality and family nursing. *Journal of Advanced Nursing*, **53** (3), 287–294.

Wilford, G. (2008) On the KOSH. *Talk About Change*. The Kosh, London.

Wintersgill, B. (2008) Teenagers' perception of spirituality – A research report. *International Journal of Children's Spirituality*, **13** (4), 371–378.

Wolff, T. & Browne, J. (2010) Minimizing crisis points in paediatric palliative care: The ACT care pathways in action. In: *Perspectives on Palliative Care for Children and Young People – A Global Discourse* (eds R. Pfund & S. Fowler-Kerry). Radcliffe Publishing, Oxford.

Wyatt Nelms, L., Hutchins, E. & Pursley, R.J. (2006) Spirituality and the health of college students. *Journal of Religion and Health*, **46** (2), 249–265.

Yust, K.M. (2007) Childhood and spiritual wisdom: Constructing a critical conversation for the 21st century. *International Journal of Children's Spirituality*, **12** (1), 5–8.

Web sites

http://www.childrenspirituality.org/

http://wordnetweb.princeton.edu/perl/webwn?s= spirituality

http://www.livingwordsofwisdom.com/definition-of-spirituality.html

http://www.livingwordsofwisdom.com/new-age-spirituality.html

http://en.wikipedia.org/wiki/Spirituality
http://www.search-institute.org/spiritual-development
http://www.spiritualdevelopmentcenter.org/Display.
    asp?Page=DefinitionUpdate
http://www.childrenspirituality.org/support/projects/
    spiritualitydays.asp
http://family.jrank.org/pages/413/Divorce.html
http://www.dcsf.gov.uk/everychildmatters/strategy/
    deliveringservices1/caf/cafframework/
http://www.dcsf.gov.uk/everychildmatters/
http://psychology.about.com/od/developmental
    psychology/a/kohlberg.htm

Suggested further readings

Feudtner, C., Haney, J. & Dimmers, M. (2003) Spiritual
    care needs of hospitalized children and their families:
    A national survey of pastoral care providers' percep-
    tions. *Pediatrics*, **111** (1), e67–72.
Roehlkepartain, E.C. (2006) *The Handbook of Spiritual
    Development in Childhood and Adolescence.* Sage
    Publication, Thousand Oaks, California.
http://www.search-institute.org/spiritual-development
http://www.google.co.uk/search?hl=en&q=search+inst
    itute+spirituality&btnG=Search&meta=

'Are you Sitting Comfortably?' Storytelling and the Power of Narratives – A Philosophical Analysis

19

Gosia M. Brykczyńska

Introduction

The aim of this chapter is to demonstrate that as an interactive species, humans are a people of the narrative: shaped, formed and healed by a narrative tradition. We are not only recognised as being *homo viator* and *homo creator* – that is, an ever-evolving, changing and developing people (literally translated as people of the way and creative people) capable of creating new realities and possibilities for ourselves and others, but also as *homo narrator* (literally translated as people of the story or people of the word) – that is, reflective, listening people. We have within our human make-up the hard-wired capacities for reflection and for being wise – hence, among other reasons, the more popular term of *homo sapiens* for our species (literally translated as *the reflective, thinking people* or *the wise people*). Moreover, one of the characteristics of truly wise people is that they are inherently good at listening to others; *really* listening and connecting with other people's narratives (Armstrong 1999; Whiting 2000; Westberg 2003).

This penultimate chapter in the book will consider to what extent we are truly listening and understanding what the child and young person have to say to us, through the stories they tell, to the stories they read and the stories that we need to learn to listen to in the course of our work. Pelander *et al.* (2006) note that much lip service is given to listening to children, but that in fact we know very little about the effect of the care we provide to children from a *child's* perspective; among other reasons because we do not listen to what children have to say – or because we don't know how to listen and hear what children have to say – something also brought up by Duncan Randall in Chapter 20.

It needs to be recognised that it is common these days to see the use of the term *narrative* applied to anything which is presented in the written or spoken form – involving the use of words – from clinical notes to newspaper reports to computer entries and many types of research studies. However, experts who have been studying and commenting upon the nature of the phenomenon of narrative and narrative-generation – especially in the context of child development – dispute this overly common usage (Pollinghorne 1988; McCabe & Peterson 1991; Cortazzi 1993; Engle 1995; Wright 1995; Stein & Albro 1997; Murphy 2000; Scarlett *et al.* 2005). As long ago as 1991, McCabe and Peterson queried the overly common use of the

Ethical and Philosophical Aspects of Nursing Children, First Edition. Edited by Gosia M. Brykczyńska and Joan Simons.
© 2011 Blackwell Publishing Ltd. Published 2011 by Blackwell Publishing Ltd.

word *narrative* and pointed out that since '… narration is fundamentally a collaborative activity' between the narrator and the listener, science and medical reports and patients' notes really do not fulfil the criteria (McCabe & Peterson 1991:xv). For these scholars, a narrative needs to engage with the reader or the listener and involves an obligatory creative dialogue between the reader or the listener, the storyteller and the story itself – something beautifully brought out in Carter's study of children in pain and their questioned and/or unheeded stories (Carter 2004). The interactive dialogue between the story, the storyteller and the story-listener is considered essential if we accept within the definition of a true narrative that the end result of the activity is to be a new story – a new creative reality (Carter 2004; DeSocio 2005). It is also a given that all true narratives will contain within themselves not only the explanatory understandings of the present story but also the predictive seeds of an unfolding future one. The term narrative is used in this way by child psychologists, educationalists and health-care workers when they employ narratives while working with autistic, troubled, distressed or language-impaired children among many others (Wright 2002; Carter 2004; Skarakis-Doyle & Dempsey 2008).

A narrative is a story which is told with and for a purpose; it is based in time and has a context, has clear internal structures and coherence and above all else is *only true* to its potential when it engages the listener or reader in a creative dialogue of recall and reflection with the narrator (Carter 2004; Skarakis-Doyle & Dempsey 2008). In this chapter, I will be using the term narrative in this sense, as the focus of the chapter is the analysis and understanding of the nature of narratives – our own narratives, those borrowed and those adopted as well as those employed by children.

Finally, it is within our intellectual capacities as humans to be able to consider the narratives of our lives, that is, to reflect on the stories of our lives. We can also generate a hypothetical life-narrative from our imagination, that is, a piece of fiction – something we will examine later in this chapter. We need above all else to accept that our own lives can be conceptualised as a narrative and that in getting to understand and accept the trajectory of our lives we are in fact, however unconsciously, putting together *the script* of our life-narrative

(Coles 1989; Korn 1998). Moreover, the outward-oriented form of my *life-narrative* is expressed in the public telling and enactment of my personal life-tale. A life-narrative is therefore nothing less than the social reflection of the privately internalised *story-of-my-life*. When I tell *my narrative*, therefore, I assume that more than just a sequence of events will be listened to, since I have in the process also revealed something about myself which is precious, unrepeatable but also non-retractable. Just as my life cannot be retracted so my tale is non-negotiable and permanent. It is here to stay. It reflects who I am.

The context of the narrative

Trisha Greenhalgh in her 2006 study about patients' tales explains to health-care professionals the main points of the scholarly literature on the subject of *telling stories*. She refers to and elaborates upon the various perspectives that narratives may take. I will base much of my analysis of storytelling on her categorisations of narratives, since in the main, she was looking at and commenting upon stories as they occur in a health-care context, a perspective that well suits our present needs.

Firstly, let us examine the context of storytelling and the genre of storytelling as this analytical process may shed some light on our quest. Trisha Greenhalgh (2006) observes, 'All narratives, although on one level personal and specific, are on another level a reflection of a particular society with a particular set of norms and values; p7'. We need therefore to acknowledge and appreciate, before anything else is said, that all narratives are embedded in a specific time frame and reflect a particular socio-cultural context – something already noted and commented upon in Chapter 1. In a recent book about children requiring palliative care and their experiences with the health services, a father tells his story about his disabled daughter, Sarah. The father, who is a First Nation Canadian, is striving to explain the story of his daughter's life (Brykczynska 2010). He is acutely aware of the cultural and social context in which he is living out his own and his daughter's tale, and he notes 'My perspective on wellness is influenced by the circle concept in my indigenous culture … The value of one is the value of all.

Failure to affirm the value of the unwell fails to affirm the value of society'. This echoes Greenhalgh's (2006) comment that '... in order to understand ... we need also to understand the "works" into which the spanner is thrown ...' p. 6. The father is well aware of this and is at pains to explain precisely this in his narrative. He is concerned that we correctly appreciate his spiritual and cultural heritage so that we can better understand and appreciate the true nature of the moral values which he professes and which guide his social interactions and give meaning to his tale.

Narratives forms

Stories as a form of representative narratives can be analysed according to their predominant themes and approaches, even according to the motivation for their telling. A *referential perspective* is one where a story is written or told basically as a report of what happened, that is, it refers back to an event which it is attempting to describe and evaluate. This type of story, unless woven into other aspects of our lives, can be superficial and the least rich in detail. It is used quite a bit, however, on an everyday basis when we are describing and recording relatively straightforward, factual and sequential events of our lives. But even here, as any historian and psychoanalyst would say, the really interesting aspect of the exercise would be to examine what is not being said in the narrative, the very order of recording the facts, the context in which the description is being offered, who is the report or narrative intended for, and so on. Even a simple story about going to the shops and tripping on a flagstone requiring hospitalisation carries within itself potential richness of insights and life-enhancing reflections!

Other stories may represent a *transformational perspective* where the story itself has the power to change what has occurred and the recounting is once again potentially transformative. Transformational stories may not only change the perceived significance of the event recounted but may also change the perspective of the storyteller and, in some cases, even the perspective of the listener. A moving account of a young boy's transformation after engaging with a transformational narrative – in this case a piece of fiction – is explained to us by Coles (1989). The narrative makes a powerful statement about the capacity for literature to change our lives. The story is about Phil (a real youngster from Boston, MA) who succumbed to the polio virus, and one of his 'softie' teachers (as the young boy describes him) who paid him a visit in the hospital and left him a copy of Mark Twain's *Huckleberry Finn* to read. Initially, Phil is not taken by the book and does not even feel the need to read it, but somehow he forces himself to read the first few pages (after all the teacher will come back and it's good to be able to say that one has read at least some of the book...). After slowly and laboriously reading a few pages the youngster said:

> ... I didn't want to stop. I read and I read, and I finished the whole book that night ... The nurse kept coming in to tell me I should put my light off and go to sleep because I needed my rest. What a joke! Are you kidding? I said to her. I'm going nowhere. I will be in bed for the rest of my life.
>
> (Coles 1989:35)

This experience of reading a book right through the night is something generations of children (and adults) have experienced and it is an enduring testament to the power of the written word that some texts can engross us to such an extent. In a similar manner contemporary children and young people have become riveted to the adventures of Harry Potter (Rowling 1997), confirming the observation that some narratives have the capacity to engage and absorb our attention totally. In popular language these books are called *page-turners*. Moreover, even when we have finished reading the book its message may linger in our mind as we process what we have read and engage with the story. Indeed, we have not finished with a book until we have thoroughly digested the tale and rearranged the furniture of our minds to accommodate the new visitors – the new concepts. As Phil noted:

> I couldn't get my mind off the book ... I joined up with Huck and Jim, we became a trio. They were very nice to me. I explored the Mississippi with them on the boats and on the land. I had some good talks with them ... they straightened me out.
>
> (Coles 1989:36)

Transformative stories are stories that have that power to straighten you out – to change you, to transform you. The story, however, may have a positive effect on a reader or a negative influence since in combination with our engagement with the text, it can influence us in a variety of ways. As Don Cupitt observes in his work on narratives and their power to influence us, 'the moral influence of stories for good and ill is ubiquitous' (Cupitt 1991:32).

While being affected and touched by the content of a book is generally considered to be a positive factor in the moral and social development of children, there is a noticeable recent increase in the level of censorship of contemporary children's literature, especially in the USA (Atkins & Mintcheva 2007). Whereas no one wishes children and young people to read gratuitously violent books or books with inaccurate content, the question society has to grapple with is, 'Who decides what is permissible for children to read and indeed what is desirable for children to read?' Cupitt is rather uncertain about the merits of literary censorship, noting that such efforts in centuries past had left children and young women '… weak, ignorant and vulnerable to exploitation' (Cupitt 1991:33). Sooner or later children want to know 'the full story' and they rightfully feel cheated and let down when they realise that they were not presented with all the facts or with less than the truth, or with a pink-tinted perspective of the world which turns out to be an illusion. Children and adults can accommodate fables, fiction and fantasy; they are on the other hand unforgiving of being served half-truths and misinformation. It is, however, the process of *reflection* upon a narrative and the *personal engagement* with the tale that is the operative catalyst – it is that activity which facilitates change in the reader. Meanwhile, Phil relates to Coles his reflections about himself:

> … I've seen a lot, lying here. I think I know more about people, including me, myself – all because I got sick and can't walk. … I like those books, and I keep reading them, parts of them, over and over.
> (Coles 1989:39)

In summary, reading and reflecting upon what one reads is one of the best ways to promote transformation and personal development.

A story may even reflect a *performative perspective*, since the story itself may represent a form of action; for example, the story may be enacted in the format of a play, such as one told in the doctor's surgery or in a courtroom as a form of testimonial, or the story itself may be the action, such as in the case of ancient ballads and poems or miracle plays. For some people, the very knowledge and narration of a story is itself a form of social enactment and what can be termed as *emplotment*. Here the storytelling becomes part of the plot itself – both the storyteller and the storyline become entwined and embedded in the unfolding plot. This has been amusingly illustrated in the legendary ballad by Flanders & Swan (1963), *The Gasman Cometh*; as Greenhalgh (2006) observes, 'Talk is not primarily about giving information to a recipient, but about the staging of dramas to an audience … p. 9'. Likewise, the amusing yet powerful poem by Fleur Adcock, *For Heidi with Blue Hair*, well illustrates the nature of an interactive drama and narrative emplotment – in this case, reflecting the life concerns of a contemporary schoolgirl (Adcock 2000:52).

Stories need to reflect internal coherence in order for sense to be made of the facts and the emotions which are recounted. In some instances, authenticity of facts and events may be called into question. Sometimes inconsistencies in the telling of the tale are of no particular consequence, but health- and social-care workers need to practice the art of attentive listening and interpretation, as it is the inconsistencies and lack of authenticity in a tale that are often the only clues to deliberate attempts at alterations of the facts as they are being retold. This caveat, however, in no way alters the validity and richness of the vast majority of tales which, depending on the context in which the tale is being retold and the mood of the storyteller at the time, often do change with each telling and are therefore endlessly embellished.

The professional narrative context

Authenticity of narratives is as much a concern about the authenticity of the content of a tale as about the authenticity and integrity of the storyteller. Could any one person have suffered so much? Is the truth of the tale consistent with the integrity and authenticity of the storyteller (Carter 2004)? Many such stories call for careful attention by the listener if harmony and a sense of purpose are to be restored. The nurse Christensen (1993:130) noted in her monograph on working in partnership with patients, over 15 years ago, that working constructively with the patient '… requires the nurse to be present with the patient, observing, listening and interpreting, in order to identify any inconsistency. Thereafter the nurse is able to use methods to help restore harmony'. This observation still holds true today.

Public narratives

There are even issues concerning the reportability of a tale. Just how *good* is the storyline and its newsworthiness? What are the relative worth and merits of the story being retold and, perhaps more significantly, being retold to whom? The latter is sometimes a point of potential dispute between the narrator and the (occasionally long-suffering) listener or reader. This would have seemed to be the case with an example presented by Dorothy Diers, the past Dean of Yale University School of Nursing. She elaborates upon an incident early in her career as Dean of the school, concerning her attempt to publish an account about the true nature of the nursing profession in the non-professional press (Diers 2004:328). After many refusals to have the piece published, she engaged the help of a journalist friend who in a relatively short period of time enabled her to have the piece published. She comments wryly, '… the point is, this piece didn't work until it got put into a form of narrative that fit the purpose'. Sometimes stories make for a good read or listen, but as already noted, in the process of embellished distortion and alteration in order to fit the taste of a particular readership or audience, they may lose something of their authenticity – and this too has implications for the nature of the tale and its structural and moral integrity.

Persuasive narratives

Stories can also persuade us to undertake certain actions and their persuasiveness can be quite astounding, as the story told by James Robertson about a 2-year-old's trip to the hospital (Bowlby & Robertson 1953). The Robertsons' interaction and engagement with the story of the 2 year old changed forever the way children in the UK were nursed in hospitals. Every time the tale is retold new resolutions are made and new decisions are undertaken to promote better care for children in hospitals. Many significant social events have come about as the result of just such interaction with persuasive stories and this narrative was both persuasive and transformative.

How often have we heard a health worker comment '… that sounds like a very good description of a bout of flue, or a pulled muscle, or of the symptoms of depression, etc.'. The patient's story is so compelling that it has persuaded the health-care worker about some inherent medical truth – not necessarily that apparent even to the storyteller. In such examples, there are aspects of persuasiveness in the patients' stories that have helped in establishing the medical diagnosis! Careful listening to the patient's narrative built up in the mind of the clinician a very clear picture of a particular human condition. The narrative was compelling evidence of a particular disease process, even without clinical tests. This type of medical narrative is engagingly presented to the public in a collection of short stories by Roueché (1991), where the physician or public health official becomes of necessity a superb listener and avid clinical detective if they are to solve the medical mysteries! In a slightly different genre, though no less engrossing, are historical narratives about diseases and medicines such as stories about the plague, or Hansen's disease, or the drug thalidomide or even the humble aspirin or quinine (Rocco 2003; Scott & Duncan 2004). Through the narrative medium, the disease or drug takes on a persona of its own and an otherwise dry account of the paleopathology of a disease comes to life and we are thoroughly engaged with the story.

Examples of the force of a personal narrative to change a situation or to bring something to the attention of the public could be John Diamond's personal account of his life with cancer, written in the form of a public diary and printed in instalments in the national press (Diamond 1999); or the far-reaching effects of the more private diary of young Anne Frank, which brought to the world's attention the typical life of an adolescent girl walled up in a secret hiding place in German-occupied Holland during World War II (Frank 2007); or the Massies' (1967) biographical account of the Imperial Russian family's struggles with their son, Tsarevitch Alexis, who suffered from haemophilia. The book, in turn, prompted the release of a film and the *subsequent* writing of the Massies' own personal narrative about their son, who also had haemophilia (Massie & Suzanne 1975). It was precisely because the Massies' had already written the biography of Tsar Nicholas and his son Alexis that the world was aware of the nature of haemophilia and were therefore primed and prepared to listen to and engage with the authors' own personal story with the disease. This example provides an interesting twist to the usual sequence of events surrounding personal narratives and public writing.

Generative narratives

Finally, the power of a narrative to prompt the creation of something new is evident in the life of Reverend Chad Varah (1911–2007). It was in 1953 that upon listening to a narrative about a 13-year-old girl who committed suicide fearing her impending death and subsequently officiating at her funeral that he was moved to found the organisation *The Samaritans*. The Samaritans can be best described as society's most expert listeners. Chad Varah's work has since passed into social and pastoral history. Interestingly, Chad Varah's own assessment of his Samaritan counsellors is that, '… They give their total attention. They completely forget themselves. They listen and listen and listen, without interrupting. They have no message. They do not preach' (Samaritan's Website; Varah 1993). What started as a a response to one specific, very sad, pastoral narrative about a young girl has resulted today in an organisation which is working in over 40 countries worldwide. There are numerous such examples of the power of narratives and they could be readily multiplied. The important principle to remember is that even a *personal* narrative can be very persuasive on a public arena and can have the potential to be transformative in ways that even the narrator could hardly have imagined. Today, children and young people can call *ChildLine* and other designated confidential telephone lines set up for them, and counsellors are reporting that

there is an ever-growing need for such services. Children want to and need to talk but they are finding it hard to find someone prepared to listen to them.

Healing narratives

Greenhalgh (2006) notes that in some cases stories are actually told in order to somehow come to terms with a painful truth, or to get some feeling of control over an adverse situation or even to help restructure society or an organisation. The art of telling political jokes in communist-occupied central Europe was a particular form of a jibed narrative having the purpose of helping entrapped people recover a sense of control over their enemy; as Greenhalgh (2006) states, '… narrative approaches seek to understand organizations, and also drive change, via the stories told within them and the stories told about them' p. 49. She continues to observe that '… the act of sense making is itself the construction of a narrative, requiring elements to be selected out, highlighted as significant or surprising, juxtaposed with another story' (Greenhalgh 2006:50). This, of course, was very evident in the case of the political joke but is also very apropos of those narratives that are of a potentially therapeutic nature.

In order to come to terms with the story of my life, at the very least I need to have some memories of my life. I only can recall at will those memories which I have, so to speak, memorised. As Gee (1991:3) explains, '… personal memories that are unrehearsed disappear, but to rehearse them means to retell them in a narrative fashion'. This would suggest that I need to keep reminding myself about events in my life and reordering and reclassifying these memories as new ones occur if I wish my recallable narratives to truly reflect my life. It could be argued that if I do not remember something occurring, it cannot have been that significant, but such an idea has only limited validity. It is a well-known phenomenon that we may not be able to consciously recall an event for many years, but as soon as we hear snatches of a particular song, experience the sudden whiff of a specific scent such as cut grass or the smell of the underground or see the sky bathed in a curious luminosity from a late winter sun, we recollect long-forgotten memories through these externally experienced events. All of a sudden we are transposed, literally, onto and into another plane, remembering occurrences which are often referred to in popular language as coming from another lifetime! Indeed. The additional point that Gee is making refers to the notion that the very process of ordering the memories of our lives (and, of course, *memorising* some of those memories) involves the use of language skills and the use of symbolic narrative and metaphor. It is somewhat reassuring that many of our memories are safely stored away in our subconscious and that 'like pictures, our memories can fade, and even disappear altogether, but they cannot radically change' (Gee 1991:1).

Scholars have looked quite closely at these aspects of narrative formation. McCabe and Peterson undertook a large longitudinal study in 1991 examining the effects of parenting style on children's ability to recall events and package them in narrative forms. Much has already been and is still being written about social class and poverty in regards to language acquisition and its use by children and their abilities to tell stories. It is not within the remit of this chapter, however, to elaborate on this developmental task; suffice to say that all children have the potential cognitive abilities to structure and, even more crucially, to restructure their memories and to create their own life-narratives, but that the more rich and creative their vocabularies, the easier the task will be for them. In fact, McCabe & Peterson (1991) noted in their research that the more social interaction the parents had with their child, the better the language skills acquisition of the child and the more sophisticated became the development of structure in the child's narrative. For a child to be able to recount events in a sensible and recreatable narrative fashion, the child needs to have a developed sense of self, time, sequencing of events and purpose. Of course, this also holds true for adults. As Polkinghorne noted, 'Narrative is the fundamental scheme for linking individual human actions and events into interrelated aspects of an understandable composite' (Pollinghorne 1988:13). It brings to mind reflections on the necessary level of narrational skills required of a 4-year-old child to be able to give testimony in the Old Bailey against her rapist (Bennett & Fresco 2009).

Teachers, and more recently nurses, have long realised that among the many results of promoting the use of the narrative form – both spoken and written – is its capacity to help educate the child to foster the exchange of information, its ability to entertain the child and those around and, possibly most importantly, its ability to help the child articulate and share its personal feelings and values (Isbell *et al.* 2004; Rennick *et al.* 2008). When we help children in school or at home to create narratives we do more than just contribute to the promotion of their literacy skills. In encouraging children to tell their stories, we are also helping them to articulate their emotions and feelings, to reflect upon the values and perspectives experienced in their own lives and to appreciate the lives of those around them. We are helping them to be reflective individuals in the present moment and to develop into engaged members of society in the future (Wright 1995). But asking a child to tell us a story presupposes, of course, that there is someone out there who is willing to listen to what the child has to say.

Some narratives, however, are presented in a simply chaotic fashion. This is most likely to be the case where the story is incoherent and unintelligible even to the storyteller. This is often because it is an incomplete story and we are only privy to one aspect of it, or because it is in fact someone else's story – for example, where the narrator is caught up in someone else's narrative and is still trying to find their way. This might occur with the siblings of children with malignancies and is well documented in the professional literature (McGrath 2001; Houtzager *et al.* 2004; Carr-Gregg & White 2006; Woodgate 2006). Or finally, the story may simply represent a muddled mind! We may see this clinically in the narratives of some children who cannot find their place in the world and retreat inwards where they feel more comfortable – for example, autistic children many of whom are being helped via the therapeutic use of storytelling (Dwivedi 1997; Wright 2002). A story may also be chaotic because it is the story of a person who has been profoundly hurt. Frank (1995:98) in a most insightful monograph even goes as far as to query if such people are capable of telling a straightforward narrative:

The teller of chaos stories is preeminently, the wounded storyteller, but those who are truly living the chaos cannot tell in words. To turn the chaos into a verbal story is to have some reflective grasp of it …

Many angry, disillusioned and emotionally disturbed children find reflected in contemporary poetry their innermost thoughts and feelings, as do many other young people. Moreover, children and young people like playing with words and enjoy the pleasures and music of poetry, as the enduring use of nursery rhymes, playground songs and popularity of children's narratives written in poetry attests to (Opie & Opie 2001; Wolf 2006).

Narratives (both in prose and poetry) can serve and reflect a myriad of functions and formats but what they all have in common, to varying degrees, is a sense of drama and action, suspense and engagement and, finally, especially in the clinical context, a recognition of interpersonal humility. To hear other people's stories can be a humbling experience. However, unwittingly, even in the very act of listening to a tale one is intruding in a sacred space – we are intruding into the stranger's world via the narrative. This is so even where there had been an invitation to share the narrative experience.

The imagined narrative

The pleasure of stories, then, is the pleasure of the metaphors that make us intelligent and the metonymies that enable us to live meaningful lives in time.

(Cupitt 1991:15)

Naturally, narrative can also have an aesthetic appeal, and this is most commonly seen in tales of literary merit and tales told specifically for the delight and pleasure of a wider audience and readership. For this reason, the humanities and especially artistic tales are often used to illustrate a particular point about patients and diseases or in the teaching of health-care ethics to nursing and medical students (Darbyshire 1994; Vezeau 1994; Moyle et al. 1995; Stowe & Igo 1996; Brykczynska 1997; Smith et al. 2004). It is debatable whether nursing educators provide enough space for the inclusion of a humanities thread within the curriculum – but there is nothing to stop instructors and leaders of the profession to keep reminding nurses and students to go back to the riches contained in the arts and humanities for insights, relaxation and moral development (Bruderle & Valiga 1994; Moyle et al. 1995; Davis 2003).

Thus, the classical work of Tolstoy, *The Death of Ivan Illych*, or Chekhov's enigmatic short story, *Sleepy-head*, are often cited as facilitating an understanding of the necessary care due to patients and in order to widen student's perspectives and understanding of the virtue of compassion and tolerance (Tolstoy 1960; Chekhov 2002). It is far easier to read tales and remember their message when it is couched in beautiful language; this tends to encourage more reflection than otherwise. This is one of the main reasons for the promotion of literature and the humanities in medical and nursing education (Begley 1995; Brykczynska 1997). What one can read and reflect upon at ease tends to affect us more positively and stay with us longer than ethical and professional imperatives thrown at us during dreary lectures on moral philosophy on a Friday afternoon, something noted by many medical and nursing educators who have tried to introduce more creative ways of teaching health-care ethics and moral development (Corri 2003; Donohoe & Danielson 2004; Shapiro et al. 2005; Davis et al. 2006). Finally, as Greenhalgh (2006:50) observes, stories can serve as both an anchor for issues raised and provide a springboard for further discussion, activities which we are about to examine.

Stories about children

Since it is adults who write stories (even if they are very young adults, like Anne Frank), the narratives which involve children will be written necessarily from an adult perspective. Somehow the adult writer needs to get into the mind of the child and needs to recall what it was like to be a child, think and reason like a child and so on. The better and more insightful the author, the closer to the reality of childhood and adolescence will be the description of children and their affairs (see Chapter 1). In a recent collection of short stories about children and childhood, the novelist Margaret Atwood makes the observation that if adults don't understand certain aspects of children's lives, they will never understand anything – in this case commenting on why children like to make poisons: '... I can remember the glee with which we stirred and added, the sense of magic and accomplishment. Making poison is as much fun as making a cake. People like to make poison ...' (Atwood 2008:3).

It is authors' ability to capture such truths which give credibility to their statements.

Sometimes, author's comment on their own childhood such as Ahlberg's (2007) biography written with both adults and older children in mind, about growing up in England in the 1950s. Here the story is only as authentic as the memories and insights of the author (see Chapter 1). The most commonly encountered narrative is where children are incidental or tangential to the tale, such as in Solzenitsyn's internationally acclaimed biographical novel *Cancer Ward* in which several adolescents with cancer play minor parts in the story but are presented with the same ferocious clarity of detail and sensitive perception as all the other characters (Solzenitsyn 2003).

Occasionally, adults write about children with a specific agenda in mind – for example, to alert readers to the plight of working children or young chimney sweeps; this was the case with the Victorian reformers Charles Kinglesley (1819–1875) and Charles Dickens (1812–1870). Some contemporary books written with the aid of cartoons, although originally aimed at adults, have found a faithful following among children and young people also, for example, the *Asterix* series by Goscinny and Uderzo (2004).

Meanwhile, stories written specifically with children in mind have been found to be delightful and thoughtful also for adults – as in the case of *Alice in Wonderland* (Carroll 1998) or *The Wind in the Willows* by Grahame (2008). Wilde (2001) wrote several very touching and memorable short stories for children such as *The Happy Prince*, which many adults also find moving and highly readable.

Occasionally books for adults, such as *The Three Musketeers* by Alexandre Dumas, *The Scarlett Pimpernel* by Baroness Orczy and various other detective stories, are also read by children, albeit older children and young people (Orczy 2002; Dumas 2008). Likewise, no one would want to stop an adolescent from reading Saint Exupery's *The Little Prince* or Leo Tolstoy's *War and Peace* or Victor Hugo's *The Hunchback of Notre Dame* – none of which were written specifically with young people in mind! Today young people like to read biographies of their heroes (celebrities), which again are not necessarily written with these young people in mind – a fact which sometimes gives rise

for concern among parents, as has already been noted (St Exupery 1995; Hugo 2007; Tolstoy 2007).

Stories for children

Adults also write stories specifically for children, either targeting particular age groups with special messages such as illustrated storybooks on potty training (Bedford and Worthington 2009; Genechlen 2009), or better eating habits (e.g. *The Very Hungry Caterpillar* (Carle 1995)) or helping the child adjust to going to hospital or to school for the first time (e.g. *Curious George Goes to Hospital* (Ray & Ray 1995) and Child's (2004) *I Am Absolutely Too Small for School*). Sometimes they simply write a tale that they know will appeal to children as it illustrates the very *spots-of-bother* the children themselves often get up to, such as the tales of *Paddington Bear* by Michael Bond (Bond 2007) or the Seuss's (2003) *Cat in the Hat*.

Additionally, a truly good story written for children will also often find sympathetic echoes in the adult psyche, and this is most likely to be the case where the book is read aloud to the child by an adult. Stories such as *Alexander and the Terrible, Horrible, No Good, Very Bad Day* by Judith Viorst resonates well among many if not most adults who read the story to their children! Meanwhile, Dr Seuss's *Cat in the Hat* stories are perceived as delightful fantasy – but situated just safely enough within familiar territory – since which child has not left a mess in the dining room or knocked over that precious plant or, God forbid, overfed the fishes (Viorst 1987). Here is a cathartic tale all children have waited for and the fact that the tale is most often recounted to them by their parents is not lost on them either. But even here the narratives, however outlandish and absurdly superficial, always have a gentle moral message, such as the message of faithfulness and loyalty in *Horton Hatches an Egg* (Seuss 2004). Such stories present truths and values to children in small, amusing and palatable doses. Dr Seuss's (Theodore Seuss Geisel 1904–1991) memorable poem *Oh the Places You'll Go* originally written in 1957 is probably as stirring as Kipling's poem *If* – which is one of the nation's favourite poems, according to the *BBC Poetry Please* series (Seuss 1990; Kipling 2001). Dr Seuss comments wisely to the children in the rambling ballad, and it is rightfully considered a modern classic.

These poems and tales are written specifically to help children adjust to the adult world and very often to help them form (unapologetically) sustainable and appropriate value systems, which they do since the child so readily engages with the narrative (Guroian 1998). Reading aloud is a great skill and a wonderful art well worth fostering, one which many parents become quite adept at. Even the weary readings of an exhausted parent or carer will be happily listened to by children tucked up in bed, hanging on every last word. Children explore and come to understand their world by firstly looking, then tasting and finally listening, and they become very good at listening – something any carer or parent will attest to when a favourite tale or poem is misquoted or a page missed out or something inadvertently added. In a delightful response to a letter from some children, Lewis wrote: 'I have done lots of dish-washing in my time and I have often been read to, but I never thought of your very sensible idea of doing both together. How many plates do you smash in a month?' (Lewis 1986:39).

Authors may also write for children about serious issues. Wilson (2009) in her books about *Hetty Feather* (the totally disorganised and scatty chambermaid) brings to the attention of contemporary children the plight of previous generations of young girls who had no choice (especially if orphaned and/or abandoned) but to be sent to foundling hospitals and then into 'service' (see Chapter 1). Here, the author is retelling the story for today's children about the Foundling Hospital in central London which was supported by philanthropists and activists like the painter Hogarth (1697–1764) and Captain Thomas Coram (1668–1751). To this day, adults can only enter Coram Fields Garden if accompanied by a child – and there lies yet another tale. Likewise, Michael Morpurgo's book – *The Amazing Story of Adolphus Tips* – about a cat, a young girl and the effects of war on a sleepy English village is a recent story with a recognisable moral content, which is fast becoming a great success with children (Morpurgo 2005).

There is (in almost all European countries) a genre of narrative written for older children and adolescents, specifically about their lives. Such tales in English include classics like *Little Lord Fauntleroy* and *Ballet Shoes* to *Just William* stories

and the girl-oriented equivalents like Elinor M. Brent-Dyer's and Angela Brazil's stories about life in girls' boarding schools and the many Enid Blyton series such as *Mallory Towers* – all of which are being reprinted and are making a literary comeback (Burnett 1994; Crompton 1999; Streatfield 2004; Blyton 2006; Buckeridge 2009). These stories have a new generation of followers and captivate the young reader and for a while, transporting them into another safer world, where the heroes and heroines are normal children like themselves and where goodness and social justice usually prevail – not that dissimilar in essence to the more contemporary *Harry Potter* stories and other fantasy tales, very many of which are geared specifically at young people.

There are, of course, modern narratives written for adolescents looking at contemporary issues. In the past, premature death and abandonment were real issues for children and were widely addressed in children's literature, while today events at school, parental divorce, bullying over the internet and lifestyle issues may be the young person's concern, and so, alongside the old classics, are new books like Elizabeth's Scott's *Stealing Heaven*, about a young person who shoplifts, or Siobhan Dowd's *Solace of the Road* about a runaway teenager or the powerful story about a young person's impending death by Jenny Downham (Downham 2008; Dowd 2009). Ahlberg (1991) in a collection of whimsical but very poignant poems addresses just such contemporary issues for the younger child while the rap poet Bejamin Zephaniah articulates them for the adolescent. Zephaniah writes:

> I used to think nurses
> Were women
> I used to think police
> were men,
> I used to think poets
> Were boring,
> Until I became one of them.
> (Zephaniah 1995:48)
> © Benhamin Zephaniah 1995

Increasingly, books and poems are trying to help children cope in what for many of them is a very strange and all-too-often (unfortunately) malignant world. Reading these narratives not only helps children to come to terms with their lives but also helps in shaping those lives and stepping out of stereotypes. As Marian Whitehead notes: 'Narrative is concerned with values and choices and most typically speculates on the human condition' (Whitehead 2002:32). Cupitt, on the other hand, noted that some powerful children's stories '... concentrate especially on preparing children to cope with the cruelty and incomprehensibly malignant power-games of adults' (Cupitt 1991:14).

As in the past, children still find safety and solace in the natural world around them, and many a child's tale is told through the lives and adventures of animals. This was the case in Rudyard Kipling's *Just so Stories*. New classics are *Charlotte's Web* by White, which was first published in 1952, and *Stuart Little*, which was published in 1945, both of which have been recently made into films (White 2007). In *Charlotte's Web*, Wilbur the piglet says of Charlotte the spider:

> ... I got a new friend all right ... Charlotte is fierce, brutal, scheming, bloodthirsty – everything I don't like. How can I learn to like her?
> (White 1963:39)

It is working through these allegorical narrative relationships which help younger children face up to the realities in the world outside of their bedrooms. The classic story of self-sacrifice in the *The Giving Tree*, which is aimed at older children (and the child in each adult), by Silverstein (1964) or Lewis' *Narnia* series (Lewis 2004) both attest to the fact that children (and adults) enjoy tales told in an allegorical fashion and on the whole have no problem sorting out metaphors and allegories – as CS Lewis observed in a letter to a child: '... It is a funny thing that all the children who have written to me see at once who Aslan is, and grown-ups never do' (Lewis 1986:114). Sometimes stories are simply whimsical tales about creatures and people who represent nothing else but themselves, such as the river bank creatures in *Wind in the Willows*. As Lewis replied to another fan: '... You are mistaken when you think that everything in the books "*represents*" something in this world. Things do that in The Pilgrim's Progress but I am not writing in that way' (Lewis 1986:44).

It is interesting to note that parents introduce their children to books and stories which they themselves enjoyed reading as a child and adoles-

cent – thus embedding even more certain stories into the cultural myths of a country, which in turn helps to shape the social values and mores of a people (Guroian 1998). Finally, many if not most of the stories and poems written for children and young people are richly decorated and much of the power of the narratives lies in the beauty of the illustrations. The world of children's literature is by far the richer for the illustrations of Quinton Blake and it is almost impossible to conceptualise the life of the river animals in the *Wind in the Willows* without the fine drawings of E. H. Shephard. As is well appreciated, many pictures have a narrative quality to them and children and young people are taught not only to appreciate art through the medium of translating these narrative pictures, but they also learn to get in touch with their emotions when describing these paintings, pictures and illustrations. Certainly, for many years now narrative art has been used with children to help them articulate their worries and concerns and to help them come to terms with the world in which they live.

Conclusion

The stranger's story (this includes narrative fiction) would appear to change its focus in the process of being told and in the course of its very retelling can start to become a reflection of *everyman's* story. It is the process of telling and retelling of a narrative which begins to give meaning to *my* life events, *my* story. Narratives are transformative not only for the narrator of the original story but also for those who are engaged in listening to and reflecting upon the story. It is the curative and restorative power of narratives that keep children and young people reading and reflecting on what they have read.

We have examined in this chapter the extent to which being in touch with our own unfolding life-narratives through stories and written tales has the potential to bring about change and personal growth, as much as it facilitates the social and moral development of children and young people. However, as noted, in order to be able to be in touch with the narratives of our lives – which is a prerequisite to understanding other people's lives – we need to learn how to listen and learn how to interpret the dramas of our own unfolding life-narrative. Interacting and engaging with metaphors, allegories and fables can help us achieve this end, something more commonly undertaken with children than with adults and maybe something that needs to be addressed and re-examined (Bettelheim 1976; Coles 1989; Dwivedi 1997). It is clear that we need to listen to ourselves and our personal narratives in the first instance if we are to be able to listen to and understand others, especially children, who are far more insightful and perceptive than most adults give them credit for (Lewis 1986; Carter 2004).

In the meantime, we need to ask ourselves are we in fact truly listening to children's narratives? We will learn nothing about children if we do not learn how to listen and engage in their life's dialogue. Perhaps, therefore, the real questions to ask ourselves should be, do we really wish to know about children and do we really wish to be a wise people? As Cupitt points out 'To learn about all this is to learn a practical wisdom of life – and that is what stories teach' (Cupitt 1991:21).

References

Adcock, F. (2000) For Heidi with Blue Hair. In: *The Nations Favourite Poems of Childhood*, (ed. A. Warwick). BBC Worldwide Ltd., London.

Ahlberg, A. (1991) *Heard it in the Playground*. Puffin Books, London.

Ahlberg, A. (2007) *The Boyhood of Burglar Bill*. Penguin/Puffin Bks. Ltd., London.

Armstrong, M. (1999) Face to face with child abuse: Towards an ethics of listening. *Law & Critique*, **10** (2), 147–173.

Atkins, R. & Mintcheva, S. (2007) *Censoring Culture – Contemporary Threats to Free Expression*. The New Press, New York.

Atwood, M. (2008) Making Poison p3. In: *The Children's Hours – Stories of Childhood*, (eds R. Zimler & R. Sekulović). Arcadia Books Ltd., London.

Bedford, D. & Worthington, L. (2009) *Potty Time*. Little Hare Publ., Surry Hills, NSW.

Begley, A.M. (1995) Literature, ethics and the communication of insight. *Nursing Ethics*, **2**, 287–294.

Bennett, R. & Fresco, A. (2009) Trial ordeal of girl, 4. *The Saturday Times*, 2 May 2009, p. 1.

Bettelheim, B. (1976) *The Uses of Enchantment: The Meaning and Importance of Fairy Tales*. Alfred A Knopf, New York.

Blyton, E. (2006) *Mallory Towers*. Egmont Books, London.

Bond, M. (2007) *Paddington Bear*. Harper Collins Children's Books, London.

Bowlby, J. & Robertson, J. (1953) A film preview; (Nov 28 1952) – A two-year-old goes to hospital. *Proceedings of the Royal Society of Medicine*, **46** (6), 425–437.

Bruderle, E.R. & Valiga, T.M. (1994) Integrating the arts and humanities into nursing education. In: *Art and Aesthetics in Nursing* (eds P.L. Chinn & J. Watson), pp. 117–144. National League for Nursing, New York.

Brykczyńska, G. (1997) Art and literature nursing's distant mirror? In: *Caring – The Compassion and Wisdom of Nursing* (ed G. Brykczyńska), pp. 35–70. Edward Arnold Publ., London.

Brykczyńska, G. (2010) Commentary on a father's tale. In: *Palliative Care of Children and Young People*. (eds R. Pfund & S. Kerry-Fowler). Radcliffe Publ., Abingdon.

Buckeridge, A. (2009) *The Best of Jennings*. Prion Books, London.

Burnett, F. (1994) *Little Lord Fauntleroy*. Puffin Classics, London.

Carle, E. (1995) *The Very Hungry Caterpillar*. Puffin Books, London.

Carr-Gregg, M. & L. White (2006) Siblings of paediatric cancer patients: A population at risk. *Medical and Pediatric Oncology*, **15** (2), 62–68.

Carroll, L. (1998) *Alice's Adventures in Wonderland*. Penguin Classics, London.

Carter, B. (2004) Pain narratives and narrative practitioners: A way of working 'in-relation' with children experiencing pain. *Journal of Nursing Management*, **12** (3), 210–216.

Chekhov, A. (2002) *Forty Stories*. Vintage Classics/Random Hse, New York.

Child, L. (2004) *I am Absolutely too Small for School*. Orchard Publ., London.

ChildLine, www.childline.org.uk.

Christensen, J. (1993) *Nursing Partnership – A Model for Nursing Practice*. Churchill Livingstone, Edinburgh.

Coles, R. (1989) *The Call of Stories – Teaching and Moral Imagination*. Houghton Mifflin Company, Boston, MA.

Corri, C. (2003) Medical humanities in nurse education. *Nursing Standard*, **17** (33), 38–40.

Cortazzi, M. (1993) Literary models of narrative. In: *Narrative Analysis*, pp. 84–99. Routledge Falmer Press, London.

Crompton, R. (1999) *Just William*. Macmillan Children Books, London.

Cupitt, D. (1991) *What Is a Story?* SCM Press, London.

Darbyshire, P. (1994) Understanding caring through arts and humanities: A medical/nursing approach to promoting alternative experiences of thinking and learning. *Journal of Advanced Nursing*, **19**, 856–863.

Davis, C. (2003) Nursing humanities: The time has come. *American Journal of Nursing*, **103** (2), 13.

Davis, A.J., Tschudin, V. & de Raeve, L. (2006) *Essentials of Teaching and Learning in Nursing Ethics – Perspectives and Methods*. Churchill Livingstone/Elsevier, Edinburgh.

DeSocio, J. (2005) Accessing self-development through narrative approaches in child and adolescent psychotherapy. *Journal of Child & Adolescent Psychiatric Nursing*, **18** (2), 53–61.

Diamond, J. (1999) *Because Cowards Get Cancer Too*. Vermillion Publ./Random Hse, London.

Diers, D. (2004) *Speaking of Nursing: Narratives of Practice, Research, Policy and the Profession*, Jones Bartlett Publ., Sudbury, Massachusetts.

Dwivedi, K.N. (ed.) (1997) *The Therapeutic Use of Stories*. Routledge, London.

Donohoe, M. & Danielson, S. (2004) A community-based approach to the medical humanities. *Medical Education*, **38**, 204–217.

Dowd, S. (2009) *Solace of the Road*. David Fickling Books, Oxford.

Downham, J. (2008) *Before I die*. David Fickling Books, Oxford.

Dumas, A. (2008) *The Three Musketeers*. Penguin Classics, London.

Engle, S. (1995) *The Stories Children Tell: Making Sense of the Narratives of Childhood*. W H Freeman/Henry Holt &Co., New York.

Flanders, M. & Swann, D. (1963) Record. *The Best of Flanders and Swann: A Transport of Delight*, EMI Records, Audio CD.

Frank, A.W. (1995) *The Wounded Storyteller: Body, Illness, and Ethics*. University of Chicago Press, Chicago.

Frank, A. (2007) *Diary of a Young Girl*. Puffin Classics, London.

Gee, J.P. (1991) Memory and Myth: A perspective on narrative. In: *Developing Narrative Structure* (eds A. McCabe & C. Peterson), pp. 1–26. Lawrence Eribaum Assoc. Publ., Hillsdale, New Jersey.

Genechlen, G. (2009) *What's in Your Nappy?* Bloomsbury Paperbacks, London.

Goscinny, R. & Uderzo, A. (2004) *Asterix the Gaul*. Orion Publications, London.

Grahame, K. (2008) *The Wind in the Willows*. Egmont Press, London.

Greenhalgh, T. (2006) *What Seems to be the Trouble? Stories in Illness and Healthcare*. Radcliffe Publishing, Oxford.

Guroian, V. (1998) *Tending the Heart of Virtue: How Classic Stories Awaken a Child's Moral Imagination*. Oxford University Press, New York.

Hugo, V. (2007) *The Hunchback of Notre Dame*. Penguin Classics, London.

Houtzager, B.A., Grootenhuis, M.A. Caron, H.N. & Last, B.F. (2004) Quality of life and psychological adaptation in siblings of paediatric cancer patients, 2 years after diagnosis. *Psycho-Oncology*, **13** (8), 499–511.

Isbell, R., Sobol, J., Lindauer, L., & Lowrance, A. (2004) The effects of storytelling and story reading on the oral language complexity and story comprehension of young children. *Early Childhood Education Journal*, **32** (3), 157–163.

Kipling, R. (2001) *Collected Poems of Rudyard Kipling*. Wordsworth Editions Publ., London.

Korn, C. (1998) How young children make sense of their life stories. *Early Childhood Education Journal*, **25** (4), 223–228.

Lewis, C.S. (1986) *Letters to Children*. Collins Fount Paperback, London.

Lewis, C.S. (2004) *Chronicles of Narnia*. Harper Collins, New York.

Massie, R.K. (1967) *Nicholas and Alexandra*. Atheneum Publ., New York.

Massie, R. & Suzanne, M. (1975) *Journey*. Victor Gollancz Ltd., London.

McCabe, A. & Peterson, C. (1991) Getting the story: A longitudinal study of parental styles in eliciting narratives and developing narrative skills. In: *Developing Narrative Structure* (eds A. McCabe & C. Peterson), pp. 217–254. Lawrence Eribaum Assoc. Publ., Hillsdale, New Jersey.

McGrath, P. (2001) Findings on the impact of treatment for childhood acute lymphoblastic leukaemia on family relationships. *Child & Family Social Work*, **6** (3), 229–237.

Morpurgo, M. (2005) *The Amazing Story of Adolphus Tips*. Harper Collins, London.

Moyle, W., Barnard, A. & Turner, C. (1995) The humanities and nursing: Using popular literature as a means of understanding human experience. *Journal of Advanced Nursing*, **21** (5), 960–964.

Murphy, F. (2000) The enigmas of story. In: *Story-Telling; The Woodford Forum* (eds B. Levy & F. Murphy), pp. 1–22. University of Queensland Press, Woodford.

Opie, I. & Opie, P. (2001) *The Lore and Language of Schoolchildren*. The New York Review of Books, New York.

Orczy, B.E. (2002) *The Scarlett Pimpernel*. Bantam Classics/Random House, New York.

Pelander, T., Leino-Kilpi, H. & Katajisto, J. (2006) Quality of pediatric nursing care in Finland – Children's perspectives. *Journal of Nursing Care Quarterly*, **22** (2), 185–194.

Pollinghorne, D.E. (1988) *Narrative Knowing and the Human Sciences*. State University of New York Press, Albany, New York.

Ray, H.A. & Ray, M. (1995) [1947] *Curious George Goes to Hospital*. Houghton & Mifflin, New York.

Rennick, J., McHarg, L., Dell'Appi, M., Johnston, C. & Stevens, B. (2008) Developing the children's critical impact scale: Capturing stories from children, parents, and staff. *Pediatric Critical Care Medicine*, **9** (3), 252–260.

Rocco, F. (2003) *The Miraculous Fever-Tree – The Cure That Changed the World*. HarperCollins, London.

Rowling, J.K. (1997) *Harry Potter and the Philosopher's Stone*. Bloomsbury Publ. Co., London.

Roueché, B. (1991) *The Medical Detectives*. Penguin Books, London.

Samaritans, The www.samaritans.org.uk.

Saint-Exupery, A. de (1995) *The Little Prince*. Wordsworth Editions Ltd., Ware, Herts.

Scarlett, S., Naudeau, S. & Salonius–Pasternak, P.I. (2005) *Children's Play*. Sage Publ., London.

Scott, E. (2008) *Stealing Heaven*. Harperteen Books, New York.

Scott, S. & Duncan, C. (2004) *Return of the Black Death – The World's Greatest Serial Killer*. John Wiley & Sons Ltd., Chichester.

Seuss, Dr. (1990) [1957] *Oh, the Places You'll Go*. Harper Collins, London.

Seuss, Dr. (2004) [1940] *Horton Hatches the Egg*. Random House Books for Children, New York.

Seuss, Dr. (Geisel, Theodore Seuss) (2009) [1957] *The Cat in the Hat*. Harper Collins Children's Books Publ., London.

Shapiro, J., Duke, A., Boker, J. & Ahearn, C.S. (2005) Just a spoonful of humanities makes the medicine go down: Introducing literature into a family medicine clerkship. *Medical Education*, **39**, 605–612.

Silverstein, S. (1964) *The Giving Tree*. Harper Collins, New York.

Skarakis-Doyle, E. & Dempsey, L. (2008) Assessing story comprehension in preschool children. *Topics in Language Disorders. Narrative Abilities: New Research and Clinical Implications*, **28** (2), 131–148 (April/June).

Smith, R.L., Bailey, M., Hydo, S.K., Lepp, M., Mews, S., Timm, S. & Zorn, C. (2004) All the voices in the room – Integrating humanities in nursing education. *Nursing Education Perspectives*, **25** (6), 278–283.

Solzenitsyn, A. (2003) *Cancer Ward*. Vintage Classics/ Random House, London.

Stein, N.L. & Albro, E.R. (1997) Building complexity and coherence: Children's use of goal-structured knowledge in telling stories. In: *Narrative Development – Six Approaches* (ed. M. Bamberg), pp. 5–44. Lawrence Erlbaum Assoc. Inc. Publ., Mahwash, New Jersey.

Stowe, A.C. & Igo, L.C. (1996) Learning from literature: Novels, plays, short stories, and poems in nursing education. *Nurse Educator*, **21** (5), 16–19.

Streatfield, N. (2004) *Ballet Shoes*. Puffin Books, London.

Tolstoy, L. (1960) *The Death of Ivan Ilyich and Other Stories*. Penguin Bks., London.

Tolstoy, L. (2007) *War and Peace*. Penguin Classics, London.

Varah, C. (1993) *Before I Die Again: The Autobiography of the Founder of the Samaritans*. Constable Publishing Hse, London.

Vezeau, T.M. (1994) Narrative in nursing practice and education. In: *Art and Aesthetics in Nursing*, pp. 163–191. National League for Nursing, New York.

Viorst, J. (1987) *Alexander and the Terrible, Horrible, No Good, Very Bad Day*. Atheneum Book for Young Readers/Shuster & Shuster, New York.

Westberg, R. (2003) Real stories: Aspiring to become a nurse: "Children Remember". *Pediatric Nursing*, **29** (1), 63,64,79.

White, E.B. (1963) [1952] *Charlotte's Web*. Penguin/Puffin Bks., London.

White, E.B. (2007) [1945] *Stuart Little*. Penguin/Puffin Bks., London.

Whitehead, M.R. (2002) *Developing Language and Literacy with Young Children*, 2nd edn. Paul Chapman Publ., London.

Whiting, J.B. (2000) The view from down here: Foster children's stories. *Child & Youth Care Forum*, **29** (2), 79–95.

Wilde, O. (2001) *The Happy Prince and Other Fairy Tales*. Dover Publications Ltd., Mineola, New York.

Wilson, J. (2009) *Hetty Feather*. Doubleday/Random House Children's Books, London.

Wolf, S.A. (2006) The Mermaid's purse: Looking closely at young children's art and poetry. *LanguageArts*, **84** (1), 10–20.

Woodgate, R.L. (2006) Siblings' experience with childhood cancer: A different way of being in the family. *Cancer Nursing*, **29** (5), 406–414.

Wright, A. (1995) *Creating Stories with Children*. Oxford University Press, New York.

Wright, A. (2002) Using story telling as a therapeutic tool with children. *Child & Adolescent Mental Health*, **7** (3), 150–151.

Zephaniah, B. (1995) *Talking Turkeys*. Penguin/Puffin Bks., London.

Suggested further reading

Begley, A.M. (2003) Creative approaches to ethics: Poetry, prose and dialogue. In: *Approaches to Ethics – Nursing Beyond Boundaries* (ed. V. Tschudin), pp. 125–135. Butterworth, Edinburgh.

20 Who is Shaping Children's Nursing?

Duncan Randall

Introduction

The idea for this chapter came from empirical research observing community children's nurses in their practice. This was part of a study into children's views of being nursed at home (Randall 2008, 2009). Observing the practice of nurses and listening to the children, it was difficult to determine what shaped the care offered to children. I was left asking where is the clinical care? Occasionally, clinical reasoning seemed to be present, but on the whole it seemed that other agendas were shaping the care delivered to children. Agendas were based in consumerism and professional rhetoric rather than philosophical principles or theoretical perspectives. I was left with the impression that the nursing care children received was adrift, buffeted by forces greater than those controlled by the child, their carers or nurses themselves. This chapter explores those forces and attempts to outline how nurses may be able to employ Christensen & Prout's (2002) ethical symmetry and Walker's (2007) conception of expressive collaborative morality to develop philosophical principles which, although they may not stop the storms that rage around health care and child care, may give nurses a

better sense that they can influence the direction that children's nursing is taking.

The chapter begins by considering Liaschenko's (1997) concept of landscapes and the position of children's nursing in the gendered landscape of the health-care industry. Then aspects of this landscape are explored in greater detail starting with the professional landscape moving to consumerist views and finally exploring the gendered landscape of child care and nursing. The chapter concludes by proposing that Christensen & Prout's (2002) ethical symmetry and Walkers (2007) ideas on expressive collaborative morality may offer a starting place from which nurses could take stock and develop philosophical principles to guide their practice, the main anchor of which would be working with children to facilitate children shaping their own nursing care.

Landscapes: where is children's nursing situated?

Liaschenko's work (1997) based on empirical research has conceptualised nursing as being situated in a gendered landscape of health care. From the position of nursing, Liaschenko argues that some aspects of health-care work are more visible

Ethical and Philosophical Aspects of Nursing Children, First Edition. Edited by Gosia M. Brykczyńska and Joan Simons.
© 2011 Blackwell Publishing Ltd. Published 2011 by Blackwell Publishing Ltd.

than others. In this landscape, the male-orientated work of medicine looms large almost blotting out other aspects of nurses' work. This less visible work is often more collaborative and nurturing and Liaschenko and others have argued, more female in orientation (Witz 1992; Davies 1995; Bjorklund 2004). As Liaschenko (1997) has pointed out, nurses tend to recognise the interpersonal landscapes in which they work, their relationships with children's carers, with children and with colleagues more than they acknowledge the wider landscapes in which they are situated. Liaschenko (1997) suggests that these wider landscapes are made up of structural social factors which are determined by the ways in which social relationships on a larger scale are organised.

This conception of children's nursing, as situated in a landscape, is in effect a thought experiment where one places oneself in the place of children's nursing and views the landscape. This perhaps assumes that there is one unified position of children's nursing from which to view the landscape. Whether this geographic thought experiment gives us anything more than a picturesque way of talking about the social structural influences on children's nursing seems open to debate. It seems possible to discuss the effects of gender, or the power of medicine without the analogy of a landscape. However, the idea of a viewpoint within a landscape such that some aspects are more visible and others less visible does seem useful in considering the relationships between various structural social factors that affect children's nursing.

Rhetoric of professional care

From the vantage point of nurses, the claims of professionalism and the concerns of the profession of children's nursing may appear highly visible. In Randall's (2009) study, the nurses seemed to focus on the technical therapeutic interventions which could be argued support the practice of medicine:

> RESEARCHER *OK so how would you characterise your relationships with children? [pause]. What would be the basis upon which they are built I suppose?*
>
> CCN *Well we only go in to a child if there is a nursing , clinical nursing need, so that would be the*

> *basis of our interaction with a child, that it had a clinical nursing need that would be the first reason why we entered the house.*
>
> RESEARCHER *Can you give me some examples of what you mean by clinical nursing needs.*
>
> CCN *Dressings, entral feeding, what else do we do? Injections, central lines.*
>
> CCN Group interview area 1.

While nurses providing play, or helping in applying for financial support, were seen as debatable areas for nurses to be involved in, administering medication and monitoring health for medical practitioners were uncontested nurses' roles for those taking part in the study. However, the nurses often alluded to how the delivery of nursing care was dependent on interpersonal factors, their relationships with parents (often mothers) or other family members. The nurses regularly contextualised the care they offered often starting their remarks with an *it depends* clause. The nurses suggested that how clinical care was delivered was dependent on their relationships with parents and to a lesser extent the children: the context of care, who was present and the place where care was delivered were all integral.

What did not seem to be evident was what principles of care the nurses were using. This does not mean that they were not using principles, they may be as Meleis (2007) puts it, 'silent knowers' (p. 21), nurses who rely on voices of authority, who use their understanding in their practice but cannot articulate that understanding. It is also possible that nurses' actions were not underpinned by principles, but contingent on the interpersonal and contextual factors. While this latter explanation may allow children's nursing to be flexible and respond to the complexities of the lives of children, it is also vulnerable, if applied uncritically, to drifting into discriminatory and arbitrary practice.

If practice is shaped purely on relationships, how can nurses be certain that their relationships with parents (often mothers) are not influenced by factors such as the relative social positions of parents and nurses, their genders or racial backgrounds? People who share values are perhaps more likely to establish and maintain relationships.

If context is to shape care, how is this constructed and influenced by the people concerned? Context can be a nebulous concept. However, the context of delivering and receiving care seems to be influenced by a number of factors such as gender, race and religion; often these factors are influenced by many groups in communities. Much of what is discussed below could be considered the context in which care is delivered. However, an uncritical and unprincipled approach to the context of care would seem to allow for arbitrary practice, where the care delivered to children would be contingent on factors over which children, their carers or nurses have little control. Assuring quality in such practice would become impossible. The care of children would be abandoned to the fates!

To avoid discriminatory and potentially arbitrary practice, nurses may turn to their professional literature to provide guiding principles. Unfortunately, as Lee (2003) has commented, children's nursing has a poor theoretical basis, often borrowing concepts from adult nursing which are based on epistemologies and conceptions of people relevant to adults, but not to children. Children's nurses are perhaps left with the mid-range theory of family-centred care. This is, as Coleman (2002) has argued, perhaps more of a professionally constructed concept, and one that has not been translated into practice (Coleman 2002). There also seems to be an ontological problem – what is meant by *family*? The term family seems to be used by nurses to mean children, parents and extended family members, although definitions in a cultural and social sense seem difficult. The different generational groups that are present in families are likely to have a different perspective on most aspects of nursing and child care (Mayall 2002). Practice shaped by *family* seems destined to confusion, and given the political position of children within societies (Robinson & Kellett 2004), such practice is perhaps inevitably bias towards adult concerns.

Although the nurses I spoke to used the rhetoric of professional practice, my observation of their practice suggested that this professional rhetoric had little influence over how the practice was shaped. The discussion outlined above may suggest that this is no bad thing. The current state of theory development does not seem to provide children's nurses with philosophical principles to guide their practice. Instead, nurses seem to rely on interpersonal relationships and their judgments about the context of care. It has been argued here that an uncritical acceptance of these factors, in shaping practice, may permit discriminatory and arbitrary practice. However, I shall return to explore a more critical approach to interpersonal relationships and contextualisation of care in the final section of this chapter.

Consumerism

Rather than professional rhetoric, the practice I observed seemed in part to be based on consumerism. Parents, and occasionally children, were asked to shape the care delivered. Appointments for interventions were made at the parents and sometimes the child's convenience rather than when clinically suggested (see data quoted below). Parents were asked what treatments were required, and sometimes they were the only link between the child and their medical practitioner; for example, parents (mothers) told the nurse what blood tests were required for children with oncology conditions.

This consumerist approach was complex, with aspects of professional and occupational agendas which contradicted the consumerist approach, for example, nurses' visits to children were negotiated not only to suit children/parents, but also to fit into the nurses' visiting pattern which were partly determined by the team they worked in and partly by their own domestic arrangements. Parents were more likely to secure a visit towards 4 p.m. if they lived on the nurses' route home and the team had no meeting that afternoon:

RESEARCHER   *When you are making appointments or deciding what to do when you visit the child what drives that do you think?*

CCN   *The needs of the child, whether they fit the criteria for the case load so they can be accepted on the caseload in the first place.*

RESEARCHER   *So if the child says I want for you to visit on Thursday you visit on Thursday?*

CCN   *We do our up most to.*

CCN   *While being flexible to the staff available I mean the whole team is completely flexible within their working time ... It is about that we will try and meet your needs [the child and family] but ultimately we need them to be flexible as well ... because its not an endless pot of resources that we have got, it's a limited resource that is stretch, shared quite thinly.*

CCN   *It is also making families aware that there will be times when we aren't able to do those visits due to circumstances within the team.*
CCN Group interview area 1.

There may be a case for a consumerist approach to the shaping of children's nursing. Recent health policy in Britain has embraced a consumerist approach (DoH 2008). The National Service Framework (DoH 2004) arguably sets out what children and their carers can expect of the health services as a service contract between policy makers, commissioners of services, health professionals and children and their carers. The evidence from expert patient programmes (Bodenheimer *et al.* 2002) and from Public Patient Involvement programmes (IIED 2001; DoH 2007) would seem to suggest that a consumerist approach may challenge professional agendas and lead to improvements in health-care services. However, this work has, until very recently, been done with adults rather than children, although some projects have started to address young people's needs (Salinas 2007).

Consumerism, like family-centred care, holds a central problem for children's nurses. Just as we asked above, in relation to family-centred care, what do we mean by *family*, for consumerism we could ask: Who is the customer? As customers, children's needs will be different from those of their carers. Knutsson *et al.*'s (2006) study of post-operative pain management shows that children have different perceptions of the effectiveness of treatment in comparison to their parents and to nurses.

I would argue that the political position of children in society as subordinate to adults (Qvortrup 2000; Robinson & Kellett 2004) means children's voices as consumers struggle to be heard. For instance, there has only been one national young patients' survey (Ramm *et al.* 2004) while adult surveys are carried out each year (Garratt & Boyd 2008). Even in the 2004 young patients' survey, only 16% of responses were from young people on their own, with 83% being completed by parents or parents with their children, although the final report rarely distinguishes between adult views and those of young people. The National Service Framework despite being influenced by consultations with children and young people contains no standards which aim to meet children's needs alone; each of the clauses that mention children

(0–19 years old) are accompanied by the phrase 'and their families' or 'and their parents', or equivalent phrases. While standard 2 clearly sets out a parental agenda, there is no standard for promoting children's rights in health care, no standard to promote children's independence in managing their own health, or health care.

Standard 2:
Parents and carers are enabled to receive the information, services and support which will help them to care for their children and equip them with the skills they need to ensure that their children have optimum life chances and are healthy and safe.
(DoH 2004)

I do not, however, want to advocate for a purely children's consumerist approach, although I would argue that listening to children about the care they receive is very important. The consumerist approach seems to have some logical flaws. If we assume for a moment that all parents have their children's best interests in mind all of the time, and prioritise their child's needs above their own, it could be argued that a parental consumerist approach would hold some merit.

However, there remain some major difficulties with the consumerist approach, even with our assumed *rose tinted* view of parenting. Children or parents as customers would need to consume a product – in this case, health services for children. These services have become highly technical and professional, such that it is very difficult for anyone other than health-care professionals to know whether the product (health services for children) is good or not. Normally consumers have a desired outcome in mind on purchasing a product, in this case returning the child to their previous health status, or growth and development equivalent to the child's peers. However, even good quality health care may not be able to deliver this outcome. As customers, the product that children or parents think they are consuming may not be possible, although they may continue to desire a healthy outcome. For example, parents of a child with a brain tumour may find it difficult to accept that instead of a full recovery, the product on offer has changed to death with dignity and a reduction of suffering.

Further consumerism relies on a certain degree of generalisation. Consumers know the expected outcome, which is expected to be the same each time a customer consumes the product. We buy coffee expecting it to taste of coffee just like the last time we tasted it. As Edwards (2001) has pointed out, this sort of generalisation cannot be applied to nursing. The interactions of people, illness and health care are different each time and generalisations are impossible to make between people, and across time and space; thus, even if parents know of other parents whose children had similar health problems, this will not necessarily help them to make judgements about the specific health care they receive.

A parental consumerist approach assumes that parents are responsible for their children's welfare, including the promotion of their child's health. This view, however, does not account for the role of communities and, through the action of communities, the state. As Mayall (2002:147–9) has pointed out, states have responsibilities to their future citizens. The role of parents is then limited by the state: while states often encourage *parental responsibility* they also assume overarching responsibility for children, taking it away from parents (UN Convention on the Rights of the Child (United Nations 1989) Article 9). Arguably, then, parental consumerism is only permitted within the limits of what the state will allow. In practice, in the British context, this has meant that the state, acting through courts of law, has consistently supported health-care professionals and not parents, in making decisions about children's health.

Consumerism seems to be unable to respond to the complexities of health care and is logically flawed as health care is not generalisable, so a consistent product is not available to be consumed and assessed in terms of quality or performance. Nor does consumerism account for the role of the state in providing for children. The division of labour in relation to child care, which is sanctioned and through policy promoted by states, is gendered. It is to these aspects of gender that we now turn.

Gendered agendas

Nursing is dominated in almost all regions of the world by women (Purnell 2007); as a part of the family of nursing, children's nursing is equally dominated by women. Gender then may be presumed to be a factor in the shaping of children's nursing. Mayall (2002) has argued that women's standing in societies is linked to the division of child-care responsibilities between the sexes. This division is socially constructed; for instance, Mayall offers a comparison between British and Finnish societies' approaches to child care. This social construction of gendered responsibilities for children's care means that issues of women's social positions and rights are interwoven with those of children. It also suggests that in societies where women are seen as primarily responsible for child rearing and care, that is, in most societies (Mayall 2002), it may be presumed that children's nursing will be heavily influenced by women.

The aspects of gender that shape children's nursing may be subtle, but they are pervasive. The arguments of Liaschenko (1997) outlined above may apply to children's nursing, that is, that nursing is situated in a landscape dominated by medicine, where masculine characteristics of objective dispassionate rationalism are valued over feminine characteristics of subjective collaborative nurturing. Thus, aspects of children's nursing which are easily portrayed as objective, where the nurse works autonomously (nurse-led clinics) and which support the practice of medicine, are more visible and therefore rewarded. Other aspects of nurses' work that are less visible go unrecognised, and unrewarded, by the bureaucracy or profession. Although Liaschenko's work and the work of others (Witz 1992; Davies 1995; Bjorklund 2004) were based on empirical studies, there is little empirical evidence that these gender issues actually affect the nursing care delivered to children. Liaschenko suggests that the poor visibility of some aspects of nurses' work makes these less visible aspects vulnerable, with resources directed to more visible aspects at the cost of these less visible ones. Whether this actually occurs in practice seems open to debate. As Liaschenko suggests, there may be a price to pay for some of nurses' work being less visible, but nurses may pay the price. For example, Liaschenko describes nurses' knowledge on *how to get things done*: this might be seen when a nurse takes on advocating for a child with the local authorities to have their house adapted for their needs. This work may be unrecognised by managers or health-care colleagues and may not feature in job evaluations. In doing this work which is often time consuming, the nurse may find that she has no time left for other aspects of her work, such as paper work, which documents care, or her own activities. This paper work has then to be done in her own time. Thus, the nurse may sacrifice her own time in order to help a child to a better living arrangement. Such practice may become an accepted norm perhaps hidden from management, but a practice into which new nurses are introduced as being *part of the job*. However, not all nurses may be willing or able to pay this price. It follows that some families would receive the help from a nurse and others would not, some children would win, while others would lose out.

Thus, the gendered landscape of health care, which does not value the less visible aspects of nursing that do not conform to masculine medical conventions of objective dispassionate and autonomous work, shapes the care delivered exacting a cost not only from nurses, but also from children and their carers. Moreover, as indicated by the data quoted above, there is a danger that by focusing on medical understanding, children become in a sense no more than a set of symptoms or a medical condition. As Liaschenko (1998) has commented, people are dehumanised by this gendered view.

The conception of a profession of children's nursing arises from gendered understandings about profession (Davies 1995). The idea of a profession involves the exclusion of those outside the profession from the area of work, the establishment and maintenance of a body of *expert* knowledge and a vocational-social contract, such that professionals provide value to society in exchange for social privileges (Abbott & Meerabeau 1998). For children's nursing, profession would seem to hold some ontological difficulties. As outlined above, the state and nurses as employees of the state are not wholly responsible for the health care of children. Parents under the United Nations Convention on the Rights of the Child (United Nations 1989) and according to UK health policy (DoH 2004) are also responsible. It seems impossible then for children's nursing to be a profession, for to do so would be to exclude parents and carers of children from the work of caring for children. It would also seem immoral for children's nurses to hold *expert* knowledge which they would not share freely with children or their carers. A vocational-social con-

tract may be possible with rewards for those willing to be children's nurses, but without the claims to exclusivity over work and expert knowledge, nurses' claims to profession for children's nursing seem weak at best.

From within nursing, there are voices which reject the idea of profession instead of proposing that nursing is seen as work (Lister 1997; Liaschenko & Peters 2004). This, they argue, would allow the emotional and intellectual labour of nursing to become more visible and allow nurses to renegotiate their position in the landscape of health care. I would also argue that viewing nursing as work would allow for nurses to negotiate with children and their carers, the allocation of areas of work and responsibilities. How such negotiation might be conducted and how this would shape children's nursing is the subject of the last section of this chapter.

Care around the child

Thus far in this chapter, I have attempted to analyse the factors which shape children's nursing, starting from empirical observation of community children's nursing and broadening the debate to include children's nursing policy and literature. Although much of this debate has focused on community children's nursing, I would argue that these can easily be applied to nursing children in hospital or other settings.

In this final section, I want to propose some ideas for how children's nursing might be shaped in the future. Following on from the arguments above, what I want to propose are some starting points to develop philosophical principles which would be available to children's nurses to guide their practice. Such principles would allow nurses to be critical about their practice and perhaps avoid their practice becoming discriminatory or arbitrary. Faced with problematic situations, children's nurses should be able to consider these philosophical principles and question their practice.

The first idea I want to put forward is that children's nursing should be shaped by children, for children. At first, this may seem like a highly simplistic statement. However, as the arguments detailed above indicate, putting such a philosophy into action will neither be simple, nor easy. The political and social position of children in society means that often the concerns of adults are put above those of children. Adults will argue that children do not have the cognitive ability to shape their own nursing care. However, a great deal of work in education, social and now health disciplines would suggest that, given appropriate opportunities, children are willing and able to contribute to healthcare development (Prout 2001; Sloper & Lightfoot 2003; Coad & Houston 2006; Coad & Shaw 2008).

Adults may argue that as adults they are responsible for children and should take decisions for them (Shields *et al.* 2003). In this debate, it may be useful to consider the concept of ethical symmetry as suggested by Christensen & Prout (2002) in relation to researching with children and applying it to health care. Christensen and Prout use the ideas of Bauman to consider how much of the responsibility adults should take *away* from children and how the adults should judge when to take responsibility *for* children. They use three principles: Firstly, adults should reject the assumptions they make about children and children's abilities based on age as these are often inaccurate. Secondly, judgements are made on the abilities of children studying their *cultures of communication*; this is not just the words used by children but how they communicate with others in non-verbal ways through behaviour and patterns of interactions. Lastly, adults take account of the social context of the child, their social environments and networks. In the health context, it may also be useful to take account of the child's health state. Thus, in considering the participation of children in their health care one would not rely on ideas about children's cognitive development or age-related abilities, but consider instead the abilities of the individual child and how they might participate. Many children given this opportunity will speak for themselves and take responsibility for their health. For some children, their social context and networks may not allow or encourage such participation. Some children may be too ill to take this responsibility; in these cases, adults may have to take some responsibility for children and work with them to encourage and enable them to take on appropriate levels of responsibility. Ethical symmetry would suggest that the participation of children should be symmetrical with that of adults as members of a society; however, this does not mean that children need to be treated the same as adults.

Allowing children's nursing to be shaped by children and for children would ensure that the nursing care received by children was based on their needs and not on the perceptions and requirements of their parents, or other adult carers. However, using ethical symmetry would allow nurses to work with adults in the child's social networks in the interests of the child. This could include working with parents to improve the child's health, but would also involve work in the broader communities in which children live. It could include working with the child's peers or their teachers. A by children, for children approach would clarify who are the customers of children's nursing, that is, the children. Conflicts between the interests of adults and children would be solved by considering the social context of the child and referring adults to appropriate agencies, allowing children's nurses to focus on the needs of the child.

A second concept which may assist nurses in meeting the first is to consider Walker's (2007) expressive collaborative morality. What I propose here is that children's nurses abandon their claims to profession. The discussion above indicates that these claims to exclusively care for ill children and the maintenance of *expert* knowledge are damaging to the relationships between nurses and others who care for children, such that children suffer, because the demands of a profession limit the ways in which nurses can work with others to facilitate children living with illness and their attainment of health (or dignity in death). Instead, nurses would consider children's nursing as work and seek to use Walker's morality to determine what children's nursing should aim to do – what good children's nursing is.

Walker (2007) rejects a theoretical judicial approach to morality, which she argues is biased towards powerful groups in society. Instead, she argues that morality is produced and reproduced in collaboration between people, with moral practices being an expression of identity and relationships.

> In the ways we assign, accept or deflect responsibilities we express our understandings of our own and others' identities, relationships and values.
>
> Walker (2007:16)

Of particular use to children's nurses may be Walker's conception that morality cannot be purified of its social context. In the main, cultures are stratified and power relationships are hierarchical. In such structures, what people are responsible for and who they are responsible to are not distributed evenly. Rather, the morality of people is different within and between social groups. Thus, moral understanding, and therefore practices, are different between generations (children and adults), but are also different within generations (both for children and adults). Certain groups are privileged by factors such as class, race or gender and of course by age. Walker suggests that expressive collaborative morality, although complex, allows for a critical approach, where the moral practices of less powerful groups are exposed and the practices of more powerful groups are challenged. Thus, for children's nurses, expressive collaborative morality may allow for a critical review of responsibilities and division of the work of caring for children living with illness. It allows nurses to consider their moral practices as health-care workers, but also those of children living with illness and or disability as well as the moral practices of carers such as parents, grandparents, teachers, etc. Debating the responsibilities of children for their health care and those of carers, including health-care workers, should allow for repositioning of children's nursing which would support children in coping with illness and living with it in their communities.

The use of Walker's morality would allow us to consider the factors discussed in this chapter, which seem to shape children's nursing. The focus on the practice of medicine and the lack of visibility of collaborative boundary work of nurses would be challenged as expressions of moral practices derived from professional elites and maintained by health bureaucracies and industry. The interpersonal relationships between nurses, children and their carers would be part of the social context of the moral understanding. Walker's morality would prompt nurses to consider the effects of race, gender and class on these relationships and how they assign, accept or deflect responsibilities for the care of children according to how these factors affect their relationships. Using ethical symmetry and Walker's morality would allow for a critical understanding of the social context of children's care, and open debates about how nurses should respond to these social contexts, which may lead to the establish-

ment of philosophical principles to guide practice. A part of recognising the moral practices of generations, as well as social groups within generations, would be to listen to *their* voice, which would allow for a child's consumer view. The pervasive affects of gender would be accounted for as part of the moral practices of different groups and the division of labour of child care could also be challenged.

While expressive collaborative morality does not provide easy answers or discreet philosophical principles, it does provide, however, an understanding from which to explore the factors shaping children's nursing, which recognises both the social position of children and the differences between social groups of children.

Conclusion: shaping children's nursing

In this chapter, I have tried to explore some of the factors which, it seemed to me, shape children's nursing, based on empirical studies and reviews of the literature. How children's nursing was delivered by nurses and received by children seemed to be based on a professional rhetoric that made aspects of nurses' work which supported medical practice more visible than other aspects of nurses' work. Nurses reported that their care was influenced by their relationships with parents and to a lesser extent with children. They also conceptualised care as being contextualised. It was argued that children's nursing literature does not provide philosophical principles which could guide nurses' practice. From my observation of community practice, it seemed that a consumerist approach was influencing practice. This approach was critiqued and it was pointed out that children's voices are often ignored in the development of health services, although this may now be changing. However, the consumerist's approach does not seem to account for the social position of children and has some ontological flaws, which may make it less useful in children's nursing. Lastly, the effects of gender were discussed. This was seen to be a pervasive factor which influenced the delivery of children's nursing on a number of levels.

The lack of philosophical principles to guide practice was seen as potentially dangerous, in that practice may drift into discriminatory or arbitrary ways. Such shaping of children's nursing would call into question its moral value and make quality assurance impossible.

In response to these critiques of how children's nursing is being shaped, two concepts were advanced which may help nurses to construct philosophical principles for practice. The first was ethical symmetry which suggests that nurses as adults reflect on their assumptions about children often based on cogitative development and age, and move to a position of relying on children's individual abilities. Ethical symmetry demands that children are subject to the same ethical considerations as adults; however, it recognises that adults may be called upon to take responsibility for children contingent on the social context in which the child lives. I suggest that in relating this to health, responsibilities of children and adults are also contingent on the health status of the child, such that there may be occasions when adults need to take responsibility for children, who due to their health status cannot take responsibility for themselves.

The second concept is that of expressive collaborative morality as defined by Walker (2007). This suggests that morality occurs as practices between people in a social context where responsibilities are not evenly distributed. It was argued that Walker's morality would allow children's nurses to negotiate the work of caring for children while recognising the social positions of children, their carers and themselves as health-care workers.

Using ethical symmetry and expressive collaborative morality, it may be possible for children's nurses to navigate their way to a landscape, no longer dominated by the masculinity of medical practice, but where children's nursing is shaped by children, for children and where children's voices are heard at last.

References

Abbott, P. & Meerabeau, L. (1998) Professionals, professionalization and the caring professions. In: *The Sociology of the Caring Professions*, 2nd edn. (eds P. Abbott & L. Meerabeau. UCL Press, London.

Bjorklund, P. (2004) Invisibility, moral knowledge and nursing work in the writings of Joan Liaschenko and Patricia Rodney. *Nursing Ethics*, **11** (2), 110–121.

Bodenheimer, T., Lorig, K., Holman, H., & Grumbach, K. (2002) Patient self-management of chronic disease in primary care. *JAMA*, **288** (19), 2469–2475.

Christensen, P. & Prout, A. (2002) Working with ethical symmetry in social research with children. *Childhood*, **9** (4), 477–497.

Coad, J. & Houston, R. (2006) *Voices of Children and Young People*. Action for Sick Children, London.

Coad, J. & Shaw, K. (2008) Is children's choice in health care rhetoric or reality? A scoping review. *Journal Advanced Nursing*, **64** (4), 318–327.

Coleman, V. (2002) The evolving concept of family centred care. In: *Family-Centred Care: Concept, Theory and Practice* (eds L. Smith, V. Coleman & M. Bradshaw). Palgrave, Basingstoke.

Davies, C. (1995) *Gender and the Professional Predicament in Nursing*. Open University Press, Buckingham.

DoH (2004) *Core document, National Service Framework for Children, Young People and Maternity Services*. The Stationery Office, Department of Health, London.

DoH (2007) *The Health Committee's Report on Patient and Public Involvement in the NHS*. The Stationery Office, Department of Health, London.

DoH (2008) *High Quality Care for All: NHS Next Stage Review Final Report*. Department of Health, London.

Edwards, S.D. (2001) *Philosophy of Nursing: An Introduction*. Palgrave MacMillan, Basingstoke.

Garratt, E. & Boyd, J. (2008) *Key Findings Report: Adult Inpatients Survey 2007*. Picker Institute, London.

IIED (2001) *Children's Participation-Evaluating Effectiveness*. International Institute for Education and Development, London.

Knutsson, J., Tibbelin, A. & Von Unge, M. (2006) Postoperative pain after paediatric adenoidectomy and differences between the pain scores made by the recovery room staff, the parent and the child. *Acta Oto Laryngologica*, **126** (10), 1079–1083.

Lee, P. (2003) Children's nursing: Can it justify a separate existence in the UK? *Journal of Clinical Nursing*, **12**, 762–769.

Liaschenko, J. (1997) Ethics and the geography of the nurse-patient relationship: Spatial vulnerabilities and gendered space. *Scholarly Inquiry for Nursing Practice*, **11** (1), 45–59.

Liaschenko, J. (1998) The shift from the closed to the open body-ramifications for nursing testimony. In: *Philosophical Issues in Nursing* (ed. S.D. Edwards), pp. 11–30. Macmillan Press, Basingstoke.

Liaschenko, J. & Peter, E. (2004) Nursing ethics and conceptulisations of nursing: Profession, practice and work. *Journal of Advanced Nursing*, **46** (5), 488–495.

Lister, P. (1997) The art of nursing in a "Postmodern" context. *Journal of Advanced Nursing*, **25** (1), 38–44.

Mayall, B. (2002) *Towards a Sociology for Childhood: Thinking from Children's Lives*. Open University Press, Birmingham.

Meleis, A.I. (2007) *Theoretical Nursing: Development and Progress*, 4th edn. Lippincott Williams and Wilkins, Philadelphia, Pennsylvania.

Prout, A. (2001) Representing children: Reflections on the children 5–16 programme. *Children & Society*, **15**, 193–201.

Purnell, L.D. (2007) Men in nursing: An international perspective. In: *Men in Nursing: History, Challenges and Opportunities* (eds C.E. O'Lynn & R.E. Tranbarger), pp. 219–235. Springer Publishing Company, New York.

Qvortrup, J. (2000) Marcoanalysis of childhood. In *Research with Children Perspectives and Practices* (eds P. Christensen & A. James), pp. 77–98. Falmer press, London.

Ramm, J., Reeves, R. & Graham, C. (2004) *The Patients Survey Report 2004 – Young Patients*. Healthcare Commission, London.

Randall, D. (2008) Children's views of being nursed at home. In: *Community Children's Nursing Forum Conference 2008*. Royal College of Nursing 13/03/08. Children's version available online from http://www.abpn.org.uk/Portals/_Rainbow/Documents/87299 ChildViewsbook.Pdf. Accessed 17/4/09.

Randall, D. (2009) *They just do my dressings: Children's perspectives on community children's nursing*. Unpublished thesis, The University of Warwick Conventry.

Robinson, C. & Kellett, M. (2004) Power. In: *Doing Research with Children and Young People* (eds S. Fraser, V. Lewis, S. Ding, M. Kellett & C. Robinson), pp. 81–96. Sage/Open University, London.

Salinas, E. (2007) *Evaluation study of the staying positive pilot workshops: A self management programme for young people with chronic conditions*. Expert Patient Programme, University of Oxford, Oxford.

Shields, L., Kristensson-Hallstrom, I., Kristjansdottir, G. & Hunter, J. (2003) Who owns the child in hospital? A preliminary discussion. *Journal Advanced Nursing*, **41** (3), 213–222.

Sloper, P. & Lightfoot, J. (2003) Involving disabled and chronically ill children and young people in health service development. *Child Care Health and Development*, **29** (1), 15–20.

United Nations (1989) *United Nations Convention on the Rights of the Child*. United Nations, Geneva.

Walker, M.U. (2007) *Moral Understandings: A Feminist Study in Ethics*. Oxford University Press, Oxford.

Witz, A. (1992) *Professions and Patriarchy*. Routledge, London.

Suggested further readings

Lee, P. (2003) Children's nursing: Can it justify a separate existence in the UK? *Journal of Clinical Nursing*, **12**, 762–769.

Liaschenko, J. & Peter, E. (2004) Nursing ethics and conceptualisations of nursing: Profession, practice and work. *Journal of Advanced Nursing*, **46** (5), 488–495.

Shields, L., Kristensson-Hallstrom, I., Kristjansdottir, G. & Hunter, J. (2003) Who owns the child in hospital? A preliminary discussion. *Journal Advanced Nursing*, **41** (3), 213–222.

Appendix I

Summary of Possible Situations for Withdrawal and Withholding Treatment in Children According to the *Royal College of Paediatrics and Child Health* Guidelines

(1) *The 'brain dead' child situation*: In the older child where criteria of brain-stem death are agreed by two practitioners in the usual way it may still be technically feasible to provide basal cardio-respiratory support by means of ventilation and intensive care. It is agreed within the profession that treatment in such circumstances is futile and the withdrawal of current medical treatment is appropriate.

(2) *The 'permanent vegetative' state situation*: The child who develops a permanent vegetative state following insults, such as trauma or hypoxia, is reliant on others for all care and does not react or relate with the outside world. It may be appropriate to withdraw or withhold life-sustaining treatment.

(3) *The 'no chance' situation*: The child has such severe disease that life-sustaining treatment simply delays death without significant alleviation of suffering. Treatment to sustain life is inappropriate.

(4) *The 'no purpose' situation*: Although the patient may be able to survive with treatment, the degree of physical or mental impairment will be so great that it is unreasonable to expect them to bear it.

(5) *The 'unbearable' situation*: The child and/or family feel that in the face of progressive and irreversible illness further treatment is more than can be borne. They wish to have a particular treatment withdrawn or to refuse further treatment irrespective of the medical opinion that it maybe of some benefit.

RCPCH (2004) *Withholding or Withdrawing Life Sustaining Treatment in Children*. Royal College of Paediatrics and Child Health, London. Used with permission.

Ethical and Philosophical Aspects of Nursing Children, First Edition. Edited by Gosia M. Brykczyńska and Joan Simons.
© 2011 Blackwell Publishing Ltd. Published 2011 by Blackwell Publishing Ltd.

Appendix II

United Nations Convention on the Rights of the Child (Abridged)

Everyone under the age of 18 has all the rights in the Convention.

The Convention applies to every child whatever their ethnicity, gender, religion, abilities, whatever they think or say, no matter what type of family they come from.

The best interests of the child must be a top priority in all actions concerning children.

Governments must do all they can to fulfil the rights of every child.

Governments must respect the rights and responsibilities of parents to guide and advise their child so that, as they grow, they learn to apply their rights properly.

Every child has the right to life. Governments must do all they can to ensure that children survive and grow up healthy.

Every child has the right to a legally registered name and nationality, as well as the right to know and, as far as possible, to be cared for by their parents.

Governments must respect and protect a child's identity and prevent their name, nationality or family relationships from being changed unlawfully. If a child has been illegally denied part of their identity, governments must act quickly to protect and assist the child to re-establish their identity.

Children must not be separated from their parents unless it is in the best interests of the child (for example, in cases of abuse or neglect). A child must be given the chance to express their views when decisions about parental responsibilities are being made. Every child has the right to stay in contact with both parents, unless this might harm them.

Ethical and Philosophical Aspects of Nursing Children, First Edition. Edited by Gosia M. Brykczyńska and Joan Simons.
© 2011 Blackwell Publishing Ltd. Published 2011 by Blackwell Publishing Ltd.

Governments must respond quickly and sympathetically if a child or their parents apply to live together in the same country. If a child's parents live apart in different countries, the child has the right to visit both of them.

Governments must take steps to prevent children being taken out of their own country illegally or being prevented from returning.

Every child has the right to say what they think in all matters affecting them, and to have their views taken seriously.

Every child must be free to say what they think and to seek and receive information of any kind as long as it is within the law.

Every child has the right to think and believe what they want and also to practise their religion, as long as they are not stopping other people from enjoying their rights. Governments must respect the rights of parents to give their children guidance about this right.

Every child has the right to meet with other children and young people and to join groups and organisations, as long as this does not stop other people from enjoying their rights.

Every child has the right to privacy. The law should protect the child's private, family and home life.

Every child has the right to reliable information from the mass media. Television, radio, newspapers and other media should provide information that children can understand. Governments must help protect children from materials that could harm them.

Both parents share responsibility for bringing up their child and should always consider what is best for the child. Governments must help parents by providing services to support them, especially if the child's parents work.

Governments must do all they can to ensure that children are protected from all forms of violence, abuse, neglect and mistreatment by their parents or anyone else who looks after them.

If a child cannot be looked after by their family, governments must make sure that they are looked after properly by people who respect the child's religion, culture and language.

If a child is adopted, the first concern must be what is best for the child. The same protection and standards should apply whether the child is adopted in the country where they were born or in another country.

If a child is a refugee or seeking refuge, governments must ensure that they have the same rights as any other child. Governments must help in trying to reunite child refugees with their parents. Where this is not possible, the child should be given protection.

A child with a disability has the right to live a full and decent life in conditions that promote dignity, independence and an active role in the community. Governments must do all they can to provide free care and assistance to children with disability.

Every child has the right to the best possible health. Governments must provide good quality health care, clean water, nutritious food and a clean environment so that children can stay healthy. Richer countries must help poorer countries achieve this.

If a child has been placed away from home (in care, hospital or custody, for example), they have the right to a regular check of their treatment and conditions of care.

Governments must provide extra money for the children of families in need.

Every child has the right to a standard of living that is good enough to meet their physical, social and mental needs. Governments must help families who cannot afford to provide this.

Every child has the right to an education. Primary education must be free. Secondary education must be available to every child. Discipline in schools must respect children's human dignity. Wealthy countries must help poorer countries achieve this.

Education must develop every child's personality, talents and abilities to the full. It must encourage the child's respect for human rights, as well as respect for their parents, their own and other cultures, and the environment.

Every child has the right to learn and use the language, customs and religion of their family whether or not these are shared by the majority of the people in the country where they live.

Every child has the right to relax, play and join in a wide range of cultural and artistic activities.

Governments must protect children from work that is dangerous or might harm their health or education.

Governments must protect children from the use of illegal drugs.

Governments must protect children from sexual abuse and exploitation.

Governments must ensure that children are not abducted or sold.

Governments must protect children from all other forms of exploitation that might harm them.

No child shall be tortured or suffer other cruel treatment or punishment. A child shall only ever be arrested or put in prison as a last resort and for the shortest possible time. Children must not be put in a prison with adults and they must be able to keep in contact with their family.

Governments must do everything they can to protect and care for children affected by war. Governments must not allow children under the age of 15 to take part in war or join the armed forces.

Children neglected, abused, exploited, tortured or who are victims of war must receive special help to help them recover their health, dignity and self-respect.

A child accused or guilty of breaking the law must be treated with dignity and respect. They have the right to help from a lawyer and a fair trial that takes account of their age or situation. The child's privacy must be respected at all times.

If the laws of a particular country protect children better than the articles of the Convention, then those laws must stay.

Governments must make the Convention known to children and adults.

For the full CRC see UNICEF website: www.unicef.org.uk/crc. Reproduced with permission.

Appendix III

Summary of the International Council of Nurses Ethical Code

Nurses and people

The nurse's primary professional responsibility is to people requiring nursing care.

In providing care, the nurse promotes an environment in which the human rights, values, customs and spiritual beliefs of the individual, family and community are respected.

The nurse ensures that the individual receives sufficient information on which to base consent for care and related treatment.

The nurse holds in confidence personal information and uses judgement in sharing this information.

The nurse shares with society the responsibility for initiating and supporting action to meet the health and social needs of the public, in particular those of vulnerable populations.

The nurse also shares responsibility to sustain and protect the natural environment from depletion, pollution, degradation and destruction.

Nurses and practice

The nurse carries personal responsibility and accountability for nursing practice, and for maintaining competence by continual learning.

The nurse maintains a standard of personal health such that the ability to provide care is not compromised.

The nurse uses judgement regarding individual competence when accepting and delegating responsibility.

The nurse at all times maintains standards of personal conduct which reflect well on the profession and enhance public confidence.

Ethical and Philosophical Aspects of Nursing Children, First Edition. Edited by Gosia M. Brykczyńska and Joan Simons.
© 2011 Blackwell Publishing Ltd. Published 2011 by Blackwell Publishing Ltd.

The nurse, in providing care, ensures that use of technology and scientific advances are compatible with the safety, dignity and rights of people.

Nurses and the profession

The nurse assumes the major role in determining and implementing acceptable standards of clinical nursing practice, management, research and education.

The nurse is active in developing a core of research-based professional knowledge.

The nurse, acting through the professional organisation, participates in creating and maintaining safe, equitable social and economic working conditions in nursing.

Nurses and co-workers

The nurse sustains a co-operative relationship with co-workers in nursing and other fields.

The nurse takes appropriate action to safeguard individuals, families and communities when their health is endangered by a co-worker or any other person.

International Council of Nurses (2006) *ICN Ethics Code*. International Council of Nurses, Geneva. Reproduced with permission.

Appendix IV

Summary of the Principles for the Ethical Conduct of Medical Research Involving Children

(1) Research involving children is important for the benefit of all children and should be supported, encouraged and conducted in an ethical manner.
(2) Children are not small adults; they have an additional, unique set of interests.
(3) Research should only be done on children if comparable research on adults could not answer the same questions.
(4) A research procedure which is not intended directly to benefit the child subject is not necessarily either unethical or illegal.
(5) All proposals involving medical research on children should be submitted to a research ethics committee.
(6) Legally valid consent should be obtained from the child, parent or guardian as appropriate. When parental consent is obtained, the agreement of school age children who take part in research should also be requested by researchers.

Royal College of Paediatrics and Child Health: Ethics Advisory Committee (2000).
Guidelines for the ethical conduct of medical research involving children. *Archives of Disease of Childhood*, **82**, 177–182.
Reproduced with permission.

Ethical and Philosophical Aspects of Nursing Children, First Edition. Edited by Gosia M. Brykczyńska and Joan Simons.
© 2011 Blackwell Publishing Ltd. Published 2011 by Blackwell Publishing Ltd.

Index

Page numbers in *italics* denote figures and tables.

The Abortion Act, 49
adolescent care
  attitudes, young people
    Child Poverty Action Group, 101
    ephebiphobia, 101
    ethical issues and dilemmas, practitioners, 102
    health issues, 102
    media, 101
    policy, 102–3
  Connexions Direct, 101
  health, 100
  phases, 100
  pressure groups, champions and young people voice
    education, 106–7
    information source, 103
    11 MILLION, 103
    participation, 105–6
    protection, 104–5
    provision, 104
    reflection, 107
    rights, 104
  Social Exclusion Unit, 101
  transition patterns, 101
aiming high for disabled children (AHDC), 91, 94, 96
assessment, children and young people
  ADHD, 116
  approach, 115–16
  core and specific skills, 116
  developmental
    child's function, 117
    factors, 117

family needs
  parental interview, 117
  strengths and barriers, 117
fluid and dynamic process, 116
information
  nursing aim, 117
  presenting concerns, family, 116–17
NICE guidelines, 116
attention-deficit hyperactive disorder (ADHD), 116, 117
attitudes, young people
  Child Poverty Action Group, 101
  ephebiphobia, 101
  ethical issues and dilemmas, practitioners, 102
  health issues
    diabetes and asthma, 102
    direct engagement, clinical services, 102
    dramatic strides, 102
  media, 101
  policy
    Every Child Matters, 103
    NSF, 103
    social investment strategy, 102
autonomy, school-aged children
  beneficence
    description, 70
    sex education, 70
    unintended pregnancy, 71
  confidentiality
    advice, 72
    drop in services, 72
    trust and duty of confidence, 72

Ethical and Philosophical Aspects of Nursing Children, First Edition. Edited by Gosia M. Brykczyńska and Joan Simons.
© 2011 Blackwell Publishing Ltd. Published 2011 by Blackwell Publishing Ltd.

definition, 70
disclosure/sharing information, 72
informed consent
    developmental stages, 72–3
    Gillick competent, 73
    HPV vaccination programme, 73–4
    Lord Fraser's guidance, 73
    vaccine programmes, 73
    written information, 74
justice
    Bichard inquiry, 71
    Sexual Offences Act 2003, 71–2
non-maleficence, 71
school nurse, 70

beneficence
autonomy, school-aged children
    description, 70
    sex education, 70
    unintended pregnancy, 71
children's pain, paediatric nurses management
    ethical management, 161
    fundamental nature, 161
    nurses and parents perceptions, 161
    nursing skills, 160–161
    pain-assessment tools, 161
    principles, 160
Bolam test, 177

CAMHS. See child and adolescent mental health
        services
cancer care, children and young people (CYP)
    autonomous decisions, 165
    day-to-day practice, 165
    ethical and legal issues, 165
    futility, treatment
        bone-marrow transplant, 169
        haematology and oncology, 169
        open communication, 169
    informed consent
        clinical interventions, 166
        fertility preservation, 166
        sequenced approach, 166
    models, 164
    open communication, 164
    refusing treatment
        burdens and risks, 168
        emotional responses, 167
        own health-care decisions, 168
        radical surgery, 168
    resource allocation
        private funding, 169
        timely therapy, 169
    rights and responsibilities, 165
    truth telling
        clinician-patient relationship, 167
        oncology, 167
        principle, 167
    withdrawing treatment
        end-of-life decisions, 169
        life-threatening effects, 168

child and adolescent mental health services (CAMHS)
    assessment, 116
    description, 113–14
    family needs, 117
    life outcomes, mental health problems, 68
childhood philosophies and histories
    craft/evidence, historians
        diets nature, 6
        'forgotten boredom,' 5
        games and songs, 5–6
        Historic Iowa Children's Diaries Project, 6–7
        Latin definitions, 4
        legal obligation, 6
        maturation process, 5
        posterity memories, 4–5
        Slumdog Millionaire, 7
        societal and cultural differences, 7
        space nature, 6
        suboptimal conditions, 4
    European review (see European childhoods review)
    past generations, 4
    public domain, 3
    The Sunday Observer, 3
    thoughts
        antisocial behaviour, 17
        children images, 15–16
        compromise position, 16
        contemporary society, 15
        counterculture behaviours, 17
        ethical and medical issue, 17–18
        innocent players, 16
        life, quality, 18
        medieval society, 16
        orphaned and poor, 18
        political and sociocultural context, 18
        potentials, 17
        sick child convalescence, 18
        societal values and moral education, 16
        UK legal system, 17
        violence, 18
The Children Act (1989)
    health-care policy, 104
    mental health problems, 118
    parental responsibility, 50
children's community nurses (CCN)
    end-of-life-care, 196
    model, 97
    training, 93
    beneficence
        ethical management, 161
        fundamental nature, 161
        nurses and parents perceptions, 161
        nursing skills, 160–161
        pain-assessment tools, 161
        principles, 160
    cues
        assessment tool, 160
        post-operative analgesia, 160
    description, 155
    justice, 157
    non-maleficence, 155–7

children's community nurses (CCN) (*cont'd*)
    UN convention, child rights
        effective pain management, 157
        fairness and equality, 158
        narrative approach, 159
        non-pharmacological management, 159
        nurses documentation, 158
        principles, 158
        self-report tool, 157–8
children's rights
    cartoons, 40
    commissioner introduction, 39–40
    consultation mechanisms, 40
    criminal responsibility age, 36
    dependence and independence, 39
    ethical principles
        autonomy, 37
        beneficence and non-maleficence, 37
        justice, 38–9
        respect, 37–8
    medical and nursing care, 39
    positive and negative, 37
    responding ability, 37
    UKCRC
        participation, 41–2
        protection, 40–41
        provision, 41
    UNCRC, 36–7
    Welsh Assembly Government aims, 39
    youth parliaments, 40
community settings nursing, children's view
    definition, 77
    ethical symmetry
        Bauman's conceptions, 79
        cultures of communication, 79
    hospital-based care, 77
    listening
        interviews, 78
        isolated children, 78
        power relationships, 79
        services, 78
    passing strategy
        attempts, rights, 83
        disclosure, information, 82–3
        living with illness, 82
        social sanctions/stigma, 83
        social trick, 82
    social actors, 78
    support, implications
        dilemma, nurses, 83
        education, 84
        policy, 85
        practice, 83–4
        research, 84–5
    'to be like the others'
        Clark's mosaic approach, 80
        Coyne's study, 81–2
        nurse visit, home, 80
        parents, 82
        summary statements, 80
        task-orientated approach, nurses, 81
        teaching role, nurses, 81

DCSF. *See* department for children, schools and families
department for children, schools and families (DCSF)
    disabled children, 88
    guidance, 105
    palliative care services, 92
    redesigning services, 94
department for education and skills (DfES)
    disabled children, 91
    leaving school, 66
DfES. *See* department for education and skills
disabled child care
    adult care transition
        community matron, 97
        difficulties, 96–7
        health practitioners, 97
        paediatric system, 97
    children's and parents concerns
        communication, 96
        ECDM, 95
        ECM outcomes, 96
        elements, core offer, 96
        employment, 95
        housing, 96
        income and expenses, 95–6
    definition, disability, 88
    education, paediatric nurses
        CCN training, 93
        drawback, 93
        placements, 93
    groups, 88–9
    low birth weight babies, 88
    needs
        homes and long-stay hospital units, 89
        parents and skills, 89–90
        technological equipment dependency, 89
        Warnock report, 89
    paediatric hospices, issues
        Children's Hospice movement, 92
        fund-raising, 92
        health and social service budgets, 92
        Icelandic Bank scandal, 92
        nursing staff recruitment and retention, 92–3
    technology and medical science, advances, 88
    throwaway mentality, 88

ECT. *See* electroconvulsive therapy
electroconvulsive therapy (ECT), 120
emotional and psychiatric health needs
    assessment
        ADHD, 116
        approach, 115–16
        core and specific skills, 116
        developmental, 117
        family needs, 117
        fluid and dynamic process, 116
        information, 116–17
        NICE guidelines, 116
    legal issues (*see* legal issues)
    mental health
        CAMHS, 113–14
        early investment, 113
        engaging families, 114–15

epidemiological research, 113
   problems and disorders, 112
   psychological building blocks, 112
   psychotic disorder, 113
   rates, 112–13
end-of-life care
   acute decisions
      ethical challenges, 193
      PICU, 193
      positive and negative implications, 193
   bereavement care
      CCN practice environment, 196
      training, skills and resources, 195
   children's involvement
      decision-making process, 194
      Fraser guidelines, 194
      UNCRC, 194
   community-based care
      professionals negotiate care, 195
      symptom management, 195
   death rate, 192
   life expectancy, 192
   life-sustaining medical treatment, 192–3
   potential issues, 193
ESRC. See European Social Research Council
ethical principles
   acknowledging rights, 207
   bedrock, 207
   beneficence, 206
   conduct, 267
   distributive justice, 206–7
   human subjects, 207
   moral dilemmas, 208
   non-maleficence, 206
   qualitative study, 209
   risks and burdens, 207
ethics committees role, neonatology
   nursing staff
      clinical knowledge and experiences, 52
      curative and palliative care, 52
      NMC, 52
      nurses identification, 53
   partnership decision making
      doctors responsibility, 51–2
      family-centred care, 50–51
      intolerability, 52
      maternal cultural background, 51
      NCOB, 52
      POPPY, 51
   RCPCH, 52
European childhoods review
   acceptance ritual, 8
   baptism, 9
   child labour, 13
   civilisation, 7
   councils and professionals, 15
   and development stages, 9
   early social maturation, 11
   economic
      and social significance, 13
      solution, 14
   employees, 13–14

Factory Act, 1802, 14
   groups, 14
   Industrial Revolution, 13
   knighthood and warfare, 11
   medieval
      schools, 10
      theology, 10–11
   Mines Regulation and Inspection Act, 1860, 15
   moral labour theory, 14
   new steam-propelled technology, 13
   open-minded parents, 10
   and parent bond, 12
   physical immaturity, 9
   postoral teaching, 9
   Registration Act, 1837, 15
   Roman law, 8
   royal commission, 14
   rural poverty, 12
   society
      and legal implications, 7
      responsibility, 8
   St Augustine writings, 8–9
   supposition and historians, 12
   Thomas Aquinas writings
      medieval theology, 11
      parental preferences, 10
      respect, 10
      tasks, parenthood, 10
      volition and intellectual reflection, 9
   Thomas More formal education, 11–12
   working conditions, mills, 14
European Social Research Council (ESRC), 78

Factory Act (1802), 14
family-centred care (FCC)
   beauchamp and childress paradigm
      autonomy, 148
      justice, 149
      non-maleficence, 149
   breastfeeding mothers, 145
   care-by-parent, 146
   childhood and parenting, 146
   child–parent separation, 145–6
   children's rights, health care, 148
   child's social and psychological needs, 145
   debate and contention
      defensive parenting, 147
      description, 147
      ethical principles, 148
      managerial efficiency, 148
      parent–nurse relationship, 147
      phenomenology, 147
      socialisation, 148
   definition, 148
   deontology
      consequentialism, 151
      health services, 150
      moral guides, 150
      negative consequences, 150
   description, 144–5
   health-care facilities, 147
   IFCC definition, 144

family-centred care (FCC) (*cont'd*)
   infectious diseases and cross-infection, 145
   internet-based organisation, 148
   negotiated care, 146
   negotiation and effective communication, 145
   partnership-in-care, 146
   Platt report, 146
   utilitarianism
      act and rule, 151
      care model, 152
      consequentialism, 151
      implementation, 151
      types, 151
   virtue ethics, 149

Gilligan-Kohlberg debate, 33

hospitalisation, health-care decision-making
   autonomy level, 137–8
   children care
      care-by-parent, 128
      environments, 128
      experiences and needs, 128
      paediatric health services, 128
      perceptions, 128
   communication process, 127
   effects
      adverse aspects, 128
      family life and powerlessness, 129
      fears, 128–9
      self-determination loss, 131
      treatments and procedures, 130–131
      ward environment, 129–30
   free-for-all approach, 138
   philosophical beliefs, 137
   right to be heard
      benefits, 134
      contributory factors, 135
      doctor-parent-child communication, 136
      health-care matters, 135
      incident technique, 136
      non-government and voluntary
         organisations, 134
      parenting style, 137
      public health system, 136
      truth telling, 136
Human Rights Act (1998), 49, 50, 118

International Council, nurses ethical code
   co-workers, 266
   people, 265
   practice, 265–6
   profession, 266
interprofessional education (IPE), 106

justice, ethical principles
   babies, Down's syndrome, 38
   child poverty, 38
   guiding principles, 38–9
   post-code lottery, 38
   truth-telling, 38

Kantian theories, 177

legal issues
   advocacy, 121–2
   Children Act (1989), 118
   children under 16, 118
   competence and capacity evaluation
      ability, child/young person, 119
      maturity and understanding, 119
   confidentiality, 120
   consent, 118
   ECT, 120
   human rights
      decision-making process, 118
      guiding principles, 118
   Mental Capacity Act 2005, 121
   Mental Health Act 1983, 120
   parent involvement, treatment
      expressed permission, 119
      responsibility, 120
   SCT, 120
   treatment without consent, 119
   young people, 16/17 age, 118–19
   ZPC, 121

Mental Capacity Act (2005), 121
mental health
   CAMHS
      description, 113
      multidisciplinary teams, 114
      NHS health advisory tiered model, 114, *115*
      service provision, 114
      specialist, 114
      Tier 1 professionals, 114
      training and consultation, 114
   emotional health and well-being
      Backing the Future, 113
      developmental trajectories, 113
      investment, 113
   engaging families
      holistic assessment, 115
      philosophical, theoretical and therapeutic
         approach, 114
   epidemiological research, 113
   problems and disorders, 112
   psychological building blocks, 112
   psychotic disorder, 113
   rates, 112–13
Mental Health Act (1983), 119, 120
Mines Regulation and Inspection Act, 1860, 15
moral philosophy, paediatric nursing
   apprenticeships, 23
   caring and nursing ethics
      emotional drain, 33
      gendered perspective, theories, 32
      Gilligan-Kohlberg debate, 33
      guide, moral decision-making, 33
   categorical imperative I, 25
   categorical imperative II
      fertilisation cases, 25
      intrinsic rights, 25

categorical imperative III
    biomedical principles, 26
    professional codes, 26
cultures, 23
deontology, non-consequentialism
    behaviour, 24
    categorical imperatives/maxims, 25
    intrinsic value, 24–5
    religion and theology, 24
    word meaning, 24
European tradition, 23–4
rights and theories
    basic human needs, 29
    children, 30
    haves and have-nots, society, 28
    human and political, 28
    human existence and happiness, 29
    interwar period, Poland, 29–30
    moral reasoning, 30
    socio-political, 28
    UNCRC, 29
    UNDHR, 30
    women, 29
utilitarianism - consequentialism
    description, 26
    ethical reasoning, 26–7
    happiness, 27
    moral integrity, 27
    principle of utility, 27
    qualified health-care professionals, 28
    shortened working hours, health-care workers, 27–8
    universal education, 27
virtue ethics
    Aristotle's theory, 31
    and education, 32
    philosophical approach, Europe, 30–31
    practical wisdom, 31, 32
    virtuous behaviour, 31–2

National institute for health and clinical excellence
        (NICE)
    guidelines, psychological conditions, 116
    maltreatment, 59
    post-code lottery, 38
national service framework (NSF), 103, 134
NCOB. See Nuffield Council of Bioethics
neonatal intensive care unit (NICU)
    ethical decisions, 47–8
    medical and nursing staff, 47
neonatology nursing
    ethics committees role
        nursing staff, 52–3
        partnership decision making, 50–52
        RCPCH, 50
    framework
        The Abortion Act, 49
        The Children Act, 50
        gestational age, 48–49
        health-care practitioners, 50
        Human Rights Act, 49, 50
        legal guidance, 49

NCOB, 49–50
        no-purpose and unbearable situation, 49
        RCPCH, 49
    NICU, ethical decisions
        babies treatment, 48
        long-term outcome, 47–8
        parents, 48
        ways, 48
    rules and guidelines
        BAPM, 48
        feature, 48
    unilateral decision making, 48
NMC. See Nursing and Midwifery Council
non-maleficence
    distressing symptoms, 156
    optimal pain, 156
    postsurgical pain relieving methods, 156
    principles, 157
    profound and long-lasting effects, 155–6
    under-medication, 155
Nuffield Council of Bioethics (NCOB), 49–50
Nursing and Midwifery Council (NMC)
    ethical principles, 56
    guidance, 52
    health visitors, 62
    information, disclosure, 72
    NMC code (2008)
        childrens pain, 161
        confidentiality rights, 72
        consent, patient/client, 73
        non-maleficence, 71
    patient risk, reporting, 61
    principle of autonomy, 56
    professional code, conduct, 24
    public health practice, 68
    public safety, 61
    record keeping, 58–9
    school nursing, 67
    SCPHN, 67
    veracity, 57

paediatric intensive care nursing
    ethical, legal and professional considerations
        Bolam test, 177
        cornerstone principles, 177
        deontology, 177
        Kantian theories, 177
        non-maleficence, 177
        patient autonomy, 178
        Toby's perspective, 177–8
        utilitarianism, 176
    RCPCH framework, 174–6
    withhold/withdraw treatment, nurse role
        decision-making process, 179
        end-of-life decision, 181
        final decision-maker, 180
        futile care, 178
        knowledge and patterns, nursing, 179–80
        life-sustaining treatment, 181
        limitation, 182
        loss of control, 182

paediatric intensive care nursing (*cont'd*)
    managerial roles, 180
    moral distress, 181
    nursing programmes, 181
    one-to-one basis, 178
    quality-of-life issues, 179
    RCPCH guidelines, 180
    responsibility and accountability, 180
paediatric intensive care units (PICUs)
    death, 173
    holistic care, 181
    UK, 177
    withdrawal, treatment, 175
pain in children, paediatric nurses management
    autonomy
        communication skills, 160
        definition, 159
        emotional parental support, 160
        pain management practices, 159
palliative care, children
    continuing care and life
        brain dead child, 187
        broad multidisciplinary approach, 187
        communication difficulties, 191
        decision-making process, 189
        diagnosis, 188
        disabled children, 188
        family link schemes, 192
        long-term effects, 188
        modern communication, 187
        support, family, 189–91
        tertiary care facilities, 191
    end-of-life care
        acute decisions, 193
        bereavement care, 195–6
        children's involvement, 194–5
        community-based, 195
        death rate, 192
        life expectancy, 192
        life-sustaining medical treatment, 192–3
        potential issues, 193
Parents of Premature Babies Project (POPPY), 51
permanent vegetative state (PVS), 174
personal, social and health education (PSHE), 68–9
philosophical analysis
    child development, 237
    children stories
        adolescents, 246
        allegorical narrative relationships, 247
        books and poems, 246–7
        Harry Potter stories, 246
        Kipling's poem, 245
        moral message, 245
        potty training, 245
        safety and solace, 247
        sympathetic echoes, 245
        value systems, 246
    forms, narrative, 239–40
    generative narratives, 242
    healing narratives
        functions and formats, 244

        personal memories, 242
        sense making act, 242
        symbolic narrative and metaphor, 243
    homo viator and homo creator, 237
    imagined narrative
        arts and humanities, 244
        compassion and tolerance, 244
        health-care ethics, 244
        medical and nursing education, 244
    intellectual capacities, 238
    internal structures and coherence, 238
    narrative context, 238–9
    obligatory creative dialogue, 238
    persuasive narratives, 241–2
    professional narrative context, 240–241
    public narratives, 241
    public telling and enactment, 238
    stories, children
        adult perspective, 244
        delightful, 245
Platt report, 146
POPPY. *See* Parents of Premature Babies Project
pressure groups, champions and young people voice
    education
        Adolescent Health Project, 106
        Balint method, 106
        negative feelings, 107
        principalism and narrative ethics, 106
    information source, 103
    11 MILLION, 103
    participation
        health care and surveillance transfer, 106
        IPE, 106
        self management behaviours, 105
    protection
        decision-making, 105
        ethical dilemma, definition, 105
        legislation and guidance, 105
        NMC and RCN, 105
        The Protection of Children in England, 104–5
        Sexual Offences Act, 105
    provision
        adolescent wards, 104
        health professionals training, 104
        Platt Report, 104
    reflection
        ethical map trail, 107
        MSR, 107
    rights, 104
Principle of universality, 25
Principles of Biomedical Ethics, 26

RCPCH. *See* Royal College of Paediatrics and Child
    Health
Registration Act (1837), 15
research, children and young people
    designing and undertaking, 215
    disseminating findings
        communication forms, 215
        IRB-approved consent forms, 216
    essential component, 215

ethical practice, 215
knowledge and territory
    benefits, 204
    codes and governance frameworks, 205
    functional representation, 205
    risk, *204–5*
    stages, *205–6*
making preparations
    assent, consent and dissent, 209
    ethical principles, 206–9
    financial inducement, 214
    non-clinical trial, 215
    payment types, 214
    proposals and information sheets, 209–14
vs. practice
    health-care research, *203–4*
    immediate/direct benefit, 204
respite and palliative care, disabled child
    AHDC, 91
    Children Act, 90
    Continuing Healthcare, 91
    friendship and social network development, 90
    gastrostomy feeding, 91
    government role
        AHDC agenda, 94
        autistic spectrum disorders, 94
        dedicated funding, 93–4
        eligibility criteria, lack, 95
        messages, 94
        ring-fenced budgets, 94
        service delivery improvement, 94
        short breaks implementation guidance, 94–5
    health *vs.* social care debate, 91
    home-based, 90
    models, 91
    multiple settings, 92
    risks, abuse, 90
    shared budgets and joint commissioning, 91–2
    types, 90
Royal College of Paediatrics and Child Health (RCPCH)
    adolescents ward facilities, 132
    brain stem death, 174
    compassionate and sensitive approach, 174
    disabled and non-disabled children, 189
    ethical decision making process, 50
    ethics committees role, 50
    fundamental principles, 176
    intolerable disability, 52
    life-threatening condition, 175
    minimum legal requirement, 176
    no-chance situation, 174
    no-purpose situation, 174
    PVS, 174
    unbearable situation, 174
    withdrawing and withholding treatment, 49,
        176, 261

school-aged children, health
    autonomy
        beneficence, 70–71
        confidentiality, 72

    definition, 70
    information, 72
    informed consent, 72–4
    justice, 71–2
    non-maleficence, 71
health promotion and ethics
    advocacy, 69
    alcohol and illegal drugs, 68
    emotional health and psychological well-being, 68
    empowerment, 69
    models, 69
    self-confidence and stress management, 68
    twin pillars, 69
legal constraints and professional role boundaries, 74
professional *vs.* personal values
    and ethics, 69–70
    influencers, 70
school nursing
    government document, 67
    internet, 67–8
    NMC standards, 67
    public health practice domains, 68
    SCPHN, 67
SCPHN. *See* specialist community public health nurses
Sexual Offences Act (2003), 71–2, 105
shaping children, nursing
    accept/deflect responsibilities, 258
    collaborative morality, 257
    communication cultures, 257
    consumerism
        consumerist approach, 254
        family-centred care, 254
        generalisation, 255
        parental consumerist approach, 254
        professional and occupational agendas, 254
        young patients survey, 254
    description, 251
    factors, 256
    gendered agendas
        aspects, 255
        better living arrangement, 255
        child-care responsibilities, 255
        empirical evidence, 255
        masculine medical conventions, 255
        UK health policy, 256
        vocational-social contract, 256
    landscapes, 251–2
    perceptions and requirements, 257
    philosophical principles, 258
    political and social position, 256–7
    professional care
        discriminatory and arbitrary practice, 253
        medication and monitoring health, 252
        technical therapeutic interventions, 252
        uncritical and unprincipled approach, 253
    theoretical judicial approach, 257
    Walker's morality, 258
specialist community public health
        nurses (SCPHN)
    NMC standards, 67
    school nurse, 67

spirituality, philosophical and epistemological aspects
  child-focused literature, 220
  child health care
    activities and relationships, 227–8
    adult awareness, 228
    assessment guidelines, 230
    barriers, 227
    degenerative illnesses, 228–9
    health-care facilities, 229
    life-limiting and life-shortening conditions, 229
    nursing concepts, 227
    paediatric nurses, 229
    social work and family therapy, 229
  children and young people
    balanced faith, 227
    chaotic faith, 224–5
    choosing faith, 227
    conforming faith, 226–7
    Fowler's stages, 224
    life experience, 222
    nursed faith, 224
    ordering faith, 225–6
    religion and secularity overlap, 221
  holistic care, child and family
    dynamic and ecumenical interpretation, 231
    emotional well-being, 231
    living activities, 231
    relationships and roles, 231
    systems theory, 231
  life cycle
    child's developmental stage, 222
    faith and spirituality categories, 223
    faith development stages, 223
    incremental stages, 223
    sensory approach, 222
    three-stage model, 223
  public domain, 220–221
supervised community treatment (SCT), 120

toddlers and school age children, health visitor
  domestic abuse
    gut feelings, 58–9
    multi-agency working, 59
    public awareness, 58
    reluctance, 58
    risks, 58
    vulnerability, 57
    women, 57–8
  ethical issues, 55
  immunisation
    consequence-based theory/consequentialism, 56
    ethical dilemma, 56
    information, vaccinations, 57
    measles, mumps and rubella (MMR), 55–6
    NMC, 56–7
    non-maleficence, 56
    trust, 57

management failure, 62
safeguarding
  advocacy, 60
  Baby Peter's death, 59–60
  harm, significant, 59
  money, 59
  moral and professional conduct, 60–61
  nature, harm, 60
  protection procedures, 59
  workload issues, 61–2
treatment refusal, CYP
  burdens and risks, 168
  emotional responses, 167
  own health-care decisions, 168
  radical surgery, 168

UNCRC. See United Nations Convention on the Rights of the Child
UNDHR. See United Nations Declaration of Human Rights
United Nations Convention on the Rights of the Child (UNCRC)
  child cases, 49
  fairness and equality, 158
  government, 262–4
  health care service, 29
  management
    non-pharmacological, 159
    pain, 157
  narrative approach, 159
  nurses' documentation, 158
  policy development, UK, 39
  principles, 158
  recognition age, child, 36
  rights
    organising framework, 36
    positive and negative, 37
  self-report tool, 157–8
United Nations Declaration of Human Rights (UNDHR), 30

virtue ethics
  FCC
    Aristotelian virtue theory, 31, 149
    definition, 149
  moral philosophy, paediatric nursing and education, 32
    philosophical approach, Europe, 30–31
    practical wisdom, 31, 32
    virtuous behaviour, 31–2

Women's Aid, 57, 58

zone of parental control (ZPC)
  Mental Health Act Code of Practice, updated, 121
  parental responsibility, 121